SYLLABUS 1:  CLINICAL MRI (Editor: H. Imhof)
11th Annual Scientific Meeting of the
European Society for Magnetic Resonance in Medicine
(Vienna, April 20-24, 1994)


SYLLABUS 2:  MUSCULOSKELETAL IMAGING: AN UPDATE
Categorical Course ECR '95
(Eds. A. L. Baert, P. Grenier, U. V. Willi - Invited Ed. J. L. Bloem)
(Vienna, March 5-10, 1995)


SYLLABUS 3:  CHEST, MUSCULOSKELETON, G.I. AND ABDOMEN,
URINARY TRACT (Editor: L. Dalla Palma)
5th Halley Radiological Refresher Course
(Budapest-Tihany, May 6-9, 1996)

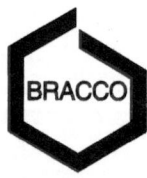

Kindly offered by BRACCO s.p.a. - Milano

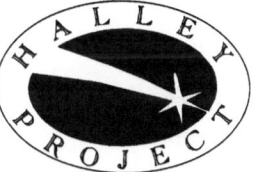

Springer
*Berlin*
*Heidelberg*
*New York*
*Barcelona*
*Budapest*
*Hong Kong*
*London*
*Milano*
*Paris*
*Santa Clara*
*Singapore*
*Tokyo*

# SYLLABUS

**5th Halley Radiological Refresher Course**

## CHEST, MUSCULOSKELETON, G.I. AND ABDOMEN, URINARY TRACT

**EDITOR: L. DALLA PALMA**

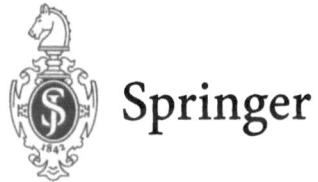 Springer

Prof. Ludovico Dalla Palma
Direttore, Istituto di Radiologia dell'Università
Ospedale di Cattinara
Strada di Fiume
I-34149 Trieste

ISBN-13: 978-3-540-75019-2        e-ISBN-13: 978-88-470-2225-6
DOI: 10.1007/978-88-470-2225-6

Library of Congress Cataloguing - in - Publication Data: applied for

© Springer-Verlag Italia, Milano 1996

## Preface

This volume brings together the papers which 33 radiologists, chosen among the leading European experts, presented at the Halley Project 1996 Refresher Course.

The project, which I promoted and co-ordinated, started out under the aegis of the European Association of Radiology in 1992 with the aim of fostering the advancement of Radiology in various countries of Eastern Europe: Bulgaria, the Czech Republic, Slovakia, Hungary, Poland and Rumania.

Thanks to the expertise and enthusiasm of distinguished colleagues from various countries in Western Europe and to the generosity of two sponsors, Bracco International and Schering A.G., it was possible to set up, in 1992, 1993, 1994 and 1995, four Faculties of Experts in Uroradiology, Gastrointestinal and Abdominal Radiology, Chest Radiology and Skeletal Radiology. These four faculties then gave a refresher course on the four radiological subspecialities in the six nations mentioned above.

The project was called Halley, after the famous comet, in a desire to express the idea of spreading Western radiological culture among Eastern radiologists who were visited in their own countries.

In these 4 years, as project leader, I accompanied the four Faculties during their tour and was thus able to experience the various local situations, not only in radiological terms but also socially, thanks to the ever warm relationships among radiologists of different nationalities and of different ages who attended the courses.

The number of participants attending the Halley Refresher course increased steadily year by year, reaching an average of 200 radiologists in the last 2 years.

The event became a national feast for Radiology, an opportunity for participants to meet each other and the various speakers who took part over the course of the 4 years. I was thus able to see first hand the culture and organisation of Radiology progressively developing in these countries, thus confirming that the project has achieved what it set out to do: bring Western and Eastern European Radiology into harmony.

This year, the fifth in our activity, I wished to celebrate the event by inviting all the 33 speakers who took part in the four previous Refresher Courses to participate in a single refresher course which would review the four subspecialities in such a way as to update progress in each branch to 1996.

For this reason I thought it was a good idea for us to all meet in a central Eastern European country: Hungary, an easily accessible venue for radiologists from the other five countries. Each Society of Radiology has chosen 50 of its members for these 4 days of radiological update.

This was possible thanks to Bracco International who generously sponsored this initiative, which has the purpose of celebrating the union of radiologists, teachers and students from all over Europe.

The European Union, which politicians have not yet achieved, is already reality in radiology! This sums up the spirit and the objective of the Executive Board of the European Association of Radiology.

This volume, to which Bracco International wished to give a particular form, and which will be distributed on a wide scale, gathers together all the 33 lectures presented at this 5th Halley Refresher Course. They are excellent papers, which focus on the most up-to-date issues in radiology of the chest, gastro intestinal tract, skeleton and urinary tract.

I would like to express my heartfelt gratitude to the authors, who are among the leading experts in their subspeciality, for their expertise and generosity and who have made it possible to print this volume in real-time alongside the refresher course. The update will thus be also made available for all those who have been unable to take part in the Refresher Course. By reading this volume they too will be able to enter the spirit of the Halley Project.

Finally thanks must be extended to the publisher, Springer-Verlag, for co-operation in keeping to our strict time limits and for the high editorial quality of the final product.

L. Dalla Palma

## Table of Contents

# G.I. and Abdominal Radiology

# Uroradiology

# FACULTY OF CHEST RADIOLOGY

## LORENZO BONOMO

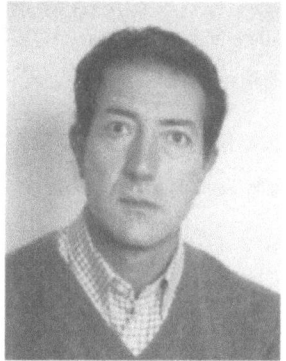

Professor of Radiology - Chairman of Department of Radiological Sciences, University of Chieti.
Medical Degree Magna cum laude, 1970.
Board Certification Magna cum laude, 1975.
Member of Italian Association of Radiology, European Society of Thoracic Imaging, Cardiovascular Interventional Radiological Society of Europe.
Previous Member of the Council of the Italian Cardiovascular and Interventional Section, Italian Society of Radiology.
Since 1992 President of Thoracic Section, Italian Society of Radiology.
Since 1994 Member of the Council of the European Society of Thoracic Imaging.
Authors of several scientific publications on radiology of the chest.

## ROBERT F. DONDELINGER

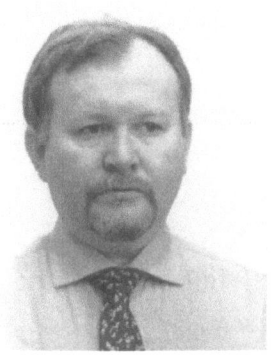

Professor of Radiology at the University of Liége.
Head of the Department of Medical Imaging of the University Hospital Sart Tilman, Liège.
Medical Degree in 1978.
Founding Meeting Chairman and Vice-President of European Society of Thoracic Imaging.
Founding Meeting Member, Annual Meeting Chairman and Chairman of Scientific Programme Committee of European Society of Gastro-Intestinal and Abdominal Imaging.
Founding Member and Chairman of Scientific Programme Committee of Cardiovascular and Interventional Radiological Society of Europe.
Author of over 150 scientific publications and of twenty chapters of books, editor of three books mainly in the field of visceral and vascular diagnostic and interventional radiology.

## CHRISTOPHER D.R. FLOWER

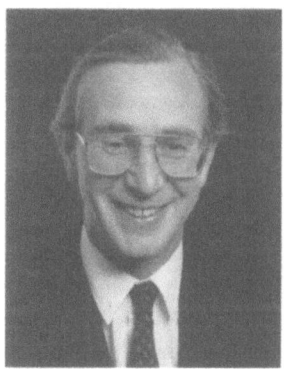

Director of the Department of Radiology, Addenbrooke's Hospital. Consultant Radiologist at Addenbrooke's Hospital and Papworth Hospital with a particular interest in thoracic radiology.
BA Cambridge, 1960 - MA Cambridge, 1963 - MB BChir Cambridge, 1963 - FRCP Canada, 1971 - FFR (FRCR) England, 1972
1978-85 East Anglian Regional Education Advisor for the Royal College of Radiologists.
1982-85 Chairman, Papworth Hospital Medical Advisory Committee.
1983-86 Clinical Tutor, Addenbrooke's Hospital, Cambridge.
1987-90 Editor, Clinical Radiology.
1990-94 Warden - Royal College of Radiologists.
President elect of the Fleischner Society.
Fellow of the Royal College of Radiologists and Member of the British Institute of Radiology.
Fellow of the European Society of Thoracic Imaging.
Member of the Association of Chest Radiologists, United Kingdom.
Honorary Member of the Canadian Association of Radiologists, French Society of Thoracic Imaging, Faculty of Radiology, Ireland, Hong Kong College of Radiology.
Reviewer of 6 journals. Author of several publications.

## PHILIPPE GRENIER

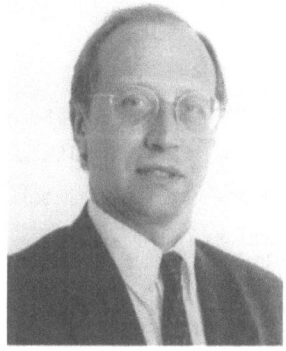

Professor of Radiology - Chairman of Department of Radiology (General Diagnosis) - Hôpital Pitié-Salpétrière, Faculté Pitié-Salpétrière, Université Paris VI, France.
Medical Degree: French Medical License, Paris 1972
Board Certification: French Board of Radiology, 1977.
Member of Fleischner Society (by election, 1990).
Member of Radiological Society of North America, European Society of Thoracic Imaging (founding member), Société Française de Radiologie, Societé d'Imagerie Thoracique (founding member), Societé de Pneumologie de Langue Française, of Société Médicale des Hôpitaux de Paris, Société Canadienne Française de Radiologie (honorary member).
Member of Editorial Boards of 7 journals.
He received several grants for research.
Author of 98 scientific papers in peer reviewed journals.

XII

## CHRISTIAN HEROLD

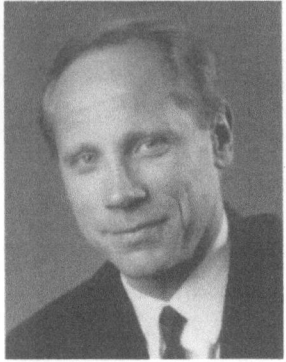

Associate Professor of Radiology - Acting-Chief of the Division of Diagnostic Radiology I - Department of Radiology, University of Vienna.
Assistant Professor of Radiology, Faculty member, Department of Radiology, The Johns Hopkins Hospital, Baltimore, USA.
Medical Degree in 1979.
Board Certification in 1989.
President of Viennese Division of the Austrian Radiologic Society.
Member of Fleischner Society.
Member of Austrian Society of Ultrasound in Medicine, European Society of Thoracic Imaging, Radiologic Society of North America, Society of Thoracic Imaging and Austrian Radiologic Society.
Founding member of Junior Radiologist Forum of European Association of Radiology.
Founding member of European working group on management in Radiology.
Member of Editorial Board and Associate Editor of European Radiology and Radiology.
He received several honors, awards and grants for research and original articles.
Co-organizer of national and international meetings.
Chairman of several international congresses.
Author of 150 papers.

## FRANÇOIS LAURENT

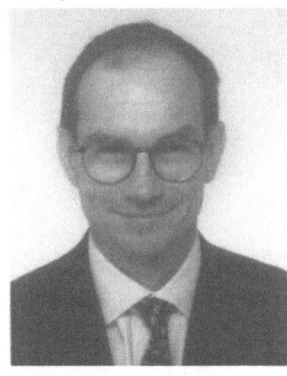

Professeur de Radiologie, Université de Bordeaux II, 1990.
Praticien Hospitalier, Départment d'Imagerie Médicale, Radiologie Diagnostique et Thérapeutique, Hôpital Cardiopneumologique du Haut-Lévêque - C.H.U. de Bordeaux.
Medical degree: Université Bordeaux II, 1980.
Author of several pubblications mostly in chest Imaging.

## PIERRE SCHNYDER

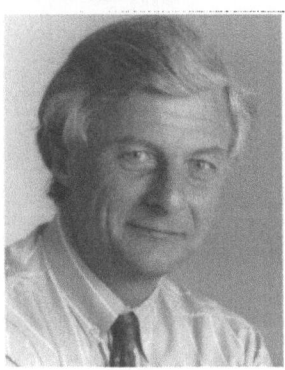

Professor and Chairman, Director of Department of Radiology, Radiooncology and Nuclear Medicine, University Hospital Lausanne.
1979-1988: Staff member, director of CT unit, University Hospital Lausanne.
1985: Privat-Docent et agrégé, University Hospital Lausanne.
1988: Professor and Chairman, Department of Radiology, University Hospital Lausanne.
Member of Swiss Society of Radiology, European Association of Radiology, American Roentgen Ray Society, Radiological Society of North America, Société d'Imagerie Thoracique, France (committee), European Society of Thoracic Imaging (treasurer), Société d'Imagerie Abdominale et Digestive, France.
Member of Editorial Board of Journal de Radiologie, European Radiology, Diagnostic Imaging.
Reviewer of several journals.
He gave 270 communications and lectures.
Author of 160 papers and of 21 book chapters.
Fields of interest: chest, abdomen, AIDS, ICU and emergency radiology, lung cancers.

## DON G. SHAW

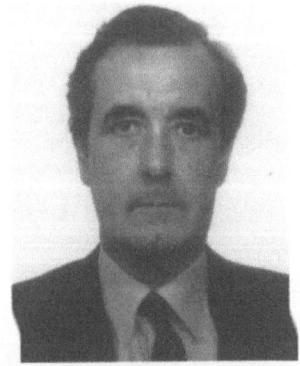

Consultant Radiologist, Great Ormond Street Hospital for Children, NHS Trust.
He qualified with First Class Honours from Oxford University in Physiology in 1958 and proceeded to a Research Degree during tenure of an MRC Scholarship in Respiratory Physiology.
Qualifying in medicine in 1962 at University College Hospital Medical School and following training in the Professorial Medical and Surgical Units, he proceeded to MRCP and FRCR.
Appointed Consultant Radiologist to the Hospitals for Sick Children and University College Hospital in 1970, he relinquished his adult sessions in 1982.
Dr. Shaw has been Examiner, Senior Examiner, member of the Faculty Board and twice member of Council of the Royal College of Radiologists of which he is the recipient of the Knox Medal. His association with the British Institute of Radiology involved many years of editorial activity with the British Journal of Radiology becoming Medical Editor.
He is a recipient of the Barclay Prize of the British Institute of Radiology and has sat on numerous committees including Council. He was president of the European Society of Paediatric Radiology in 1993 and he is now an honorary member and the treasurer of the society.

**JOHNY A. VERSCHAKELEN**

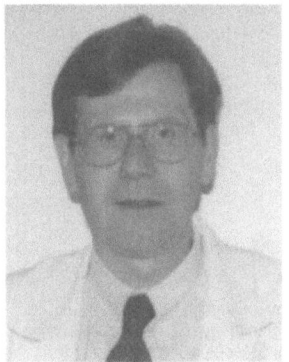

Associate Professor of Radiology and Anatomy - Catholic University of Leuven.
Senior staff member responsible for chest radiology at the Department of Radiology, University Hospitals of Leuven.
Medical Degree in 1980.
Board Certification in 1984.
General Secretary and Member of Royal Belgian Society of Radiology.
Member of Belgian Society of Pneumology, Society of Thoracic Radiology, European Society of Thoracic Imaging, European Respiratory Society, Radiological Society of North America, Société d'Imagerie Thoracique.
Member of the Board and Reviewer of Belgian Journal of Radiology, European Radiology.
Reviewer of European Journal of Respiratory Disease and Clinical Rheumatology.

# FACULTY OF SKELETAL RADIOLOGY

**MARK DAVIES**

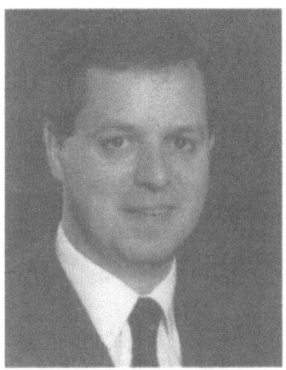

Clinical Director Imaging University Hospital Birmingham NHS Trust.
Consultant Radiologist Royal Orthopaedic Hospital, Birmingham.
Chairman of Scientific Programme Committee of British National Radiological Conference, Radiology UK '96.
Examiner in Fellowship examination of Royal College of Radiologists.
Member of Royal College of Radiologists Committee assessing UK radiology training departments.
Member joint Royal College of Radiologists and British Institute of Radiology European Committee.
Secretary British Society of Skeletal Radiologists.
Segretary European Society of Musculoskeletal Radiology.
Member of the International Skeletal Society.
Member of Editorial Board of British Journal of Radiology, Skeletal Radiology and European Radiology.

**KJELL JONSSON**

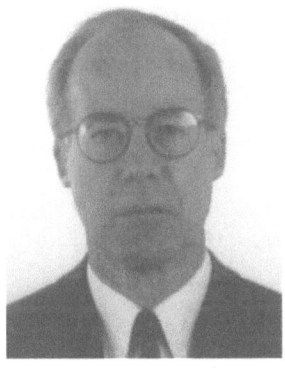

Associate Professor, Department of Radiology, University Hospital, Lund, Sweden.
Head of Section for Bone and Joint Radiology.
Visiting Associate Professor, Department of Diagnostic Radiology, MD Anderson Hospital and Tumor Institute, Houston, Texas, USA, 1976-1977.
Visiting Associate Professor, Department of Radiology, University Hospital, Ann Arbor, Michigan, USA, 1988-1989.
Member of several national and scandinavian societies, of European Society of Skeletal Radiology and International Society of Skeletal Radiology.
Author and co-author of 140 original papers.

**CARLO MASCIOCCHI**

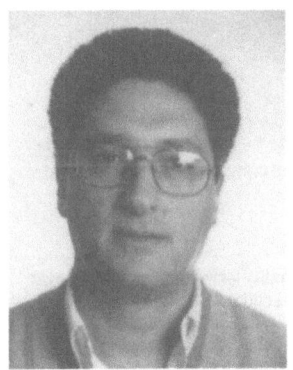

Associate Professor of Radiology at the University of L'Aquila.
President of Diagnostic Imaging in Sport Medicine Section of the Italian Society of Radiology.
Member of International Skeletal Society and cancellour of European Skeletal Society of Radiology.
Member of MuscoloSkeletal Subcommittee in the ECR '93 and ECR '95.
Lectures and workshops in Italian and international congresses mostly focused on MRI and musculo-skeletal radiology.
Organizer of 35 italian meetings in the field of MRI and musculo-skeletal radiology.
Authors of 215 papers mostly related to MRI and musculo-skeletal radiology.

## HOLGER PETTERSSON

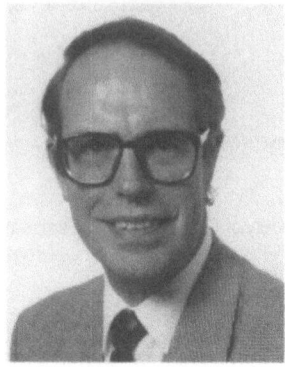

Professor of Radiology, Department of Radiology, University of Lund.
Adjunct Professor, Department of Radiology, University of Florida.
Deputy Medical Director, University Hospital, Lund, Sweden.
Chief County Radiologist, County of Malmohus.
Director WHO Collaboration Center for Continuing Education in Radiology, University Hospital, Lund, Sweden.
Educational and Scientific Director, NICER program.
Visiting Professor at several universities in Europe, USA, and Australia.
Member/Officer of the Board of Directors: Swedish Society of Medical Radiology (Treasurer), Swedish Society of Pediatric Radiology, Swedish Club for Skeletal Radiology (past president), Scandinavian Society of Radiology (General Secretary), European Association of Radiology, European Congress of Radiology, European Society for Musculoskeletal Radiology (President), International Skeletal Society (President Elect).
Editor/Member of Editorial Board of 7 journals.
Author of 13 books, 25 chapters in multi-author books, 190 original papers in international scientific journals.

## MAXIMILIAN F. REISER

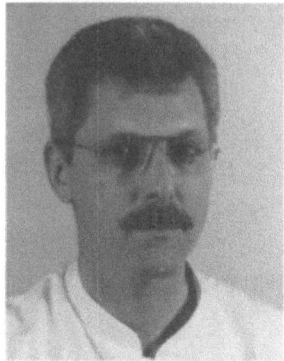

Professor of Radiology and Chairman - Department of Diagnostic Radiology - University of Munich.
Medical Degree in 1974.
Board Certification in 1981.
President of the European Society of Musculo-Skeletal Radiology.
Member of Radiological Society of North America, International Skeletal Society, German Roentgen Society, German Society of Osteology, European Seminars in Diagnostic and Interventional Radiology, Japanese-German Radiological Affiliation.
Member of Executive Board of European Society of Musculoskeletal Radiology, European Society of Abdominal Radiology, Magnetic Resonance in Biology and Medicine.
Editor-in-Chief of Der Radiologie.
Former or present member of Scientific Board of European Journal of Radiology, Radiologia Diagnostica, Angio, Osteologia, MAGMA, Skeletal Radiology, Fortschr. Rontgenstr., Surgical and Radiologic Anatomy, Osteologiai Kozlemenyek.

## DANIEL VANEL

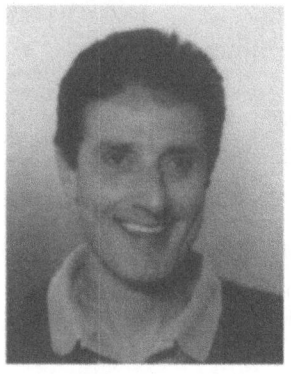

Head of the Department of Radiology of the Institute Gustave-Roussy 1976-1992.
Medical Degree in 1976.
Board Certification in Diagnostic Radiology.
Honorary Member of the Canadian Association of Radiologists.
Member of International Skeletal Society, European Musculoskeletal Oncology Society, Computed Body Tomography and Magnetic Resonance Society.
Member of Editorial Board of 5 journals.
Awarded: Prix Nycomed de Recherche en Imagerie Médicale 1992 and Prix de la Recherche en Cancérologie du Conseil Général du Val de Marne 1993.
Author of 88 full scientific publications.

## IAIN WATT

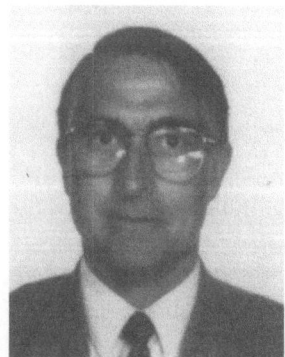

Consultant Clinical Radiologist - Bristol Royal Infirmary - United Bristol Healthcare  NHS Trust (musculoskeletal diseases).
Clinical Lecturer in Radiodiagnosis - University of Bristol.
Honorary Radiological Curator - the Bristol Bone Tumour Registry.
Dean, Faculty of Clinical Radiology - The Royal College of Radiologists.
Member, Editorial Boards of 7 journals.
Member of International Skeletal Society, Radiological Society of North America, Osteoarthritis Research Society, European Skeletal Radiology Association, Royal College of Radiologists, Royal College of Physicians London, British Orthopaedic Association (Fellow), British Orthopaedic Research Society, British Society for Rheumatology, Royal Society of Medicine.
Author of 120 scientific papers and 26 chapters and books.
He has lectured widely.

# FACULTY OF G.I. AND ABDOMINAL RADIOLOGY

**ALBERT BAERT**

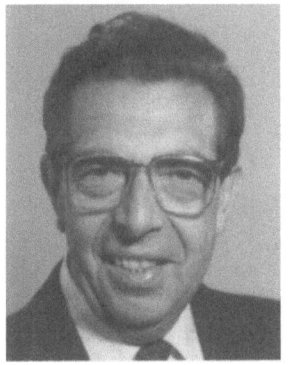

Professor of Radiology and Chairman. Department of Radiology - University of Leuven.
Doctor Honoris Causa University of Lisbon.
Past President of the European Congress of Radiology 1993 and 1995.
Past Secretary General and actual President of the European Association of Radiology.
Editor-in-Chief of European Radiology.
Honorary Member of RSNA, ISR and eight European National Societies of Radiology.
Author of several books in radiology and numerous scientific publications.
Has lectured widely in Europe and United States on angiography and computed tomograhy.

**JOHANNES LAMMER**

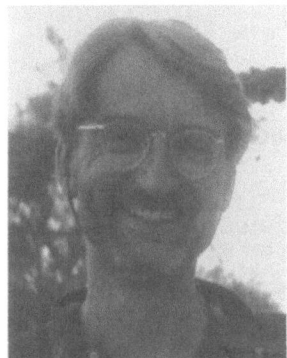

Professor of Radiology, Head of the Department of Angiography and Interventional Radiology, Univ. Klinik für
Radiodiagnostik, Universität Wien, AKH.
Board Certification: University of Vienna, 1975.
Internship, Surgery, Internal Medicine and Pathology at City Hospital Bregenz and Feldkirch, 1976-1978.
Residency in Radiology at Department of Radiology, Karl Franzens University Graz, 1978-1982.
Vice President of the Austrian Rontgen Ray Society.
Medical Director of the Academy for Rontgentechniques.
Member of the Editorial Board of Cardiovascular and International Radiology, Seminars of International Radiology, Rontgen
Fortschritte.
Visiting Professor at several universities in Europe, USA, Canada.
Publication of more than 200 manuscripts in international journals and medical text books.

**MEINHARD LUNING**

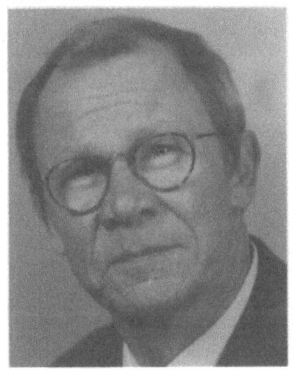

Medical degree: Humboldt-University Berlin (HUB), 1965.
Fellowships at New York Hospital, Cornell University New York and Moffit Hospital, University of California, San Francisco.
From 1980 to 1985 professor of diagnostic radiology and vice chairman at the Charite. From 1985 to 1993 chairman of the
Institute of Diagnostic Radiology. In 1993 started a privat practice MRI-CT in Berlin.
President of the Society of Radiology (Germ. Democr. Republic) 1985-1988.
Chairman of the Section of Radiodiagnosis of the European Association of Radiology 1989-1993.
Memberships on Editorial Boards: Diagnostic Imaging Europe, Rontgenpraxis, Clinical Imaging, European Journal of
Radiology, Roentgenologia Radiologia, Radiologia Diagnostica (1976-1993).
Honorary Memberships of five eastern European Societies of Radiology.
Scientific publications: approx. 400 papers on lymphography, CT, MRI; 4 books.

**PIERRE MAHIEU**

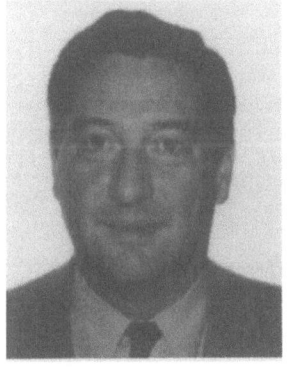

Associate Professor of Radiology - Catholic University of Louvain - Cliniques Universitaire Saint Luc - Brussels.
Medical Degree in 1972. Board Certification in 1976.
Master's Degree in Hospital Administration in 1988.
Medical Director of the Clinique de l'Europe since 1992.
Member of the Board of administrators, Clinique Europe Saint-Michel.
Secretary of the Academic Department of Radiology and Medical Imaging UCL.
Member of the Royal Belgian Society of Radiology, Royal Belgian Society of Gastroenterology, European Council for
Coloproctology, GERMAD.
Honorary member of the Société Nationale Française de Coloproctologie.
Secretary of the Belgian Union of Radiologist.
Member of Board of Consultants of the International Journal of Colorectal Disease.
Member of Editorial Board of Acta Gastroenterologica Belgica.
Author or coauthor of 69 publications. He gave 177 oral communications, lectures or invited courses.
Fields of interest: alimentary tract radiology, defecography.

XVI

## ALFEO MONTESI

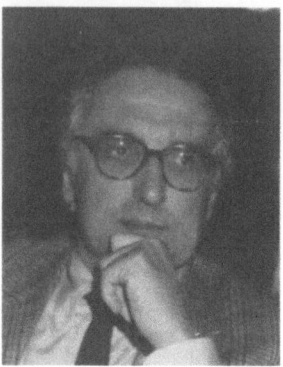

Chief of Department of Radiology, Umberto I General Hospital, Ancona.
Medical Degreee, 1967.
Board Certification in Radiology in 1970 and in Nuclear Medicine in 1974.
Member of Italian Association of Radiology.
President of the Marche Regional Group of Italian Association of Radiology.
Former active member of Gastrointestinal Radiology Section of the Italian Association of Radiology.
Member of the European Society of Gastrointestinal Radiology.
Former associate editor of the Italian Journal of Gastroenterology.
Speakers in more than 200 scientific meetings.
Organizer of 15 Residential Courses and 5 Workshops on Gastrointestinal Radiology, 3 Advanced Courses on Muscolo-Skeletal Radiology and 3 Scientific meetings on Vascular and Interventional Radiology.
Authors of 168 papers mostly related to abdominal-gastrointestinal radiology and organization and management of radiological department.

## DANIEL J. NOLAN

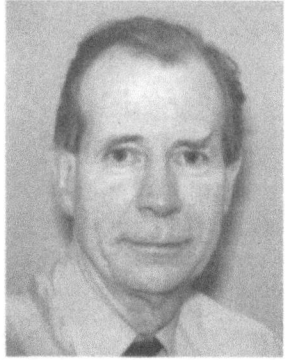

Consultant Radiologist with a special interest in gastroenterology, John Radcliffe Hospital, Oxford.
Clinical Lecturer, University of Oxford.
Chairman, Department of Radiology, John Radcliffe Hospital 1982-1991.
Director of Postgraduate Radiological Studies - Oxford Training Programme 1980-1991.
President, European Society of Gastrointestinal Radiologist (ESGR) 1989-1991.
President, Radiology Section, Royal Society of Medicine 1988-1989.
Previously Examiner in Part I and II, Fellowship of the Royal College of Radiologists.
Visiting Professorships, lectures, tutorials and workshops by invitation at university medical centres, meetings, conferences and courses in the United Kingdom, Europe, Asia and North America.
Publications: books, contributions to book, review articles and original articles on radiology of the gastrointestinal tract, mostly related to the small intestine.

## JACQUES H.T.H. PRINGOT

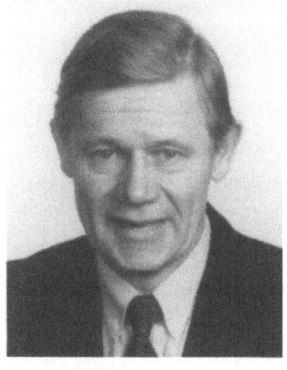

Chef de Service associé en Radiologie and Professeur ordinaire, Université Catholique de Louvain.
Medical Degree, 1953.
Board Certification, 1961.
Professor of Radiology, 1977.
Redacteur en Chef of Journal Belge de Radiologie.
Permanent Member of Bureau de la Société Royale Belge de Radiologie.
Associate Editor of the Journal of Medical Imaging (Elsevier).
Founding member and member of Bureau de la Société d'Imagerie Abdominale et Digestive.
Founding member of European Society of Gastrointestinal Radiologists.
Member of 15 national and international societies.
Member of Editorial Board of 8 international journals.
Author or co-author of 124 scientific papers and 25 books.

## ULRICH V. WILLI

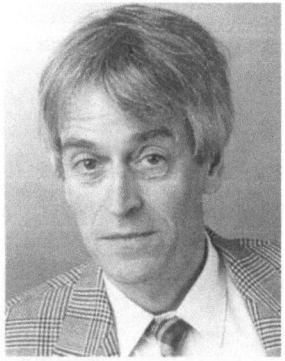

Head of Radiology Department - University Children's Hospital of Zurich.
Medical Degree, 1965.
Board Certification in pediatrics and in diagnostic radiology.
President elect 1997 of the European Society of Pediatric Radiology. In charge of the 34th Annual Congress and 20th Postgraduate Course of the European Society of Pediatric Radiology.
Organizing chairman of the first conjoint meeting of the European Society of Uroradiology and the Society of Uroradiology.
Fields of interest: ultrasonography, nuclear medicine, imaging of the genitourinary tract (vesicoureteric reflux and obstructive uropathy, pediatric gynecology), the gastrointestinal tract, endocrine disease and tumors.

# FACULTY OF URORADIOLOGY

## HELEN CARTY

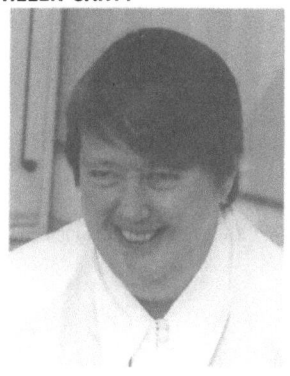

Consultant Radiologist and Clinical Director at the Royal Liverpool, Children's Hospital - Alder Hey since 1975.
Qualifications:
MB, Bch, BAO, (NUI), 2nd Hons. 3rd Place in Class. MRCPI, 1970. FRCPI, 1981. DMRD, London 1972. FFR, London 1974. FRCR on foundation of The Royal College of Radiologists.
She has a widespread interest in all aspects of paediatric radiology, with a particular interest in chest, musculoskeletal and gastrointestinal radiology and non-accidental injury.
Invited lecturer worldwide on many aspects of paediatric radiology.
Author of more than 100 papers, 10 chapters and 1 book.

## LUDOVICO DALLA PALMA

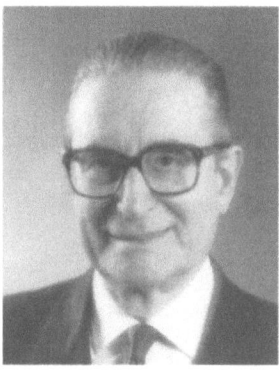

Professor and Chairman, Department of Radiology, University Hospital, Trieste.
Founding member and President of European Society of Uroradiology 1990-1994.
Past President of European Association of Radiology 1993-1995.
Member of Executive Board of International Society of Radiology.
President of Italian Society of Radiology since 1992.
Honorary Fellow of the American College of Radiology.
Honorary member of eight European National Societies of Radiology.
Member of Editorial Boards of 5 international journals.
Leader of the Halley Project Refresher Courses in east Europe since 1992.
Authors of 260 scientific publications.

## SVEN DORPH

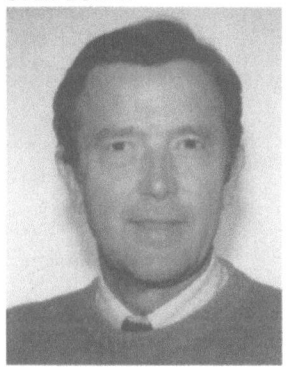

Chairman and Associate professor, Department of Radiology, University of Copenhagen.
Medical Degree 1964. Board Certification diagnostic radiology 1975.
Scolarships: United States Education Foundation, US Government Grant (Fulbright), 1975.
Pilot Grant Picker Foundation 1975.
Study travels and services abroad: 1969 United States; 1971 Marseille, France; 1975, June-September, visiting assistent professor, Department of Radiology, University of California, San Diego; 1985 West Germany; 1992 Member of faculty, Halley Project, training East European countries in uroradiology.
Pregraduate teaching: since 1970. Postgraduate teaching: since 1974.
Co-organizer of international postgraduate courses and symposia since 1983.
Associate editor of Acta Radiologica since 1986.
Active Member of Society of Uroradiology since 1980.
Founding member of European Society of Uroradiology, established 1990.
Author or co-author of about 100 papers in international journals and books.

## NICOLAS GRENIER

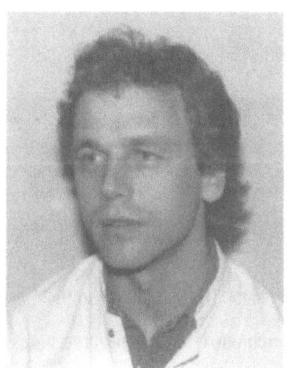

Professor of Radiology - Chef de Service of Radiology - Groupe Hospitalier Pellegrin, Bordeaux.
Resident in Radiology in Bordeaux (October 1980 - May 1986).
Fellow in Radiology (Pr Broussin, Bordeaux) (May 1986- - May 1990).
DEA de Biologie-Santé, Option Imagerie Fonctionelle, Bordeaux (June 1988).
Member of Société Française de Radiologie, Groupe de Recherche sur les Applications du Magnétisme en Médecine, Society of Magnetic Resonance, Société Francophone pour l'Applications des Ultrasons à la Médecine et à la Biologie, European Society of Uroradiology, Délégation Régionale à la Recherche Clinique, CHU de Bordeaux.
Member of Editorial Board of Revue d'Imagerie Médicale and member of Scientific Board of European Radiology.
Fields of interest: vascular radiology, uroradiology, ultrasounds.

## MICHAEL J. KELLETT

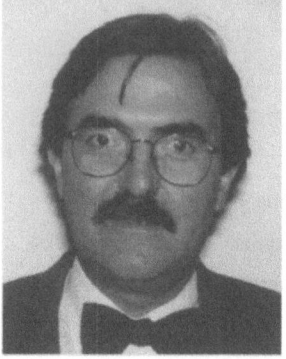

Consultant Radiologist - Director Department of Uroradiology - St Peter's Hospital - Middlesex Hospital - London.
Honorary Consultant Radiologist - Institute of Urology - University College - University of London.
Medical Degreee in 1968.
Qualifications:
MA Cambridge 1965. MBBChir Cambridge 1968. DMRD England 1972. FRCR England 1974. Honorary Member of the Hong Kong Urological Association.
Fellow of the Royal College of Radiologists, of the Royal Society of Medicine.
Member of the Society of Uroradiology, four British Societies, four European Societies.
Author of 54 scientific publications and 16 chapters in books.
Visiting Professor in many centers through the world.
Regular lectures and seminars at urological and radiological conferences in Britain and Europe.

## JEAN-FRANÇOIS MOREAU

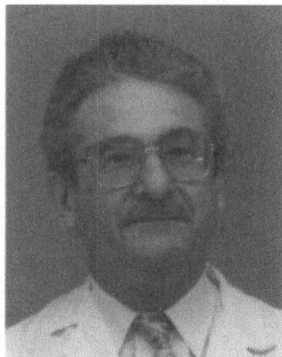

Professor of Radiology - Chairman of Department of Radiology of the Necker Hospital, Paris.
Past President of the Radiodiagnostic Section of the International Society of Radiology 1985-1989 and of the Paris International Congress of Radiology.
Treasurer of the ISR and Co-chairman of ICR '96. Land of European Federation of the Societies for Ultrasound in Medicine and Biology.
President of the European Society of Uroradiology.
Member of the International Society of Nephrology.
Editor-in-Chief of Journal de Radiologie.
Corresponding Editor of Academic Radiology.
Honorary Fellow of the American College of Radiology.
Honorary Member of the Bulgarian Society of Radiology.

## RAYMOND H.G. OYEN

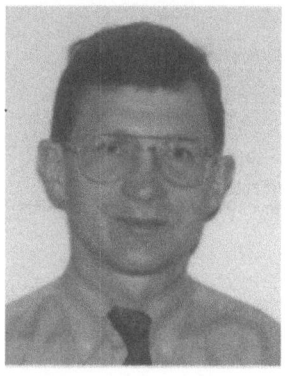

Adjunt-Clinical Head of the Department of Radiology, University Hospitals of Leuven.
Medical Degree 1981.
Board Certification diagnostic radiology 1985.
Member of the Royal Belgian Society of Radiology, Belgian Society of Ultrasound, Belgian Society of Nephrology, American Institute of Ultrasound in Medicine, European Society of Uroradiology, French Society of Genito-Urinary Imaging, American Society of Uroradiology.

## HUGH M. SAXTON

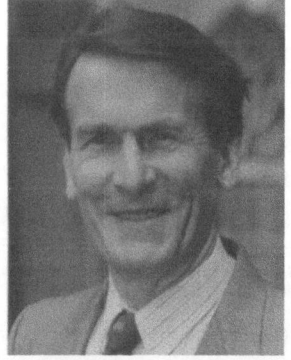

Consultant Radiologist Emeritus, Guy's Hospital, London, SE1 9RT.
Honorary Professor, Centre for Health Planning and Management, University of Keele, 1991 - present.
Clinical Director, Department of Radiology, Guy's Hospital, 1979-1988.
Chairman, Guy's Hospital Management Board, 1988-1991.
Editor: British Journal of Radiology, 1971-1981.
Author (jointly) Management for Hospital Doctors, by Burrows M, Dyson R, jackson P and Saxton H, 1994, Butterworth - Heinemann, Oxford.
Author of several publications mostly in urinary tract radiology, in particular the excretory urogram, interventional procedures involving the kidney and functional disorders of the bladder.

**FULVIO STACUL**

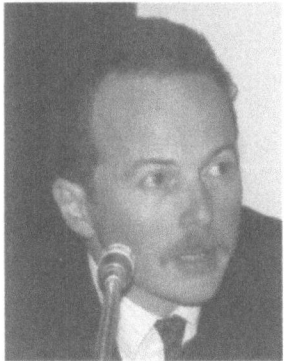

Consultant radiologist at University Hospital of Trieste since March 1981.
Medical degree with full marks and honours in Trieste on 1979.
Board Certification, Diagnostic Radiology with full marks and honours in Trieste on July 1982.
Member of the Italian Society of Radiology, European Society of Uroradiology, ESUR contrast media safety committee, ESUR membership committee.
Speaker in about 80 scientific meetings.
Author of more that 120 scientific papers.
Main fields of interest: uroradiology, ultrasonography, contrast media, interventional radiology, digital radiology.

**JUDITH A. WEBB**

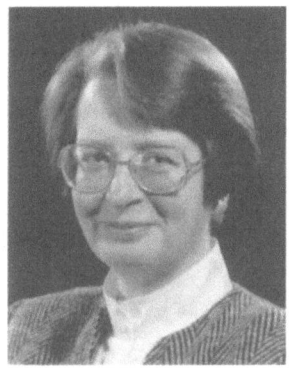

Consultant Radiologist at St. Bartholomew's Hospital, London since 1979.
President-Elect of the European Society of Uroradiology.
Her early interests were in the renal excretion of contrast media, particularly in renal failure, and the nephrotoxic effects of contrast medium.
Currently her main professional interest is in all aspects of urinary tract imaging, particularly the appropriate choice of imaging methods and imaging of the kidneys in renal failure.

# CHEST RADIOLOGY

# Haemoptysis: The Role of Radiology in Investigation and Treatment

C.D.R. Flower

Department of Diagnostic Radiology, Addenbrooke's Hospital, NHS Trust, Hills Road, Cambridge CB2 2QQ, UK

Haemoptysis, a common symptom in clinical practice, is frightening for patients and presents a diagnostic challenge to physicians and radiologists. The relative frequency of causes has changed since the turn of the century when tuberculosis was the commonest aetiology. Bronchial cancer now accounts for a large proportion of cases in most studies, although the relative frequency of the different aetiologies is dependent upon a number of factors, including patient selection, the patient population studied and the techniques used for diagnosis [1]. In a significant proportion of cases no cause for the haemoptysis will be found and these patients are labelled as having cryptogenic haemoptysis.

From the management point of view it is convenient and appropriate to differentiate between haemoptysis which is intermittent and of small volume and that which is massive and potentially life-threatening. Most patients are in the first category, coughing up small volumes of blood, a symptom which is rightly regarded as a possible indication of a serious underlying disease. A careful history and clinical examination usually excludes nonpulmonary causes of haemoptysis such as epistaxis or haematemesis. While the chest radiograph may reveal abnormalities suggestive either of cancer or tuberculosis it is frequently normal or reveals only nonspecific appearances.

## The Role of Bronchoscopy

Rigid bronchoscopy is normally reserved for patients with massive haemoptysis (see below). Fibreoptic bronchoscopy is a relatively straightforward procedure, usually well tolerated by patients, and provides excellent views of the bronchial tree. It is usually performed to confirm or exclude malignancy whether or not the chest radiograph is abnormal. However, it is an invasive procedure not without complications. Furthermore, several studies have shown that in patients with either a normal or nonlocalising chest radiograph the prevalence of bronchial cancer is extremely low. In one retrospective study of 196 patients presenting with haemoptysis and a normal or nonlocalising chest radiograph only 12 (6%) had bronchial cancer diagnosed by bronchoscopy. In another review of 110 patients there were no reported cases of malignancy. However, the incidence in five other studies ranged from 4% to 16% [2-4].

Many studies have indicated that the prognosis for patients with a normal chest radiograph and negative bronchoscopy (so-called cryptogenic haemoptysis) is good with an insignificant proportion developing cancer when followed up [5]. Resolution of haemoptysis occurs within 6 months in approximately 90% of these patients. For these reasons attention is being paid to the role computed tomography (CT) can play as an adjunct or alternative to bronchoscopy.

## The Role of CT

CT should be used as an adjunct to bronchoscopy in patients who are likely to have a carcinoma or as an alternative to bronchoscopy in patients in whom the likelihood of a bronchial carcinoma is low. The value of CT in imaging the airways is well established; not only endobronchial tumours but other causes of haemoptysis such as bronchiectasis and broncholithiasis are well demonstrated. Using conventional "thick slice" CT in the 1980s, CT was shown to have a reasonable sensitivity when compared to bronchoscopy for diagnosing bronchial abnormalities. Webb et al. demonstrated a good correlation between CT and bronchoscopy in a small number of patients without normal chest radiographs and histologically proven carcinomas [6]. Although CT failed to identify some tumours it demonstrated others, not identified by bronchoscopy, either because the tumour was beyond the range of the bronchoscope or in areas which were difficult to visualise bronchoscopically. Henschke et al. confirmed the complementary roles of CT and bronchoscopy in a retrospective study of 100 patients with suspected bronchial abnormalities [7]. Although CT missed a small proportion of tumours, it detected an equal number which were initially missed at bronchoscopy. Similar results

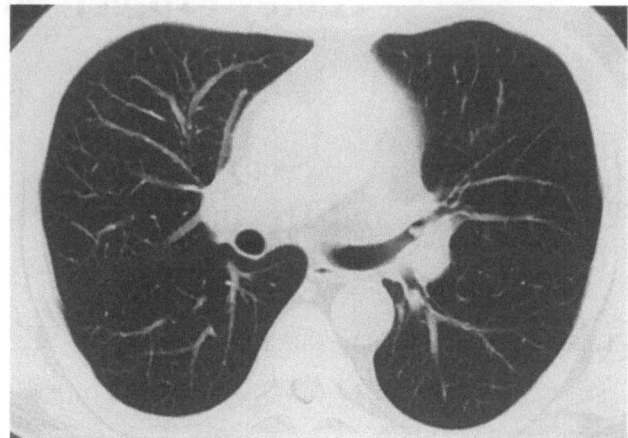

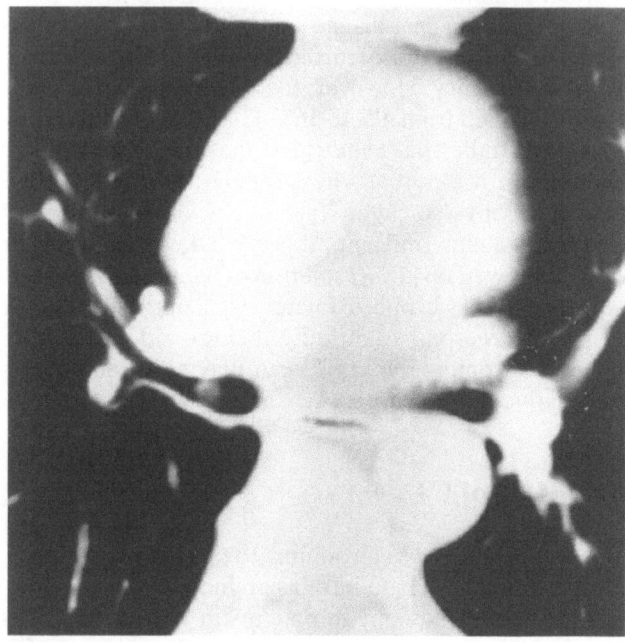

**Fig. 1. a** Small carcinoma in left upper lobe bronchus detected on computed tomography. **b** Polypoid carcinoid tumour in right upper lobe bronchus

were obtained in a study by Naidich and co-workers, with CT identifying 59 of 64 lesions detected by bronchoscopy and six lesions missed by bronchoscopy [8]. In the largest study to date, Mayr et al. achieved sensitivities for CT of 91%-95% for two observers, each of whom achieved specificities of 99%. Undoubtedly improved scanning techniques (particularly spiral scanning and the use of a high resolution algorithm) together with a precise understanding of CT bronchial anatomy are important contributing factors to the accuracy of CT [10].

The role of CT specifically in the investigation of haemoptysis has also been evaluated in a number of studies. Tumours which cause haemoptysis are usually relatively advanced when they produce this symptom and are therefore likely to be identified by CT. In an

early study using 10-mm collimation and a long exposure time CT correctly identified the source of bleeding in 85% of patients who were suspected of having cancer. Whilst these authors concluded that CT did not obviate the need for bronchoscopy Millar et al., who also used conventional CT, concluded that CT should precede bronchoscopy. In their study of 40 patients with haemoptysis, a normal chest radiograph and a normal bronchoscopy, significant abnormalities were detected by CT in 50% of cases [11].

The optimal technique for imaging the thorax in patients with haemoptysis consists of 1- to 2-mm thick sections, obtained every 10 mm from the thoracic inlet to the lung bases, with an additional spiral sequence of 5-mm thick sections from the level of the aortic arch to just below the level of the inferior pulmonary veins. All images are reconstructed using a high spatial frequency algorithm. This protocol provides good visualisation of the airways and the lung parenchyma. Using such a technique, even small lesions may be accurately detected (Fig. 1). Three recent studies which have compared the accuracy of CT and bronchoscopy in the investigation of patients with haemoptysis have all indicated the important role which high-resolution CT (HRCT) [10, 12, 13] can play. In these studies HRCT was able to identify all tumours diagnosed by bronchoscopy but, in addition, identified a small but significant additional number of tumours and, importantly, other causes of bleeding. The latter include bronchiectasis, which accounts for 15%-20% of cases (Figs. 2, 3).

The central role that CT plays in the investigation of haemoptysis has been established. In an era of concern over the best use of healthcare resources, the main issue now is whether CT can be used as an alternative to bronchoscopy in the investigative pathway of these patients. The accuracy of the technique, coupled with the low prevalence of cancer in those whose haemoptysis is not associated with any chest radiographic abnormality (approximately half of all patients presenting with haemoptysis), suggests that it may be used safely as an alternative to bronchoscopy in patients with a normal or nonlocalising chest radiograph. In these patients bronchoscopy can be reserved for those who are identified by CT as having a tumour or in those whose haemoptysis persists beyond 6 months. Patients with an abnormal chest radiograph are much more likely to have a bronchial carcinoma (30%-40%) and all will need bronchoscopy. However, by providing a road map for the bronchoscopist, CT improves the diagnostic yield from bronchoscopy and it should therefore be performed prior to the bronchoscopic examination.

→

**Fig. 2 a-c.** Patient with haemoptysis. **a** The chest radiograph reveals enlargement of the right hilum. **b** Computed tomography (CT) revelas a bulky right pulmonary artery but no evidence of a hilar mass. **c** High-resolution CT images at lung windows reveal evidence of bronchiectasis

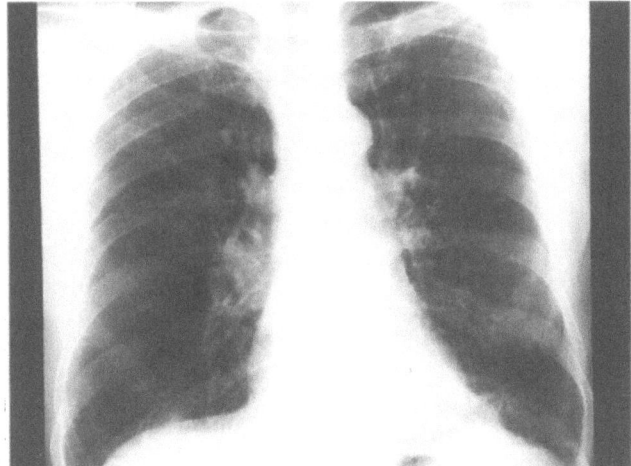

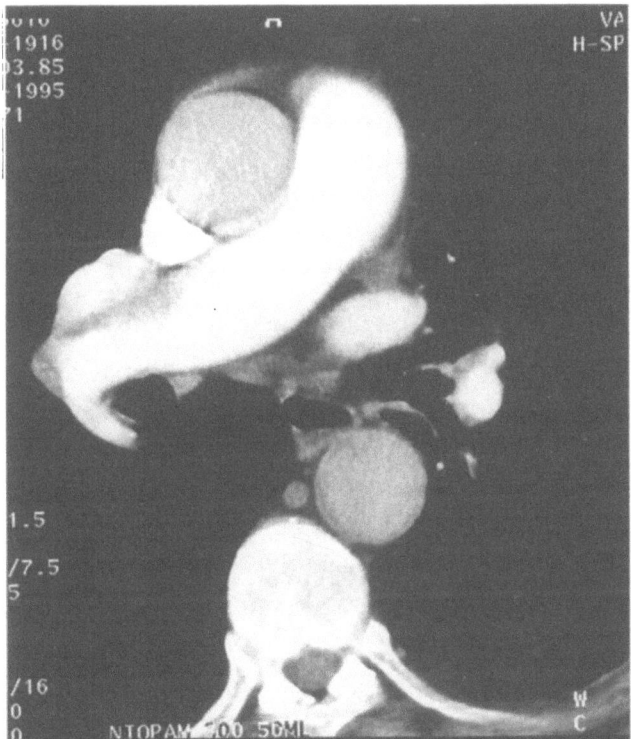

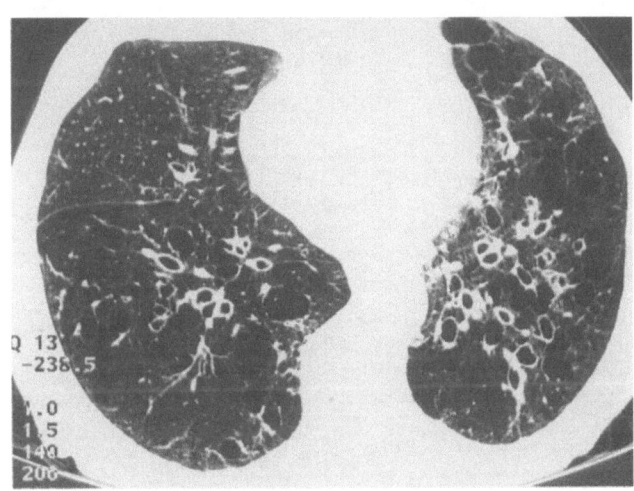

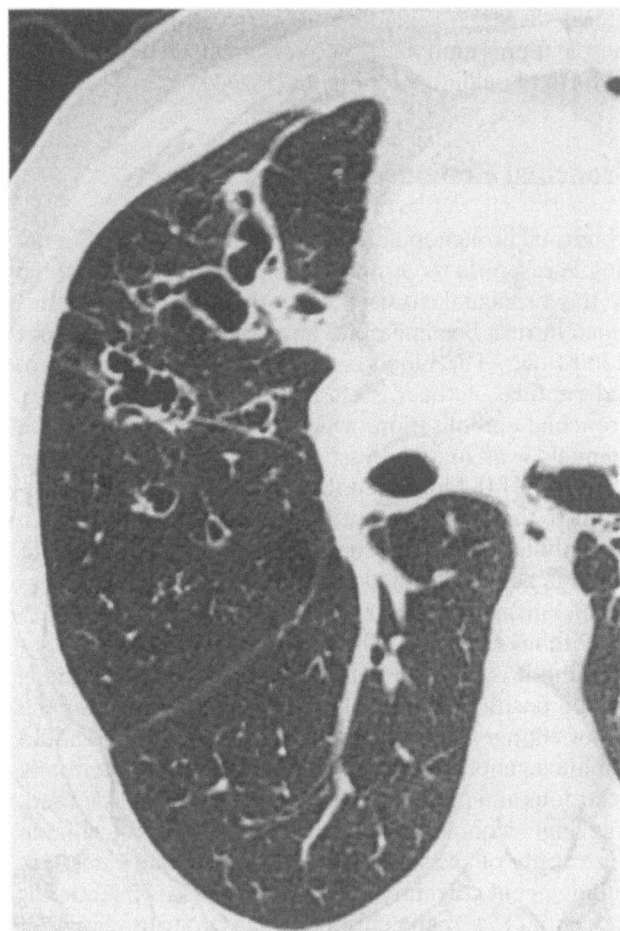

**Fig. 3.** Patient with haemoptysis and normal chest radiograph. High-resolution computed tomography reveals severe varicose bronchiectasis in the right lung

## Massive Haemoptysis

Massive haemoptysis is defined as the expectoration of greater than 600 ml of blood over a 24-h period. It is usually caused by chronic inflammatory fibrocavitary disease which is mostly related to tuberculosis or sarcoidosis, often with the additional formation of aspergillomas. In addition, patients with cystic fibrosis survive longer than they did a decade ago and this disease is also frequently associated with life-threatening haemoptysis. In patients with massive haemoptysis the chest radiograph is often nondiagnostic, frequently revealing only consolidation due to blood which has been aspirated throughout the bronchial tree. If the chest radiograph is normal, HRCT may serve to localise the disease by demonstrating a focal area of haemorrhage or other abnormality.

The mortality from massive haemoptysis is high, with around 50% of patients dying, usually from asphyxiation, when managed conservatively. Whilst surgery may be curative, it is not always feasible, either because of bilateral disease or inadequate respiratory reserve. In these patients embolisation offers an attractive and useful form of palliative treatment (Fig. 4).

## Bronchial Embolisation

Abnormal bronchopulmonary shunts develop within the lung in response to chronic inflammation. These are fed by the bronchial arteries and other systemic arteries which in turn become quite large due to the significant blood flows. The blood is at systemic arterial pressure and rupture of the vessels results in severe bleeding. Bronchial embolisation, which aims to obliterate these channels, was first successfully performed by Remy et al. in 1973 [14]. Since then there have been many refinements to the technique both in the catheters used and in the embolic agents and contrast media [15, 16]. Embolisation is best performed using digital subtraction, non-ionic contrast media, and relatively small catheters (5 Fr) with no side holes. The catheter position must be secure and it is preferable to occlude the vessels from as distal a position as possible. This often necessitates the use of slippery guidewires and coaxial systems. Liquid embolic agents such as absolute alcohol are potentially hazardous and particulate agents should always be used. Polyvinyl alcohol, a particulate agent which is available in a variety of sizes, is probably the best and safest occluding agent currently available. During its injection it is essential to screen continuously in order to recognise alternative arterial pathways which open up as occlusion of the main feeding vessels takes place. Using this technique, it should be possible to avoid occlusion of the spinal artery.

It is important to remember that a number of systemic arteries other than the bronchial arteries may be causative factors in the haemoptysis. These include the intercostal arteries, the costocervical and thyrocervical trunks, the internal mammary artery and the inferior phrenic arteries. Immediate control of haemoptysis is achieved by embolisation in 75%-90% of patients but it is only a palliative technique and rebleeding will occur in up to 20% of patients within 6 months. Early rebleeding usually results from incomplete embolisation either of one of the bronchial arteries or because nonbronchial systemic arteries have not been identified.

Aspergillomas are particularly difficult to treat, responding least well to embolisation. These patients do, however, respond quite well to the intracavitary injection of amphoteracin. This technique is usually performed under CT guidance and will control the haemop-

→

**Fig. 4 a-c.** Patient with massive haemoptysis due to chronic tuberculous cavity with an aspergilloma (right upper lobe). **a** Chest radiograph. **b** Right bronchointercostal arteriogram reveals a large mesh of abnormal vessels. Note filling of the pulmonary vein and the subclavian artery (*arrows*). **c** Post embolisation appearances

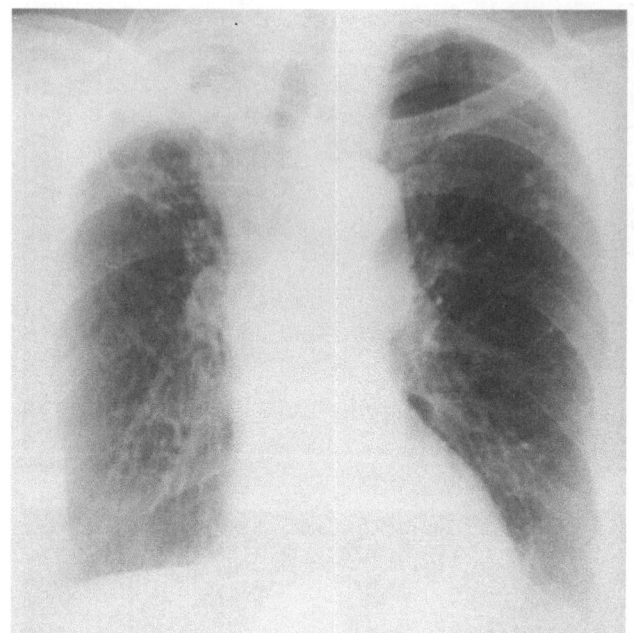

a

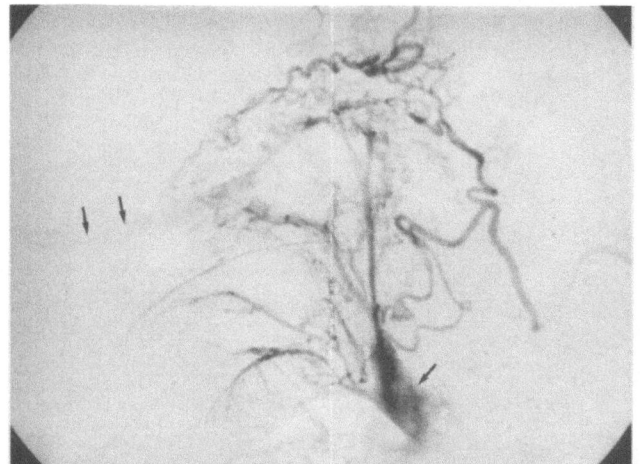

b

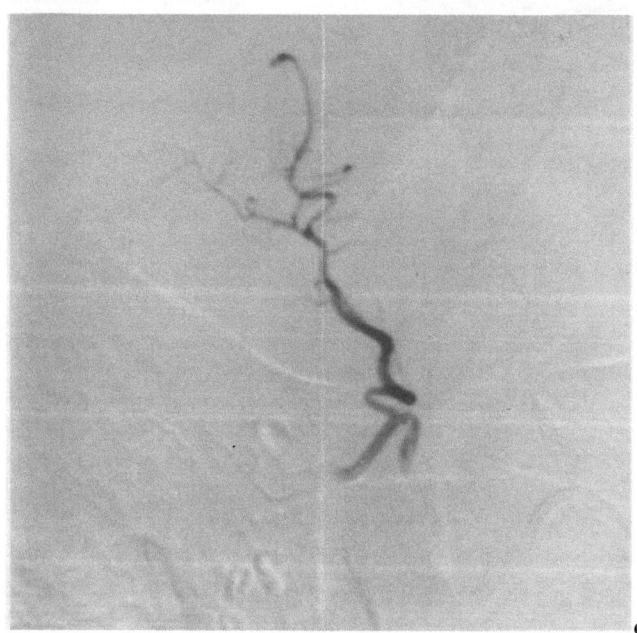

c

tysis and resolve the aspergilloma in a significant proportion of patients. It can be used as an adjunct to embolisation. Serious complications of embolisation are rare. Transverse myelitis and bronchial necrosis are the most feared complications but are extremely unlikely to occur if nonionic contrast media and appropriate embolic agents are used with a meticulous technique.

# References

1. Santiago S, Tobias J, Williams AJ (1991) A reappraisal of the causes of haemoptysis. Arch Intern Med 151:2449-2451
2. Poe RH, Israel RH, Marin MC et al (1988) Utility of fibreoptic bronchoscopy in patients with haemoptysis and a non-localising chest roentgenogram. Chest 93:70-75
3. Jackson CV, Savage PI, Quinn DL (1985) Role of fibreoptic bronchoscopy in patients with haemoptysis and a normal chest radiograph. Chest 87:142-144
4. Weaver LF, Solliday N, Cugell DW (1979) Selection of patients with haemoptysis for bronchoscopy. Chest 76:7-10
5. Snider GL (1979) When not to use the bronchoscope for haemoptysis. Chest 76:1-2
6. Webb WR, Gamsu G, Speckman JM (1983) Computed tomography of the pulmonary hilum in patients with bronchogenic carcinoma. J Comput Assist Tomogr 7:219-225
7. Henschke CI, Davis SD, Auh PR et al (1982) Detection of bronchial abnormalities: comparison of CT and bronchoscopy. J Comp Assist Tomogr 6:437-444
8. Naidich DP, Lee JJ, Garay SM et al (1987) Comparison of CT and fibreoptic bronchoscopy in the evaluation of bronchial disease. AJR 148:1-7
9. Mayr B, Ingrisch H, Haussinger K, Huber RM (1989) Tumours of the bronchi: role of evaluation with CT. Radiology 172:647-652
10. Naidich DP, Funt S, Ettenger NA et al (1990) Haemoptysis: CT-bronchoscopic correlations in 58 cases. Radiology 177:357-362
11. Millar AB, Boothroyd AE, Edwards D et al (1992) The role of computed tomography (CT) in the investigation of unexplained haemoptysis. Respir Med 86:39-44
12. Set PAK, Flower CDR, Smith IE et al (1993) Haemoptysis: comparative study of the role of CT and fibreoptic bronchoscopy. Radiology 189:677-680
13. McGuiness G, Beacher JR, Harkin TJ et al (1994) Haemoptysis: prospective high-resolution CT/bronchoscopic correlation. Chest 105:1155-1162
14. Remy J, Voisin C, Dupuis C et al (1974) Traitement des hemoptysies par embolization de la circulation systemique. Ann Radiol (Paris) 17:5-16
15. Jardin M, Remy J (1988) Control of haemoptysis: systemic angiography and anastomoses of the internal mammary artery. Radiology 168:377-383
16. Uflacker R, Kaemmerer A, Picon PD et al (1985) Bronchial artery embolization in the management of haemoptysis: technical aspects and long-term results. Radiology 157:637-644

# Small-Airway Diseases of the Lungs: Value of Expiratory CT

J. Verschakelen

Department of Radiology, University Hospitals K.U.L., Herestraat 49, 3000 Leuven, Belgium

## Introduction

Small-airway disease (SAD) is generally defined as a pathological condition in which the small conducting airways are affected. There is disagreement about which airways should be considered as small airways. Physiologists generally consider airways smaller than 2 mm as small airways, while pathologists define small airways as bronchioles and usually include terminal bronchioles, respiratory bronchioles and alveolar ducts [1, 5].

Bronchiolar involvement in SAD can be the primary finding but is more often a component of a more widespread lung disease. It is generally accepted that the lesions result from damage to the bronchiolar epithelium. Inflammation of the wall, excessive proliferation of granulation tissue and possibly varying degrees of fibrosis can lead to narrowing and obliteration of the lumen. Unfortunately there is a wide variation in histologic appearance. This variation, together with a variable clinical course and aetiology, is responsible for the different terminology that has been used to describe the syndrome: bronchiolitis, bronchiolitis obliterans, obliterative bronchiolitis, constrictive bronchiolitis, bronchiolitis obliterans with organizing pneumonia (BOOP), and BOOP reaction [3, 6].

Many attempts have been made to classify bronchiolitis but no classification scheme is widely accepted at this moment. In some studies classification is according to pathological pattern [3, 7], in others according to origin, while recently a review was published in which bronchiolitis was classified according to the radiological (computed tomographic, CT) findings [4]. It is not within the scope of this communication to discuss all the radiological features of SAD in detail. Only a brief review of the CT features of SAD will be given based on the radiological classification suggested by Müller and coworkers [4].

## CT Findings in SAD

Since CT is not able to demonstrate bronchi smaller than 2 mm, normal bronchioles cannot be seen. Part of their course, however, can be determined to a certain degree by studying the intralobular arteries. These arteries, which can be visualized with high-resolution CT (HRCT) when the diameter is larger than 0.2 mm, form together with the lobular bronchiole the core of the secondary pulmonary lobule.

Ill-defined nodules and thin branching lines are the most common HRCT findings when the syndrome is dominated by acute or chronic inflammation in the walls of the airways and by inflammatory exudate and mucus in the bronchiolar lumina. Often, some of these abnormalities are located in the centrilobular lung areas. This presentation is seen, for example, in patients with infectious bronchiolitis, asthma, chronic bronchitis, and diffuse panbronchiolitis and can be part of the syndrome in respiratory or smokers' bronchiolitis.

When there is excessive proliferation of granulation tissue within the lumina of the bronchioles and alveolar ducts or when interstitial or alveolar inflammation involves the alveoli immediately adjacent to the small airways, CT presentation is dominated by the presence of (bronchocentric) ground-glass opacity and lung consolidation. This presentation is seen in BOOP [8] and in many of the diseases in which the BOOP is a complication (BOOP reaction) [3]. These BOOP reactions may be seen in the chronic phase of bacterial, fungal or viral infection or after inhalation of toxins and can be a complication in collagen vascular diseases such as rheumatoid arthritis, systemic lupus erythematosus, dermatomyositis and mixed connective tissue disease. Areas of ground-glass attenuation are also described in patients with respiratory bronchiolitis [9].

Sometimes there is overlap between the patterns and in some cases it is difficult to identify the predominant pattern. In addition, ground-glass opacification and consolidation can be seen together with ill-defined nodules and branching lines in diseases in which bronchiolitis is only part of a chronic lung disease that primarily affects the peribronchiolar regions. These abnormalities are found, for example, in hypersensitivity pneumonitis [10] and pneumoconiosis.

Mosaic perfusion and air-trapping are generally con-

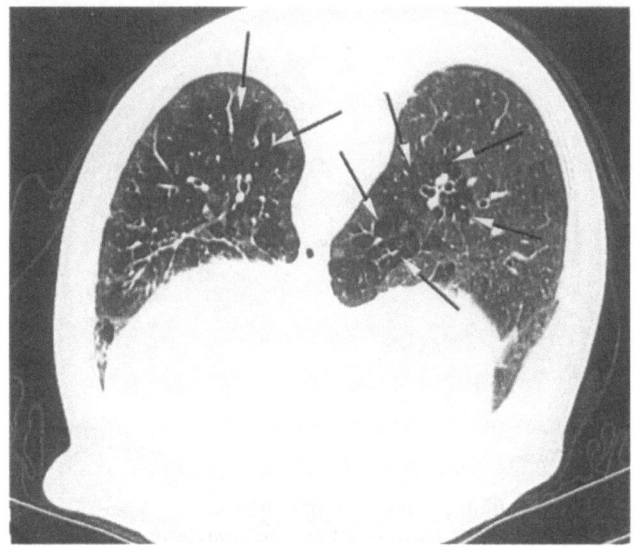 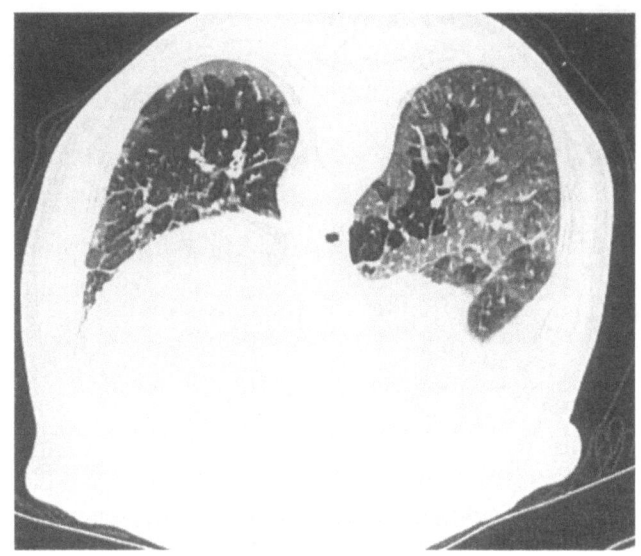

a b

**Fig. 1 a, b.** Mosaic perfusion as a sequela of mycoplasma pneumonia. **a** High-resolution computed tomography (HRCT) at suspended deep inspiration. Bronchiolar (sub)obstruction results in hypoventilation and secondary hypoperfusion. Affected areas present as zones of decreased attenuation (*arrows*). Because of vascular redistribution surrounding areas show increased attenuation (ground-glass appearance). **b** HRCT at suspended deep expiration. Because of air-trapping, areas of decreased attenuation do not show decrease in volume or increase in density and the mosaic perfusion is accentuated

sidered to be indirect CT signs of bronchiolitis. Mosaic perfusion is defined as regional differences in lung perfusion that result in visible attenuation differences on HRCT. It can reflect vascular obstruction, but in bronchiolitis it is believed to be the result of decreased perfusion of areas with bronchiolar (sub)obstruction (and hypoventilation) and flow redistribution to normal surrounding areas.

Air-trapping is characterized by the lack of lung density increase of one or more lung areas compared to the surrounding areas during expiration. Since the visualization and interpretation of both features is related to CT images performed during expiration these signs will be discussed in more detail.

## Mosaic Perfusion and Air-Trapping

Mosaic perfusion (Fig. 1) was first described on HRCT images performed after deep inspiration [11]. It was defined as areas of decreased perfusion that result in decreased attenuation surrounded by areas of increased attenuation caused by vascular redistribution. The explanation that hypoperfusion is the result of hypoventilation caused by bronchiolar obstruction suggests that the bronchiolar narrowing is important and probably chronic. That is why mosaic perfusion is predominantly found in those cases in which bronchiolitis is characterized by concentric narrowing of the bronchioles caused by submucosal and peribronchiolar fibrosis. This type of bronchiolitis is seen, for example, as a sequel of childhood viral infection, mycoplasma pneumonia or toxic fume inhalation. It is a well-known complication of bone marrow and lung transplantation and is also described in

patients with rheumatoid arthritis [12, 13].

When mosaic perfusion is caused by bronchiolar narrowing, the low attenuation areas will be accentuated on expiratory CT because they do not increase in density due to air-trapping. The surrounding areas with hyperperfusion will further increase in density during expiration and accentuate the mosaic pattern (Fig. 1b).

Since expiratory CT scans are usually not performed routinely in every patient, experience of how the lung parenchyma presents in this situation is limited. However, especially in patients with bronchiolitis, scans performed during suspended deep expiration can be interesting [5, 14, 15]. Early collapse of narrowed bronchioles during expiration or mucous plugging can cause areas of air-trapping in these patients. An interesting feature is the fact that this air-trapping sometimes comes as a complete surprise on routine CT scan during suspended full inspiration (Fig. 2). The latter suggests that expiratory CT scan can be a very sensitive tool to depict mild SAD even during the acute phase of the disease.

## Expiratory HRCT of the Normal Lung

During expiration there is an increase in lung density that is caused by the reduction of air in the lung. Due to gravity, there is a greater blood flow and a reduced expansion of air spaces in the dependent lung areas, resulting in a higher density increase in these parts of the lung [15, 16].

Although density increase is mostly homogeneous, it has been shown that small areas of air-trapping (often limited to a few lobules) can occur in healthy nonsmokers [17, 18].

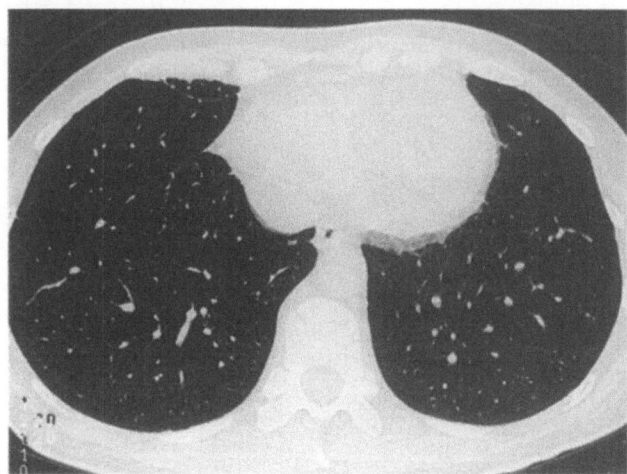
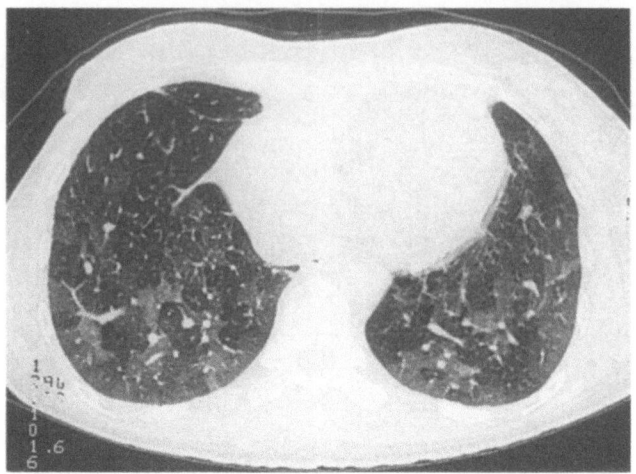

**Fig. 2 a, b.** Bronchiolitis and air-trapping caused by cigarette smoking. High-resolution computed tomography (HRCT) performed at deep inspiration. **a** shows no abnormalities. However, expiratory CT (**b**) shows multiple areas of air-trapping (areas not increasing in density)

### Expiratory HRCT in Patients with SAD

As indicated earlier, experience with expiratory HRCT performed in patients suspected of having bronchiolitis is limited, especially when no mosaic perfusion was found on inspiratory scans.

Focal areas of air-trapping were found in asthmatic patients after bronchoprovocation. Air-trapping together with diffuse micronodules, ground-glass attenuation, lung fibrosis and emphysema was demonstrated in patients with hypersensitivity pneumonitis [10].

Areas of decreased attenuation on expiratory CT scans are common in severe bronchiectasis both in lobes with and without bronchiectasis, suggesting that SAD may precede the development of bronchiectasis [19].

Bronchiolitis is a well-known feature in smokers [9]. In our experience focal areas of air-trapping are a common finding in healthy smokers and ex-smokers (Fig. 2) [17]. Although not always examined with expiratory CT, air-trapping was also suggested by the presence of multiple areas of low attenuation in patients with connective tissue disease (Fig. 3) [11, 12] and in patients who had undergone lung transplantation [13].

### Air-Trapping on Expiratory HRCT: Clinical and Functional Relevance

Knowledge of the clinical and functional relevance of the focal areas of air-trapping is limited [17, 19, 20]. Hansell and co-workers examined patients with severe

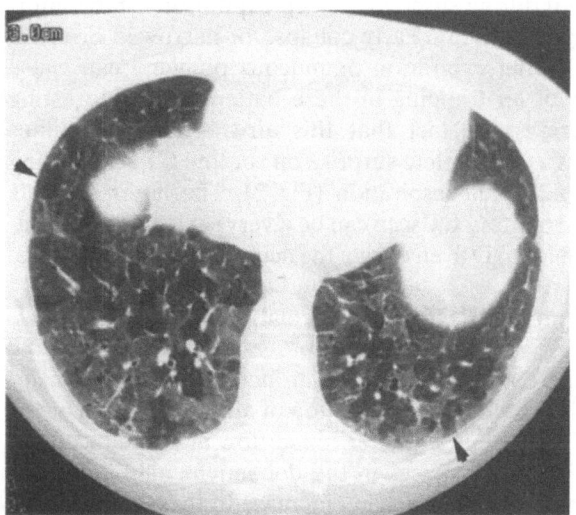
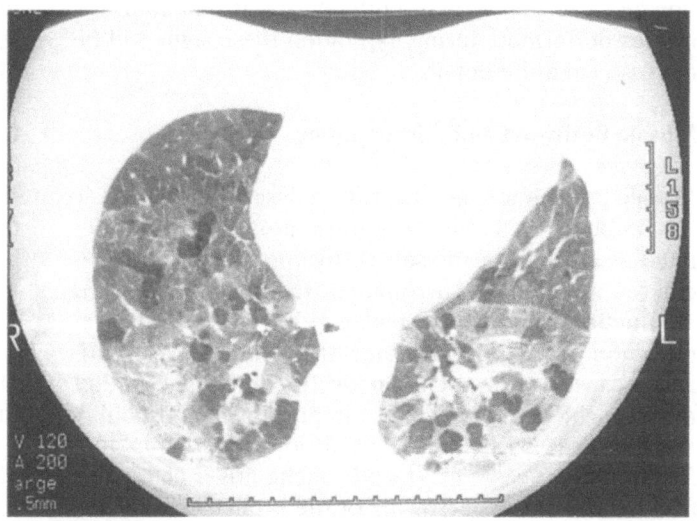

**Fig. 3 a, b.** Ground-glass opacity and air-trapping in a patient with rheumatoid arthritis. **a** High-resolution computed tomography (HRCT) at suspended deep inspiration. Multiple areas of decreased attenuation (some of these have the size of a secondary pulmonary lobule, *arrowheads*) are surrounded by areas of increased density probably not only caused by vascular redistribution but also by interstitial disease. **b** HRCT at suspended deep expiration: areas of decreased attenuation are accentuated, indicating air-trapping and small-airway disease

bronchiectasis and found significant correlations between the extent of air-trapping and some pulmonary function tests (FEV1, FEV1/FVC, RV) [19]. Because airways smaller than 2 mm account for only one quarter of the airway resistance, these airways must become severely narrowed before pulmonary function tests (PFT) become abnormal [4, 20]. For this reason, it can be expected that HRCT, and especially expiratory HRCT, will depict SAD earlier than PFT do. Yet, the exact value of this early detection needs to be determined: Perhaps CT can predict the development of more severe lung damage.

## Air-Trapping on Expiratory CT: Differential Diagnosis

Differential diagnosis with compensatory overinflation of a portion of the lung as a result of lobar collapse or resection is in most cases easy because air-trapping as a result of bronchiolitis is often patchy. Moreover, the cause of compensatory overinflation is usually easy to find.

Vascular obstruction as a cause of mosaic perfusion can be diagnosed, when the low attenuation areas show density increase on expiratory CT scans [5, 14].

## Conclusions

Air-trapping is a physiological consequence of SAD and is most often patchy and multifocal. Severe air-trapping can be diagnosed on HRCT at suspended deep inspiration and presents as mosaic perfusion. Mild to moderate air-trapping can be seen on HRCT at suspended deep expiration and is sometimes not visible on inspiratory HRCT. Hence, HRCT is able to detect air-trapping and SAD in an early stage and this technique is probably more sensitive than PFT. However, the clinical impact of these findings has not been fully determined yet.

## References

1. Grenier P, Beigelman C, Brauner M (1994) High resolution computed tomography in the study of the respiratory tract. Ann Radiol (Paris) 37:198-215
2. Hartman TE, Primack SL, Lee KS, Swensen SJ, Muller NL (1994) CT of bronchial and bronchiolar diseases. Radiographics 14:991-1003
3. King TE (1993) Overview of bronchiolitis. Clin Chest Med 14:607-610
4. Müller NL, Miller RR (1995) Diseases of the bronchioles: CT and histopathologic findings. Radiology 196:3-12
5. Webb WR (1994) High-resolution computed tomography of obstructive lung disease. Radiol Clin North Am 32:745-757
6. Lynch DA (1993) Imaging of small airways diseases. Clin Chest Med 14:623-634
7. Garg K, Lynch DA, Newell JD, King TE Jr (1994) Proliferative and constrictive bronchiolitis: classification and radiologic features. AJR 162:803-808
8. Bouchardy LM, Kuhlman JE, Ball WC Jr, Hruban RH, Askin FB, Siegelman SS (1993) CT findings in bronchiolitis obliterans organizing pneumonia (BOOP) with radiographic, clinical, and histologic correlation. J Comput Assist Tomogr 17:352-357
9. Remy-Jardin M, Remy J, Gosselin B, Becette V, Edme JL (1993) Lung parenchymal changes secondary to cigarette smoking: pathologic-CT correlations. Radiology 186:643-651
10. Hansell DM, Moskovic E (1991) High-resolution computed tomography in extrinsic allergic alveolitis. Clin Radiol 43:8-12
11. Eber CD, Stark P, Bertozzi P (1993) Bronchiolitis obliterans on high-resolution CT: a pattern of mosaic oligemia. J Comput Assist Tomogr 17:853-856
12. Aquino SL, Webb WR, Golden J (1994) Bronchiolitis obliterans associated with rheumatoid arthritis: findings on HRCT and dynamic expiratory CT. J Comput Assist Tomogr 18:555-558
13. Morrish WF, Herman SJ, Weisbrod GL, Chamberlain DW (1991) Bronchiolitis obliterans after lung transplantation: findings at chest radiography and high-resolution CT. Radiology 179:487-490
14. Stern EJ, Frank MS (1994) Small-airway diseases of the lungs: findings at expiratory CT. AJR 163:37-41
15. Stern EJ, Webb WR (1993) Dynamic imaging of lung morphology with ultrafast high-resolution computed tomography. J Thorac Imaging 8:273-282
16. Verschakelen JA, van Fraeyenhoven L, Laureys G, Demedts M, Baert AL (1993) Differences in CT density between dependent and nondependent portions of the lung: influence of lung volume. AJR 161:713-717
17. Verschakelen JA, Scheinbaum K, Bogaert JG, Lacquet L, Nemery B, Baert AL (1994) Correlation between cigarette smoking and presence of focal areas of air-trapping on expiratory high-resolution CT scans. Radiology 193(P):368
18. Webb WR, Stern EJ, Kanth N, Gamsu G (1993) Dynamic pulmonary CT findings in healthy adult men. Radiology 186:117-124
19. Hansell DM, Wells AU, Rubens MB, Cole PJ (1994) Bronchiectasis: functional significance of areas of decreased attenuation at expiratory CT. Radiology 193:369-374
20. Padley SP, Adler BD, Hansell DM, Muller NL (1993) Bronchiolitis obliterans: high resolution CT findings and correlation with pulmonary function tests. Clin Radiol 47:236-240

# CT of Chronic Obstructive Lung Disease

P. Grenier

Service de Radiologie Générale, Groupe Hospitalier La Pitié-Salpetrière, 47 Blvd. de l'Hôpital, 75651 Paris, France

Lung diseases associated with obstruction to airflow are usually grouped together under the term chronic obstructive pulmonary disease (COPD). This disparate group of diseases is defined by the presence of abnormal pulmonary function rather than specific morphologic findings and, consequently, has no characteristic and consistent radiographic appearance. Imaging studies have had a limited role in the diagnosis in evaluation of patients with COPD. The recent development of high-resolution computed tomography (HRCT), however, has significantly improved our ability to image morphologic abnormalities associated with chronic airflow obstruction [1].

## Emphysema

### CT Findings

Emphysema is characterized by permanent abnormal enlargement of airspaces distal to the terminal bronchioles, accompanied by the destruction of their walls, and without obvious fibrosis. Emphysema is classified into three main types: centrilobular, panlobular and paraseptal. In the early stages, these three types of emphysema can be distinguished using HRCT [1]. The differentiation becomes difficult or impossible when the lesions become more extensive. Centrilobular emphysema, resulting usually from cigarette smoking, predominantly affects the upper lung zones. It is characterized on HRCT scans by the presence of small, round areas of low density several millimetres in diameter grouped near the centre of the secondary pulmonary lobule without any visible wall. These conditions allow emphysema to be easily distinguished from cystic airspaces and honeycombing. The detection of centrilobular emphysema is facilitated by the contrast of density between normal and emphysematous areas in the secondary pulmonary lobule.

Panlobular emphysema is classically associated with an antitrypsin deficiency, although it may also be seen in smokers without protease deficiency, as well as in patients with bronchial and bronchiolar obliteration. Panlobular emphysema is characterized by uniform destruction of the pulmonary lobule, leading to widespread areas of abnormally low density (Fig. 1). It is almost always most severe in the lower lobes. In severe panlobular emphysema, extensive lung destruction and paucity of vascular markings are easily distinguished from normal lung parenchyma, but, in contrast, mild and moderately severe panlobular emphysema can be very difficult to detect.

Paraseptal emphysema is characterized by involvement of the distal part of the secondary pulmonary lobule. It is often associated with spontaneous pneumothorax in adults. Paraseptal emphysema is easily detected when located subpleurally. It is very easy to detect with HRCT along the peripheral, mediastinal, pleura as well as the fissures. The bullae or air cysts, commonly seen in patients with paraseptal emphysema, have visible walls but the walls are very thin. Bullae are generally defined as being larger than 1 cm.

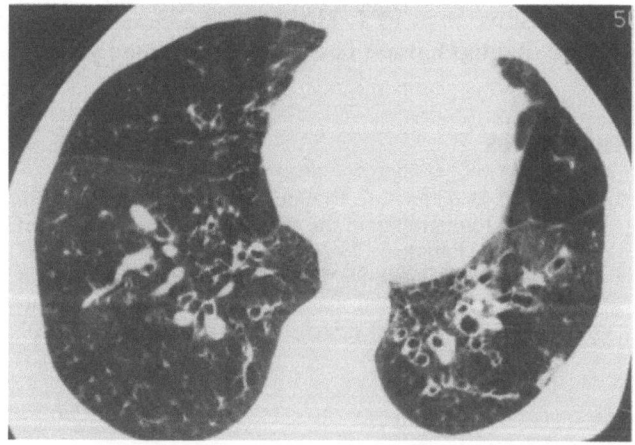

**Fig. 1.** Chronic obstructive pulmonary disease with emphysema, bronchiectasis and pulmonary hypertension. Panlobular emphysema is seen mainly in the right middle, lingula, and left lower lobes, as low attenuation and paucity of vascular markings. Cylindrical and varicose bronchiectasis involves the right and left basal segments. The segmental pulmonary arteries of the lower lobes are enlarged, occurring as a result of pulmonary hypertension

## Pathologic and Functional Correlations

The correlations between CT scores of emphysema extent and pathologic scores have been proved to be good. However, emphysema may be missed on CT scans and underestimation of the extent of emphysema is observed in most of the cases [2]. There is a considerable variability in the relationship between the loss of structure due to emphysematous destruction and the loss of function. About 20% of patients with emphysema defined by characteristic pulmonary function tests have no evidence of emphysema on HRCT, and in about 40% of the patients with emphysema at HRCT, results of pulmonary function tests are normal [3]. The presence of emphysema on CT was demonstrated in 21% of current smokers with normal results of pulmonary function tests and chest radiographs [4].

## Clinical Utility of CT

CT is undoubtedly the most sensitive diagnostic investigation of emphysema in vivo. However, as emphysema may be missed on CT, this investigation cannot be used to definitely rule out the diagnosis. In clinical practice, there are two main indications for CT in diagnosing emphysema. The first corresponds to patients having shortness of breath and low diffusing capacity without evidence of airway obstruction on pulmonary function tests and chest radiograph. If significant emphysema is found on HRCT, no further evaluation is necessary [5]. Secondly, in the preoperative assessment of patients with bullous emphysema who are being considered for bullectomy, the extent of bullous disease, the degree of compression of underlying lung, and the severity of emphysema in the remaining lung parenchyma can be assessed by CT examination [6].

## Quantification

To estimate the overall extent of the emphysema visible on CT, some authors have proposed highlighting areas of abnormally low density using a computer program. When the appropriate density value cut off is determined, areas of emphysema can be segmented and objective quantification of emphysematous changes obtained [7].

## Cystic Lung Disease

The term lung cyst is used to describe a thin-walled (usually < 3 mm), air-containing lesion. Two lung diseases, histiocytosis X and lymphangiomatosis, are commonly associated with the presence of lung cysts. Pulmonary histiocytosis X (eosinophilic granulomas of the lung, Langerhans histiocytosis) is an idiopathic, uncommon disease characterized pathologically in its early stages

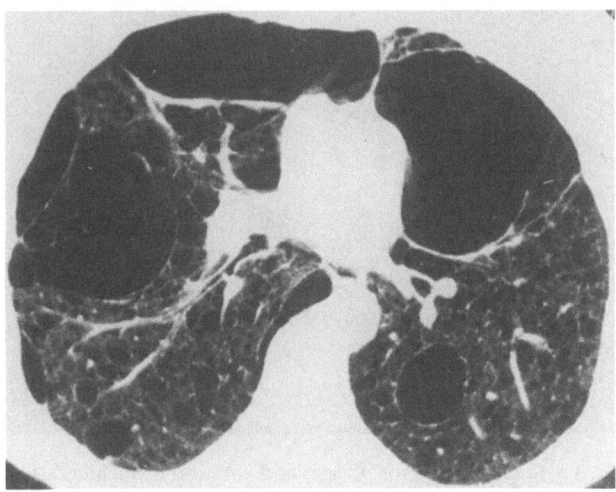

**Fig. 2.** Lymphangiomyomatosis. Multiple, thin-walled cysts are diffusely distributed throughout the lungs. Large cysts and bullae are associated in the anterior part of the lungs

by granulomatous nodules. The majority of patients are young or middle-aged adults and more than 90% are smokers. On HRCT scans, the lung cysts have walls that range from being barely perceptible to being several millimetres in thickness. They appear round, but they also can have bizarre shapes due to the fusion of several cysts. An upper lobe predominance in the size and number of cysts is common and the intervening lung parenchyma appears normal without evidence of fibrosis. Small nodules may also be present [8].

Lymphangiomyomatosis is a rare disease characterized by progressive proliferation of spindle cells in the lung. Proliferation of spindle cells along the bronchioles leads to air trapping and the development of thin-walled lung cysts. Lymphangiomyomatosis occurs only in women between 17 and 50 years of age. On HRCT, numerous thin-walled lung cysts are seen surrounded by relatively normal lung parenchyma. The cysts are distributed diffusely throughout the lungs and no lung zone is spared [9] (Fig. 2).

## Bronchiectasis

Bronchiectasis is defined as a localized, irreversible bronchial dilatation. Bronchiectasis has been classified into three types on the basis of morphology. The CT diagnosis of varicose and cystic bronchiectasis is simple. A group or cluster of multiple, air-filled cysts is a common finding in cystic bronchiectasis (Fig. 3). Air fluid levels in the dependent portions of the dilated bronchi are a specific sign of this entity. Varicose bronchiectasis is seen as dilated bronchi with a beaded appearance or as a string of pearls. The only limitation of CT in assessing bronchiectasis concerns the cylindrical pattern. Cylindrical bronchiectasis is characterized on HRCT by the

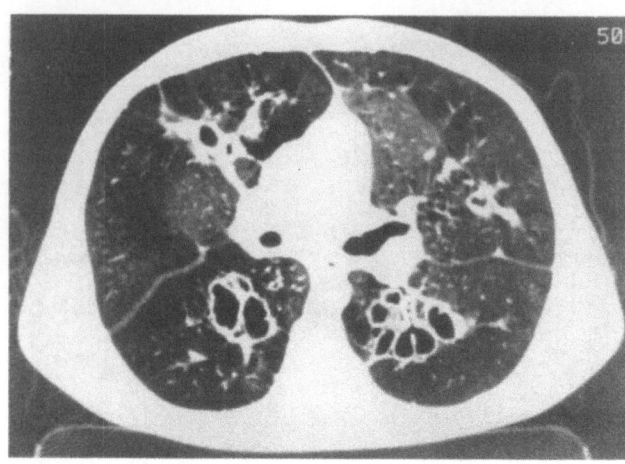
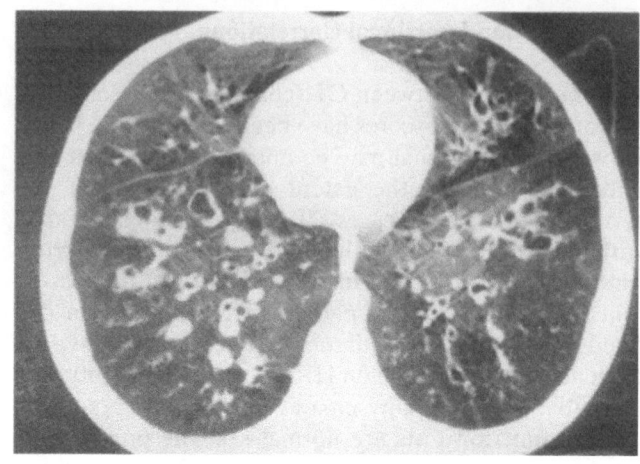

a b

**Fig. 3 a, b.** Cystic fibrosis. Cystic and varicose bronchiectasis is distributed in all lobes. Mucoid impactions in dilated bronchi are seen within the right lower lobe. Mosaic perfusion indicates the presence of abnormal regional lung ventilation

presence of thick-walled bronchi, which extend to the lung periphery and fail to show normal tapering. Depending on their orientation relative to the scan plane, they can simulate tramlines or can show the signet-ring sign in which the dilated, thick-walled bronchus and its accompanying pulmonary artery branch are seen adjacent to each other [1] (Figs. 1, 4).

HRCT has become a widely accepted technique for assessing the presence, type and distribution of bronchiectasis. Its accuracy is comparable to that of bronchography [10]. The HRCT protocol recommended for patients suspected of having bronchiectasis is based on 1.5-mm collimation scans with 10-mm interspacing over the chest from the apex of the lung to the diaphragm [11]. Slice interspacing can be reduced to 5-mm over the most suspicious pulmonary areas. In addition, the gantry can be inclined 20° cranially as it improves CT analysis of segmental or subsegmental bronchi. Surgery is still performed in some patients when bronchiectasis is localized. In such cases, accurate assessment is required on a segmental basis. HRCT is not able to definitively elimi-

nate the possibility of overlooking areas of focal bronchiectasis located exclusively in areas not visualized between thin-section scans, and bronchial dilatation of mild cylindric bronchiectasis may be difficult to perceive on successive HRCT scans. Spiral CT, using thin collimation, may contribute to reducing some of these pitfalls. Therefore, it may be helpful to use HRCT and spiral CT in combination. We recommend performing HRCT scans with 1.5-mm collimation and 10-mm interspacing over the upper and lower parts of the lungs, where segmental and subsegmental bronchi run mainly perpendicular to the scan plane. Spiral CT scanning with 3-mm collimation is selected from 15 mm above the carina, in a caudal direction, during a 20-s breath-hold over the lung areas where segmental and subsegmental bronchi run mostly parallel to the scan plane.

Dilated bronchi can be filled with fluid, mucus or pus. Mucoid impaction-filling bronchiectasis can simulate pulmonary nodules or masses on HRCT scans (Fig. 3). Complementary scans performed in prone position may help to mobilize bronchial secretion and visualize the dilated bronchial lumen. It may be helpful to use spiral CT with thin collimation over the suspicious area for multiplanar reconstruction and recognition of the tubular shape of opacities due to filled, dilated bronchi.

CT can be used to grade the severity of bronchiectasis and to monitor the response to therapy in patients with cystic fibrosis, allergic bronchopulmonary aspergillosis and primary ciliary dyskinesia [1] (Fig. 3).

## Small Airway Abnormalities

Morphologic abnormalities of the small airways in patients with COPD include wall thickening, narrowing or obliteration of the bronchiolar lumen, bronchiolar dilatation and mucous plugging. On HRCT, abnormal bronchioles filled with fluid, mucus or pus can appear as

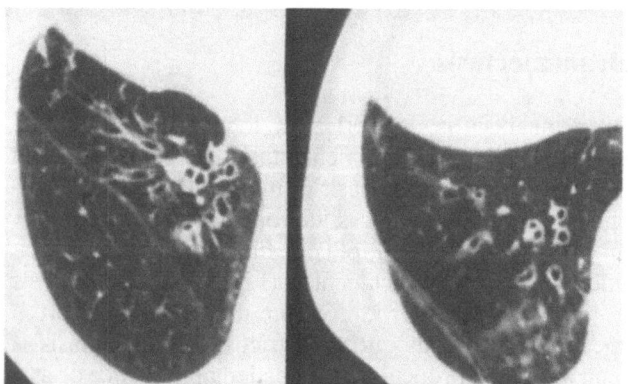

**Fig. 4.** Cylindrical bronchiectasis. Tramlines and signet rings are seen within an aerated, collapsed, right lower lobe

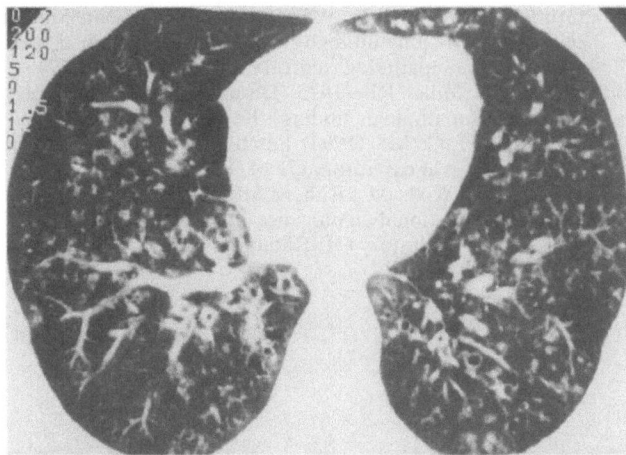

**Fig. 5.** Diffuse panbronchiolitis. Small nodular and branching linear centrilobular opacities are associated with small, ring-like centrilobular images

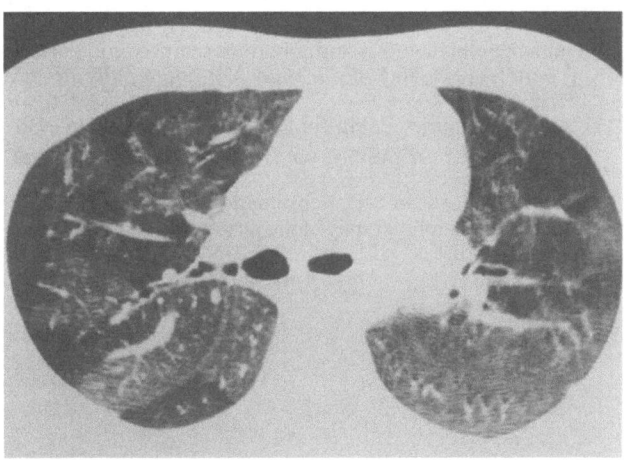

**Fig. 6.** Postinfectious bronchiolitis obliterans. Mosaic perfusion, due to air trapping is seen on high-resolution computed tomographic scans performed at end expiration

small centrilobular tubular, branching, linear or nodular structures. These can be associated with peribronchiolar, centrilobular, ill-defined nodular opacities if the adjacent lung is inflamed. If air-filled bronchioles are visible on the peripheral lung, it usually indicates a bronchiolar wall thickening and/or dilatation (Fig. 5). Diseases in which bronchiolar abnormalities are visible on HRCT include panbronchiolitis, cystic fibrosis, diseases associated with chronic bronchial sepsis, bronchiolitis obliterans, bronchopneumonia, respiratory bronchiolitis and hypersensitivity bronchiolitis [12, 13]. In many patients with small airway abnormalities visible on HRCT, bronchiectasis or bronchial wall thickening are also visible.

The diagnosis of small airway disease is challenging for the clinician, as there are no pathognomonic, clinical, functional, and radiographic features. At a functional level, the small airways contribute very little to normal airway resistance. As a result, widespread obliteration of these small airways is needed before there is any obvious functional impairment and clinical manifestations.

Patchy areas of varying lung attenuation are often visible on HRCT in patients with small airway abnormalities (Fig. 3). They often indicate the presence of perfusion abnormalities occurring as a result of abnormal regional lung ventilation (mosaic perfusion) [14]. The denser lung regions visible in these patients are better ventilated and better perfused. Air trapping contributes to this phenomenon of mosaic perfusion. This is particularly well demonstrated on HRCT scans performed at expiration. Normally at expiration, lung density increases while lung cross-section areas decrease. When air trapping is present, lung density fails to increase while lung cross-section areas fail to decrease as normally expected. Air trapping was demonstrated on HRCT scans in patients with emphysema, asthma, bronchiectasis and bronchiolitis [14]. Expiratory scans may show evidence of air trapping even in the absence of morphologic abnormalities recognizable on inspiratory scans (Fig. 6).

Although air trapping can be seen in subjects with normal pulmonary function tests, the extent and intensity of air trapping assessed on expiratory scans have been shown to correlate with the degree of airway obstruction [15]. A suggested protocol for HRCT scanning in cases of suspected small airway disease is 1.5-mm collimation at every 10-mm section in full inspiration followed by 1.5-mm/30-mm sections obtained at end expiration. Spiral HRCT may also be used to search for air trapping during active expiration.

## References

1. Webb WR (1994) High-resolution computed tomography of obstructive lung disease. Radiol Clin North Am 32:745-757
2. Miller RR, Müller NL, Vedal S, Morrisson NJ, Staples CA (1989) Limitations of computed tomography in the assessment of emphysema. Am Rev Respir Dis 139:980-983
3. Gurney JW, Jones KK, Robbins RA, Gossman GL, Nelson KJ, Daughton D, Spurzem JR, Rennard SI (1992) Regional distribution of emphysema: correlation of high-resolution CT with pulmonary function tests in unselected smokers. Radiology 183:457-463
4. Remy-Jardin M, Boulenguez C, Edme JL, Sobazek A, Wallaert B, Rémy J (1993) Morphologic effects of cigarette smoking on airways and pulmonary parenchyma in healthy adult volunteers: CT evaluation and correlations with pulmonary function tests. Radiology 186:107-115
5. Klein JS, Gamsu G, Webb WR, Golden JA, Müller NL (1992) High-resolution CT diagnosis of emphysema in symptomatic patients with normal chest radiographs and isolated low diffusing capacity. Radiology 182:817-821
6. Carr DH, Pride NB (1984) Computed tomography in preoperative assessment of bullous emphysema. Clin Radiol 35:43-45
7. Müller NL, Staples CA, Miller RR, Abboud RT (1988) "Density mark": an objective method to quantitate emphysema using computed tomography. Chest 94:782-787
8. Brauner MW, Grenier P, Mouelhi MM, Mompoint D, Lenoir S (1989) Pulmonary histiocytosis X: evaluation with high resolution CT. Radiology 172:255-258

9. Lenoir S, Grenier P, Brauner MW et al (1990) Pulmonary lymphangiomyomatosis and tuberous sclerosis: comparison of radiographic and thin-section CT findings. Radiology 175:329-334

10. Grenier P, Maurice F, Musset D, Menu Y, Nahum H (1986) Bronchiectasis: assessment by thin-section CT. Radiology 161:95-99

11. Grenier P, Cordeau MP, Beigelman C (1993) High-resolution computed tomography of the airways. J Thorac Imaging 8:213-229

12. Gruden JF, Webb WR, Warnock M (1994) Centrilobular opacities in the lung on high-resolution CT: diagnostic considerations and pathologic correlation. AJR 162:569-574

13. Müller NL, Miller RR (1995) Diseases of the bronchioles: CT and histopathologic findings. Radiology 196:3-12

14. Stern EJ, Frank MS (1994) Small-airway diseases of the lungs: findings at expiratory CT. AJR 163:37-41

15. Hansell DM, Wells AU, Rubens MB, Come PJ (1994) Bronchiectasis: functional significance of areas of decreased attenuation at expiratory CT. Radiology 193:369-374

# Imaging in Pulmonary Embolism

C.J. Herold

Universität für Radiodiagnostik, Allgemeines Krankenhaus, Waehringer Gürtel 18-20, A-1090 Vienna, Austria

## Introduction

Pulmonary embolism (PE) is an entity that is frequently encountered in the hospital environment as well as in private practice. Currently, although it is recognized as an important medical problem with a long history of extensive investigation, many fundamental questions remain unanswered. At this time, even the true incidence and mortality of PE are difficult to determine accurately. The magnitude of the problem can be demonstrated by the fact that in the United States, the number of patients who suffer from PE is estimated to reach 750 000 annually. Of these, approximately 150 000 die from this disorder [1]. While representative comprehensive numbers are not available for Europe, the significance of the problem is similar to that in the U.S.

Accurate diagnosis of PE is of paramount importance not only because untreated PE carries a significantly increased mortality risk due to recurrent massive thromboembolism, but also because of the potential complications involved with anticoagulation therapy. Among all other diagnostic tools, imaging methods play a leading role in the diagnostic work-up of patients suspected of having PE. The radiologist must be familiar with the features of PE on plain films, spiral computed tomographic (CT) angiography, and pulmonary angiography. Just as critical is the radiologist's awareness of the role of ventilation perfusion scanning. In the following summary, we will provide a basic overview on the diagnosis of PE.

## PE and Deep Venous Thrombosis

Approximately 95% of pulmonary thromboemboli originate in the deep venous system of the lower extremities, with the large leg veins above the knee being the most common source of significant PE that attracts clinical attention [2]. Other sources, responsible for the remainder of PE, are veins in the pelvis, the upper extremities and the right cardiac chamber. The incidence of PE in patients with deep venous thrombosis (DVT) is difficult to determine. This is because in approximately 50% of patients with DVT, the disease is unrecognized [3]. However, estimates of the incidence of PE in DVT range from 10% to 34%. The significance of detecting deep venous thrombosis in patients with suspected PE, however, is again emphasized by the fact that recurrent PE (from DVT) is the most significant contributor to the death toll in this disorder.

Contrast venography remains the diagnostic standard for the detection of acute venous thrombosis. Recently, however, duplex Doppler and colour Doppler sonography, because of their high sensitivity and specificity as well as their noninvasiveness, have challenged the leading role of contrast venography and, in some institutions, have become the first-line diagnostic tool in patients evaluated for DVT [1-3].

## Clinical Presentation

Whereas the pathogenesis of PE can be regarded as straightforward – a clot travels from the deep venous system into the pulmonary circulation – the clinical diagnosis of PE may be more challenging. First, only approximately 50% of patients with PE demonstrate clinical symptoms [4]. Second, the clinical manifestation of PE is variable and nonspecific. The classical clinical presentation includes signs such as unexplained dyspnoea, shortness of breath, cough, pleuritic chest pain, tachypnoea, tachycardia and fever [5]. However, these symptoms may also result from various other pulmonary disorders and are therefore nonspecific for PE.

## Chest Radiography

The role of chest radiography in the evaluation of PE has been extensively investigated during the last several decades. Currently, chest radiographs do not allow a specific diagnosis of PE or help to reliably exclude the disease. Chest radiographs show signs and symptoms compatible with PE in only about 50%-80% of cases [6]. This is at least partly due to the fact that roentgenologi-

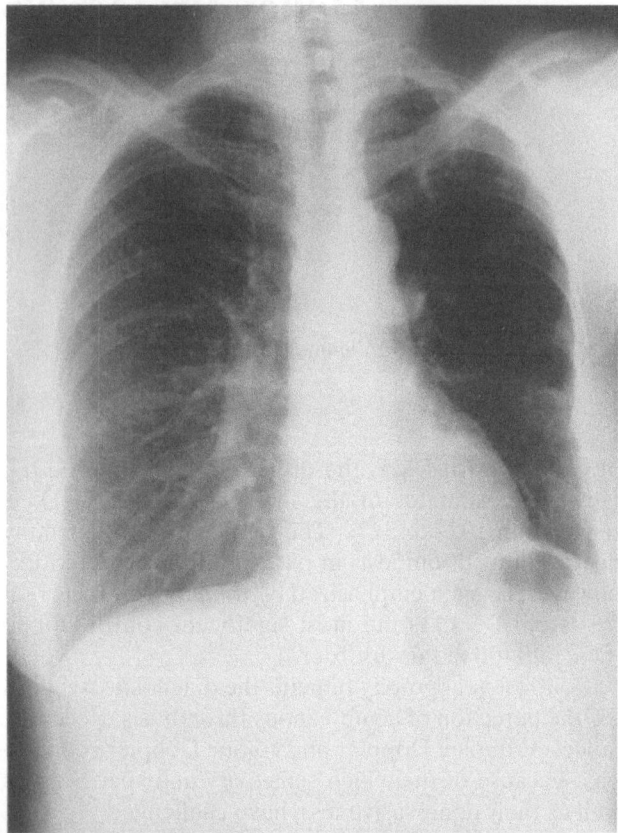

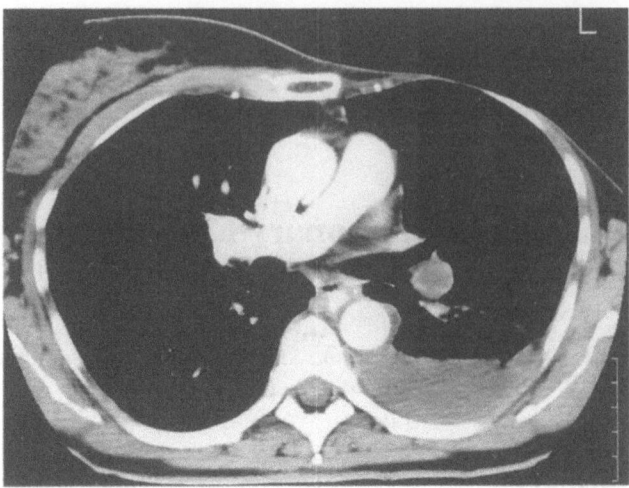

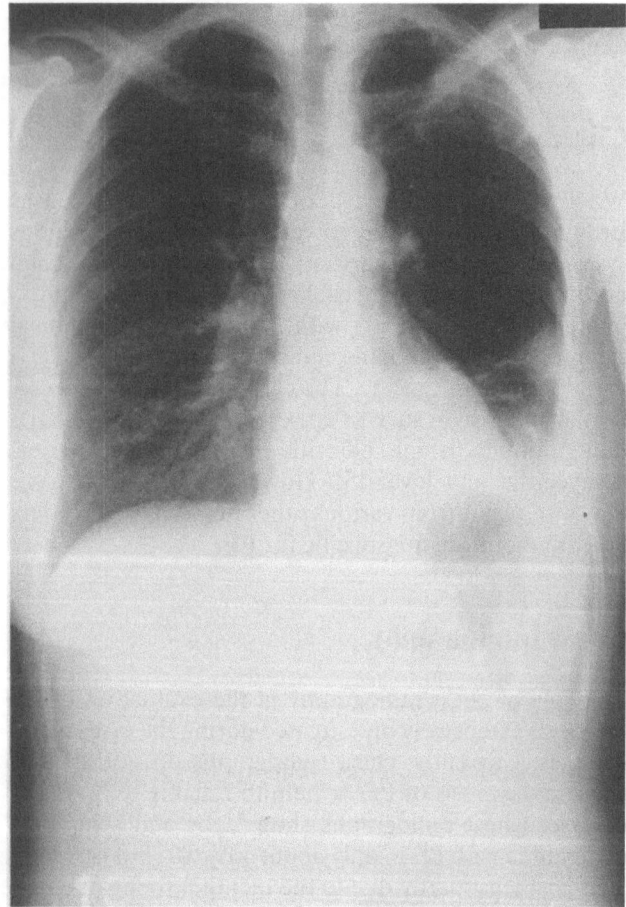

**Fig. 1 a-c.** Plain-film findings and spiral computed tomographic angiography (SCTA) in the evaluation of suspected pulmonary embolism in a patient with breast cancer. **a** Marked widespread oligemia and decreased attenuation in the left lung due to central pulmonary embolism/ The follow-up film, obtained 3 days after the initial examination. **b** demonstrates peripheral alveolar partially wedge-shaped densities in the left lower lobe and lingula combined with plate-like atelectasis, pleural effusion and elevation of the left hemidiaphragm. Note that a peripheral opacification of somewhat lower density is also present in the left upper lobe. SCTA (**c**) performed in the same patient 1 day after the initial chest X-ray demonstrates a large filling defect in the left lower lobe artery with complete luminal occlusion. The main and right pulmonary artery show regular opacification. In addition, left-sided pleural effusion is present

cally apparent changes occur only when a fairly large segmental or even more proximal artery is occluded or when obstruction of many small vessels impairs pulmonary haemodynamics. Thus, a normal chest X-ray does not exclude the diagnosis of PE.

Most commonly, roentgenographic manifestations of pulmonary embolism involve the lower lobes as a result of haemodynamic flow patterns. The right lung, particularly the posterior basal segment, is more frequently involved than the left lung. Pulmonary thromboembolism may cause a variety of different symptoms including oligemia, changes in vessel size, loss of lung volume, signs of lung infarction, pleural effusion and, finally, alteration in the size and configuration of the heart [6, 7]. These radiographic changes may be apparent as single symptoms or as a combination of different patterns.

Peripheral oligemia may be local, caused by occlusion of a fairly large lobar or segmental pulmonary artery, or general, as a result of central vascular occlusion or widespread small vessel thromboembolism (Westermark sign) (Fig. 1). This sign simply represents the obstruction of flow to a certain lung region and may be associated with a decrease in local lung density. Local oligemia may be associated with enlargement of a major hilar pulmonary artery, the latter probably representing dilatation of the vessel by the thrombus itself. Often, this

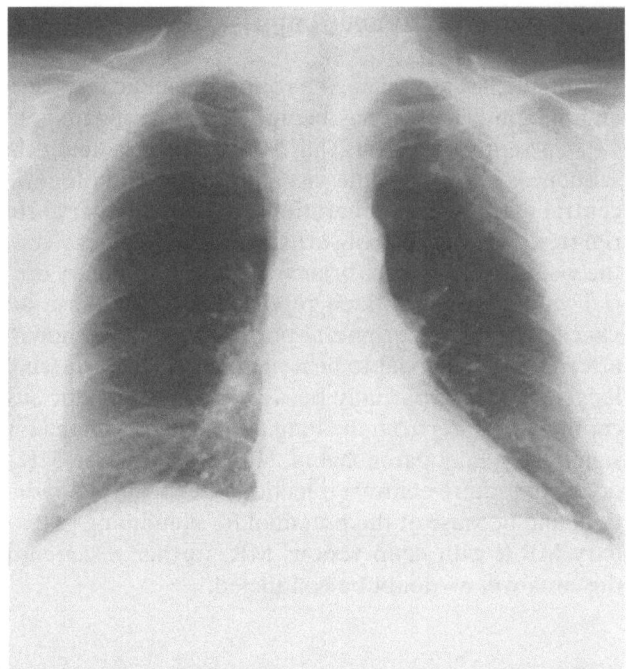

a

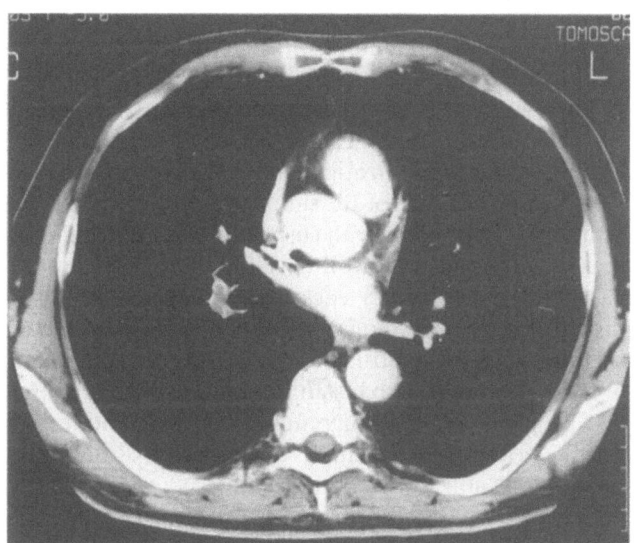

b

**Fig. 2 a, b.** Plain film findings (**a**) and spiral computed tomographic angiography (SCTA; **b**) in a patient with right upper quadrant pain and pulmonary embolism. Plain chest film (**a**) shows a discrete elevation of the right hemidiaphragm and plate-like atelectasis in the left lower lung field. Whereas the CT scan of the upper abdomen was unremarkable, SCTA of the pulmonary arteries (**b**) demonstrates filling defects in the central portion of two lower lobe vessels, partially surrounded by contrast-enhanced blood, representing pulmonary embolism. No other examination was needed to establish a specific diagnosis

dilated vessel may taper abruptly, resulting in the so-called "knuckle sign". Another characteristic sign that is frequently overlooked is loss of lung volume, manifested radiographically by elevation of the diaphragm associated with discoid or plate-like atelectasis (Fig. 2). Pleural

effusion may or may not be present. Finally, cardiac changes are only seen with massive central embolization, which results in dilatation of the right ventricle and atrium.

The term "pulmonary infarct" refers to a pulmonary opacity that has developed distal to an occluded pulmonary artery due to haemorrhage or haemorrhage with necrosis of the lung parenchyma. Pulmonary infarcts are very likely the result of ischaemic damage to endothelial and alveolar epithelial cells, which permits the passage of red blood cells and oedema into air spaces. The typical radiographic appearance of an infarct is a mostly wedge-shaped, subsegmental, segmental or even lobar consolidation (Fig. 1b). Almost invariably, infarctions relate to the visceral pleural surfaces. A classic appearance is the so-called "Hampton's hump", representing a wedge-shaped consolidation of the lung periphery with its base contiguous to the visceral pleural surface and its rounded convex apex toward the hilum. Infarcts resolve over a time period ranging from 4 days to 5 weeks (average time of resolution, 20 days).

## V/Q Scanning

During the last few decades, ventilation/perfusion (V/Q) scintigraphy has been the first-line noninvasive procedure in the evaluation of patients suspected of having PE. This is because the sensitivity of an abnormal result at scintigraphy approaches 100%, whereas a normal result more reliably excludes embolic disease [8-10]. High-probability results at scintigraphy provide a sufficiently reliable diagnosis, indicating that therapy should be instituted. Problems with V/Q scanning arise in patients who demonstrate an intermediate or low probability for PE. In these patients, who can comprise 75% of patients referred for ventilation/perfusion scanning for suspected PE, the percentage of positive pulmonary angiograms has been shown to be as high as 33% and 16%, respectively [9]. Even patients with "near normal" V/Q scans had positive angiograms in 9% of cases. Moreover, V/Q scanning is limited in patients with incomplete obstruction of pulmonary arteries. In an animal study, sensitivity of perfusion scanning was 83% for the detection of emboli that completely obstructed versus 26% for emboli that partially occluded a pulmonary vessel.

## Conventional Pulmonary Angiography

To date, pulmonary angiography served as the gold standard in the diagnosis of PE. However, despite its excellent sensitivity and specificity, the method has not gained widespread acceptance because of its invasiveness and the persisting unwillingness of clinicians to expose patients with frequently unstable cardiovascular conditions to a potentially risky procedure [11]. It has been shown that less than 50% of patients clinically suspected of having PE and in whom results of V/Q scintigraphy are indeterminant proceed to pulmonary angiography [12]. Notably, pulmonary angiography has major limitations, particularly in the evaluation of the peripheral pulmonary arteries. In animal studies, the rate of false-negative pulmonary angiograms for peripheral PE was as high as 25% [13]. In humans, the rate of false-negative examinations was estimated to range between 1% and 9% [13]. Moreover, agreement among observers about the diagnosis of small peripheral emboli is poor. Other limitations of conventional pulmonary angiography include nondiagnostic precedures, estimated to reach 3% in the PIOPED study [9], and false-negative studies at the segmental level and beyond. Despite these limitations, pulmonary angiography remains the gold standard for the evaluation of PE.

## Spiral CT Angiography

Within the last 2 years, spiral CT angiography (SCTA) has emerged as a new method to investigate the pulmonary vasculature [14, 15]. In their landmark study, Remy and co-authors [14] have demonstrated an excellent accuracy rate for SCTA and the diagnosis of PE. The notion that SCTA is suited for the demonstration of PE has been confirmed by recent presentations. Advantages of SCTA include the direct visualization of the intravascular clot in pulmonary arteries down to the fourth order (Figs. 1, 2). Remy and co-authors found an excellent correlation between SCTA and conventional angiography [14].

Currently, most SCTA protocols use a single breath-hold technique, a high-flow/low concentration (4-5 ml/s flow, 150 mg/ml iodine concentration) or a low-flow/high concentration (2-3 ml/s flow, 300 mg/ml iodine concentration) approach, with a slice thickness of 3 mm, and a table increment of 5 mm/s, which should be combined with a reconstruction index of 2 mm. With this approach, it appears that the diagnostic range of SCTA now encompasses the subsegmental vessels. However, even if peripheral emboli in subsegmental vessels are missed, the accuracy of this method does not seem to suffer because multiple emboli shower the lung when a larger embolus is fragmented in the heart. In the study of Remy et al. [14], an average of more than six emboli were found within the pulmonary arterial system in patients with proven PE.

SCTA could represent an ideal method for evaluating patients suspected of suffering from PE but also as a means to exclude PE in patients with nonspecific symptoms. However, in a recent study, Goodman and co-authors [16] reported that the sensitivity of SCTA for the detection of PE was 86% in central and only 63% in peripheral arteries. Thus, despite promising initial results, the role of SCTA in patients suspected of having PE needs to be further evaluated in a larger patient population.

## Magnetic Resonance Angiography

Within the last few years, the role of magnetic resonance angiography (MRA) has begun to be investigated [17, 18]. Currently, it appears that MRA using gradient echo sequences allows reliable visualization of emboli in the central three to four generations of the pulmonary arterial tree. With the use of surface and phased array coils, the visualization of five branches of the pulmonary arterial vasculature has been reported. Despite these advances, the more peripheral portions of the pulmonary arterial system appear to be a significant diagnostic challenge for MRA, partially because of the magnetic susceptibility effects from the lung parenchyma and the low signal from lung parenchyma. However, because MRA does not require contrast injection or exposure to radiation, and because of the potential for combining pulmonary MRA with deep venous MR, further research in this area will no doubt be conducted.

## Summary

Pulmonary thromboembolism is a common and potentially fatal disorder that is often missed or undiagnosed. Even a physician who is alert to the clinical symptoms of PE, the presence of DVT, and various risk factors (such as long-term immobilization) may misdiagnose or overlook numerous cases of PE simply because of the lack of symptoms. In patients with suspected PE, a clinical evaluation should be followed by laboratory tests, cardiovascular studies and a cascade of imaging tests. Although the chest radiograph demonstrates a very low accuracy in the diagnosis of PE and is often completely normal, its importance lies in its ability to exclude other disease processes that may mimic acute PE and in providing correlation with the V/Q scans. V/Q scanning, at this time, is still the leading noninvasive tool to assess patients with suspected PE. However, because of its limited availability and the large number of intermediate – or low – probability results, SCTA is increasingly being used as an alternative or an additional diagnostic measure to reach a specific diagnosis. The value of SCTA, which in some institutions has already emerged as a first-line method of assessment (particularly in emergency and intensive care cases), has yet to be evaluated and compared in large studies with the current gold standard, conventional angiography. MRA has shown some promising results but its clinical value has yet to be determined.

## References

1. Ferris EJ (1983) Peripheral deep venous thrombosis and pulmonary embolism, correlative diagnostic evaluation. Int Angiol 2:85-98

2. Matzdorff AC, Green D (1992) Deep vein thrombosis and pulmonary embolism: prevention, diagnosis, and treatment. Geriatrics 47:48-63
3. Bell WR, Simon TL (1982) Current status of pulmonary thromboembolic disease: pathophysiology, diagnosis, prevention, and treatment. Am Heart J 103:239-262
4. Johnsrude IS (1962) Pulmonary embolism. Curr Probl Diagn Radiol 11:1-60
5. Hoellerich VL, Wigton RS (1986) Diagnosing pulmonary embolism using clinical findings. Arch Intern Med 146:1699-1704
6. Greenspan RH, Ravin CE, Polansky SM et al (1982) Accuracy of the chest radiograph in diagnosis of pulmonary embolism. Invest Radiol 17:539-543
7. Buckner CB, Walker CW, Purnell GL (1989) Pulmonary embolism: chest radiographic abnormalities. J Thorac Imaging 4(4):23-27
8. Sostman HD, Rapoport S, Gottschalk A, Greenspan RH (1986) Imaging of pulmonary embolism. Invest Radiol 21:443-454
9. The PIOPED Investigators (1990) Value of the ventilation/perfusion scan in acute pulmonary embolism. Results of the prospective investigation of pulmonary embolism diagnosis (PIOPED). JAMA 263:2753-2759
10. Hull RD, Hirsh J, Carter CJ et al (1985) Diagnostic value of ventilation-perfusion lung scanning in patients with suspected pulmonary embolism. Chest 88:819-828
11. Newman GE (1989) Pulmonary angiography in pulmonary embolic disease. J Thorac Imaging 4(4):28-39
12. Sostman HD, Ravin CE, Sullivan DC et al (1982) Use of pulmonary angiography for suspected pulmonary embolism: influence of scintigraphic diagnosis. AJR 139:673-677
13. Wellman HN (1986) Pulmonary thromboembolism: current status report on the role of nuclear medicine. Semin Nucl Med 16:236-274
14. Remy-Jardin M, Remy J, Wattine L, Giraud F (1992) Central pulmonary thromboembolism: diagnosis with spiral volumetric CT with the single-breath – hold technique – comparison with pulmonary angiography. Radiology 185:381-387
15. Teigen CL, Maus TP, Sheedy PF II et al (1993) Pulmonary embolism: diagnosis with electron-beam CT. Radiology 188:839-845
16. Goodman LR, Curtin JJ, Mewissen MW et al (1995) Detection of pulmonary embolism in patients with unresolved clinical and scintigraphic diagnosis: helical CT versus angiography. AJR 164:1369-1374
17. Foo TFK, MacFall JR, Hayes CE et al (1992) Pulmonary vasculature: single breathhold MR imaging with phased array coils. Radiology 185:473-477
18. Alderson PO, Martin EC (1987) Pulmonary embolism: diagnosis with multiple imaging modalities. Radiology 164:297-312

# Minimally Invasive Methods for the Assessment of Solitary Pulmonary Nodules

P. Schnyder

Department of Radiology, University Hospital, CHUV, 1011 Lausanne, Switzerland

Among the noninvasive methods, the only valid proof of the benignity of a solitary pulmonary nodule (SPN) is an absence of growth for more than 2 years, documented by plain films or computed tomography (CT) [1]. A size inferior to 0.8 cm is no longer considered as a statistically reliable indicator of benignity [2], 42% and 15% of malignant SPN being less than 2 and less than 1 cm, respectively [2]. In contrast, the vast majority, over 95%, of SPN larger than 3 cm are malignant.

Calcifications, whether diffuse or focal, are strong indicators of benignity if the amount of calcium represents over 10% of the nodule, if calcifications have a popcorn pattern, if they are centrally located or if they are situated at the periphery of the SPN and present a laminated pattern. Calcifications can be safely evaluated exclusively on high-resolution CT (HRCT) sections and, even though they may be difficult to differentiate from the irregular, eccentric ones are found in up to 15% of squamous cell carcinomas evaluated by CT [1].

The use of qualitative CT patterns such as shape, edge definition, presence of satellite lesions and cavitation may contribute to the radiological assessment of benignity or malignancy of a SPN. However, radiologists have to be aware of the wide overlap in shape between benign and malignant SPNs [1-3].

Indeed, smooth edges can be seen with an equal frequency in benign or malignant SPNs. Spiculations are more frequently seen in malignant SPNs (88%) than in benign conditions. Adenocarcinomas, which are classically slow-growing lesions, can mimic a round or slightly lobulated, well-defined granulomatous lesions. If an adenocarcinoma presents a strong desmoplastic component, then its shape will become irregular with ill-defined, spiculated edges, similar to lung scar or squamous cell carcinoma [3].

CT densitometry represents a quantitative approach in the investigation of the SPN. It was used in the 1980s after Siegelmann [4] showed that SPNs with CT attenuation values over 164 Hounsfield units (HU) represented benign conditions. The inconstant reproducibility of this threshold of benignity has led Zehrouni et al. [5] to propose a phantom for qualitative analysis of the cal-

cium content of SPNs. Due to the low sensitivity of the method [6] and a threshold equivalent to 264 HU [7], this phantom was never popular, at least in Europe.

The air bronchogram, or air-bronchiologram described by Kurijama et al. [8], is found in 65% of adenocarcinomas less than 2 cm in diameter and in only 5% of benign conditions. The positive predictive value of this sign is high, around 93%.

Percutaneous biopsy or thin-needle aspiration under CT guidance is the most commonly used minimally invasive technique for the assessment of SPNs. At our institution, the success rate of thin-needle aspiration for cytological examination is much lower than that reported in the literature and does not reach the cited 95% diagnostic accuracy for malignant diseases and 88% for benign conditions [9]. For this reason, we prefer percutaneous needle biopsies, using 18 to 19 true-cut type needles, with Bard Spring, even if the related incidence of pneumothoraces reaches 20%. Contraindications are not uncommon and must be known. They include: noncompliant patients, decreased prothrombin levels and platelet counts, marked emphysema and patients who have undergone pneumonectomy.

Recently, Swensen et al. [10] showed in a series of 108 patients with 6- to 40-mm noncalcified nodules that iodinated contrast material injection induced a moderate increase of the mean attenuation value of benign lesions which does not exceed 19 HU (mean 12 HU). The behaviour of malignancies differs greatly, since their attenuation values increase over 19 HU with a mean of 40 HU. The sensitivity of this technique is 100%, although false-positive results encountered with hamartomas decrease its specificity to 70%.

HRCT has been shown to represent an excellent guide for bronchoscopy in demonstrating a bronchus "cut-off" sign or bronchus contained within a tumour [11]. This sign should convince a bronchoscopist of the 90% success rate of transbronchial forceps biopsy and brushing of the lesion, when it lies on a fourth order bronchus [11, 12]. In contrast, when the SPN is adjacent to the bronchus, a transbronchial needle aspiration is preferable. Finally, when the SPN is associated with a thickened or narrowed bronchus, both transbronchial needle aspiration and brushing should be performed [12].

When the SPN is smaller than 1.5 cm and if its distance to the pleura is 3-4 cm or less, it is now frequently removed by a wedged resection performed under video-assisted thoracoscopy, after methylene blue marking under CT control. This technique is safe and has been applied in over 60 patients during the last 2 years in our institution without any major complications and with a success rate of 95% [13] (videotape).

We recently conducted 10 CT-guided bronchoscopies in patients with SPNs located at mid-distance between the pleura and the main bronchi. None of them could be directly visualized at bronchoscopy. In all subjects, a well-trained radiologist was able to precisely guide the pneumologist via CT in the insertion of the pediatric bronchoscope and the forceps and/or brushes introduced through the bronchoscope up to the centre of the lesions located on a four- to seven-generation bronchus. In all cases, adequate material was obtained for histologic and cytological examinations. The diagnosis was assessed in all ten patients. If no complication is encountered with this new technique, precise information and close cooperation of the patient are required in order to reproduce the same inspiratory position during the successive helical CT acquisitions necessary to guide the manoeuvre. The images are interpreted in real-time by the radiologist, who transmits the exact position of forceps or brush to the operator.

In conclusion, we consider that qualitative and quantitative CT patterns are usually not sufficiently accurate to assess with certainty a diagnosis of benignity or malignancy of a SPN. Only if the SPN is totally calcified or has a fat content indicative of hamartoma, or if the SPN has remained unchanged for at least 2 years can one forego considering one of the above-mentioned minimally invasive procedures such as percutaneous biopsy, transbronchial biopsy or brushing, CT-guided bronchoscopy, or CT guided methylene blue marking before edge resection under video thoracoscopic control be adopted.

# References

1. Caskey CI, Templeton PA, Zerhouni EA (1990) Current evaluation of the solitary pulmonary nodule. Radiol Clin North Am 28:511-520
2. Zerhouni EA, Stitik FP, Siegelmann SS et al (1986) Computed tomography of the pulmonary nodule : a national cooperative study. Radiology 160:319-327
3. Rosado-de-Christenson ML, Templeton PA, Moran CA (1994) Bronchogenic carcinoma : radiologic-pathologic correlation. Radiographics 14:429-446
4. Siegelmann SS, Zerhouni EA, Leo FP et al (1980) CT of the solitary pulmonary nodule. AJR 135:1-13
5. Zerhouni EA, Boukadoun M, Siddiky MA et al (1983) A standard phantom for a quantitative CT analysis of pulmonary nodules. Radiology 149:767-773
6. Swensen SJ, Harms GF, Morin RL, Mayers JL (1991) CT evaluation of solitary pulmonary nodules. AJR 156:925-929
7. Siegelmann SS, Khouri NT, Leo FP et al (1986) Solitary pulmonary nodules : CT assessment. Radiology 160:307-312
8. Kurijama K, Tateishi R, Doi O et al (1991) Prevalence of air bronchogram in small peripheral carcinomas of the lung on thin-section CT : comparison with benign tumors. AJR 156:921-924
9. Khouri NF, Stitik FP, Erozan YS (1985) Transthoracic needle aspiration of benign and malignant lung lesions. AJR 144:281-288
10. Swensen SJ, Brown LR, Colby TV, Weaver AL (1995) Pulmonary nodule : CT evaluation of enhancement with iodinated contrast material. Radiology 194:393-398
11. Gaeta M, Pandolfo I, Volta S et al (1991) Bronchus sign on CT in peripheral carcinoma of the lung : value in predictive results of transbronchial biopsy. AJR 157:1181-1185
12. Gaeta M, Barone M, Russi EG et al (1993) Carcinomatous solitary pulmonary nodules : evaluation of the tumor bronchi relationship with thin-section CT. Radiology 187:535-539
13. Wicky S, Mayor B, Cuttat JF, Schnyder P (1993) CT-guided localization of pulmonary nodules with methylene blue injection for thoracoscopic resections. Chest 106:1326-1328

# Mediastinal Masses

F. Laurent

Service de Radiologie, Hôpital Haut Lévêque, CHU de Bordeaux, Avenue de Magellan, 33604 Pessac, France

The radiological evaluation of mediastinal masses is an important challenge in chest radiology. Although plain film is limited, cross-sectional techniques, especially computed tomography (CT) and magnetic resonance imaging (MRI), play a powerful role in the evaluation of the mediastinum. Today, a specific diagnosis is often possible and, if not, a limited differential diagnosis can be made. This review only concerns adult patients.

## Clinical Aspects

Most patients with mediastinal lesions are chronically asymptomatic. Eighty-three per cent of incidentally discovered lesions are benign and 57% of lesions in symptomatic patients are malignant [1]. Symptoms include dysphagia, cough from airway compression, superior vena cava syndrome, hoarseness from laryngeal nerve involvement or symptoms from spinal cord compression. Myasthenia gravis or, less frequently, Cushing syndrome can also reveal mediastinal masses. Approximately one third of mediastinal masses are malignant and invasion or obstruction of nearby structures on imaging studies is suggestive of malignancy. The most frequent lesions are thymoma, neurogenic tumours and benign cysts, altogether representing 60% of patients with mediastinal masses.

The radiologic compartmentalization of the mediastinum introduced by Felson helps in focusing the differential diagnosis of masses on the basis of their site. However, most tumour types can be found in any of the compartments. Today, tissue components, as shown by CT or MR scans, are, together with the precise location of the mass, the leading thread of the diagnosis. After reviewing the different imaging modalities, we will classify mediastinal masses according to their main tissue composition.

## Imaging Modalities

### Chest Radiographs

Posteroanterior and lateral chest radiographs are the first imaging modalities used when a mediastinal mass is suspected. Deformation of mediastinal contours and lines and displacement of normal structures must be present to identify a mass. Typical location and findings can help to identify lymph nodes and vascular masses and can suggest a limited differential diagnosis on the basis of age, sex and clinical findings [2].

### Computed Tomography

CT is the most important tool in the evaluation of a mediastinal mass. It is the next step after chest radiography and is often sufficient to manage the patient. Characterization on CT is based on specific attenuation of fat, air, cysts and calcifications. Vascular abnormalities and the degree of vascularization of soft tissue masses are demonstrated by dynamic incremental CT or spiral CT [3, 4].

### Magnetic Resonance Imaging

MRI has many advantages in imaging the mediastinum: excellent soft tissue contrast with spontaneous tissue-vessel contrast and multiplanar capabilities. The MRI technique includes ECG-gated spin echo T1- and T2-weighted spin echo and gadolinium-enhanced T1-weighted scans in the appropriate axial, sagittal, coronal or oblique plane. Gradient echo techniques are used to explore vascular abnormalities. MRI is used in clinical situations when CT is inadequate or after CT if unanswered questions remain. Assessment of vascular involvement, identification of cystic lesions, assessment of preoperative relationships with the pericardium, heart cavities, spinal cord and canal are the most common indications [5, 6].

### Ultrasound

Ultrasound (US) is not currently used in mediastinal mass evaluation although it does have a potential role in certain situations. The major limitation is the inadequate window, but useful information can be obtained, especially in children, in masses abutting the chest wall and in vascular abnormalities [7].

## Transthoracic Needle Biopsies

Invasive diagnostic procedures often play a valuable part in staging and providing tissue for pathological study in order to plan treatment. Mediastinoscopy and parasternal mediastinotomy have traditionally filled this role. Percutaneous fine needle aspiration and, more recently, core biopsies with large bore needles guided by CT scanning or US have also been advocated for the diagnostic examination of mediastinal lesions [4]. A definite histological diagnosis is obtained in as many as 89% of patients. Despite the excellent safety and low complication rate with this technique, the nature of the common tumours found in particular in the anterosuperior compartment tends to limit its accuracy.

As a general rule, if clinical judgement suggests a lesion that can be unequivocally diagnosed by tissue obtained with a needle, thereby avoiding an open surgical biopsy, then a percutaneous needle biopsy of the mediastinal mass is a reasonable first choice. If a lesion requiring a large amount of tissue for diagnosis is suspected clinically, then the clinician should forego the initial needle biopsy and proceed with open biopsy or possibly a complete resection.

## Imaging Findings

According to their main CT findings, mediastinal masses may be classified as fatty, cystic, solid and vascular.

### Fatty Masses

Fat is specifically recognized by its low CT numbers, which vary from –70 to 130 HU. Fat is normally present in the mediastinum and increases with age. Normal fat is unencapsulated and does not affect the normal contours of the mediastinum. With MRI, well-differentiated fat has a high signal intensity on both T1- and T2- weighted sequences, identical to subcutaneous fat.

In the majority of cases, discovery of the fatty nature of a mass indicates benignancy. True lipomatous tumours are much less common than herniation of abdominal fat.

Omental fat can herniate through the foramen of Morgagni and create the appearance of a cardiophrenic angle mass. Oesophageal hiatus herniations of perigastric fat extend along the aorta, widening the spinal line, or may appear as a retrocardiac mass. Connections with abdominal fat are demonstrated by multiplanar reconstruction with CT and sagittal and coronal acquisitions with MRI.

In mediastinal diffuse lipomatosis, overabundant amounts of histologically normal fat accumulate in the upper mediastinum, resulting in smooth mediastinal widening on chest radiographs. Locations of this overaccumulation of fat are the upper mediastinum, the cardi-

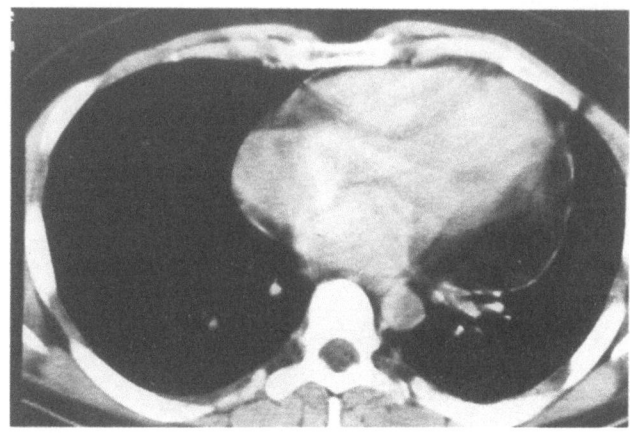

**Fig. 1.** Intrapericardial liposarcoma. Computed tomographic scan shows a fatty mass arising at the lateral aspect of the left ventricle

ophrenic angles and, less frequently, the paraspinal areas. Homogeneity and absence of compression of surrounding structures differentiate this benign condition from multiple lipomas.

Mediastinal lipomas and liposarcomas represent only 2% of all mediastinal tumours (Fig. 1). They do not produce compressive symptoms unless they are large enough. Other uncommon tumours may contain a variable amount of fat: thymolipoma and benign teratoma should be included in the differential diagnosis of a fatty lesion [3, 8].

### Cystic Masses

Cysts represent 15%-20% of all mediastinal masses. Most do not produce symptoms and become large before they are discovered, usually as an incidental chest radiograph finding. Because of their tendency to enlarge or become infected, surgical excision is recommended.

On chest radiography, cysts appear as smooth, sharply marginated mediastinal lesions. On CT, typical cysts have a similar attenuation to that of water and do not enhance with intravenous contrast material. Their margins are well defined and their wall is barely perceptible. Some cysts have a higher attenuation than that of water due to calcic, proteinaceous, mucous, and haemorrhagic content [3, 9].

On MRI, cysts containing serous fluid have a high signal intensity on T2-weighted images. However, depending on their protein or blood content, they show a varying T1-weighted appearance, from the low signal intensity of a serous fluid to the very high signal intensity of a viscous proteinaceous fluid [3].

Mediastinal bronchogenic cysts do not usually communicate with the bronchial tree, unlike intraparenchymal cysts. Half of them are of water density and the others have a CT density which varies, depending on the cyst content. Most are located along the paratracheal

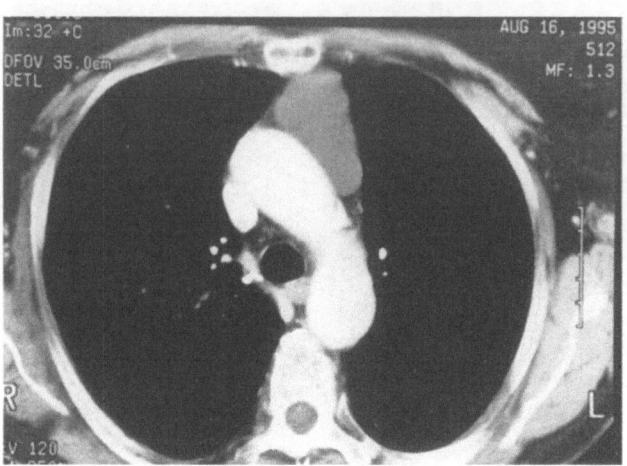

**Fig. 2.** Thymic cyst. Computed tomographic scan shows a water attenuation mass in the retrosternal space

wall near the carina or in the posterior mediastinum. Duplication cysts are indistinguishable from bronchogenic cysts except for their location because they are most often connected to the oesophagus, sometimes within its wall. Neuroenteric cysts are rare lesions connected to the meninges through a midline defect in one or more vertebral bodies. Pericardial cysts are commonly located in the right cardiophrenic angle although they may occur anywhere in relation to the pericardium. Congenital thymic cysts are rare and occur anywhere along the course of the embryonic thymus gland from the angle of the mandible to the manubrium (Fig. 2). Lymphangiomas are typical when connected with a cervical mass but they may be isolated in the mediastinum.

These true cystic lesions should be differentiated from cystic degenerative changes of thymoma, Hodgkin's disease, teratomas and nodes and from abscesses and haemotomas. Tumours with cystic degeneration have a thick irregular wall which enhances after contrast media injection.

Thymic cysts are known to occur occasionally in patients with mediastinal Hodgkin's disease. Their histogenesis is controversial. They may be treatment related or due to thymic infiltration by lymphomatous tissues either on presentation or at recurrence. The natural history of thymic cysts following treatment is not known. However, persistent relapse-free survival can usually only be achieved after complete resolution of all viable tumours. Careful observation with regular follow-up CT scans without additional treatment seems to be the management of choice for residual thymic cysts of mediastinal Hodgkin's disease.

**Solid Masses**

Most mediastinal masses in an adult population are solid. Large necrotic areas have to be differentiated from real cystic masses but this is achieved by CT in most cas-

es. Among the solid masses, clinical and CT findings and the precise location in the mediastinal compartments are essential for planning treatment and invasive procedures necessary to obtain a definite diagnosis. CT is often sufficient to distinguish invasive unresectable tumours from well-defined, resectable lesions which will be treated by complete resection. The most common masses of the anterior mediastinal compartment are thymomas, lymphomas, germ cell tumours and goitre, while neurogenic masses are mostly located in the posterior compartment.

*Thymomas*

Thymoma is the most common primary neoplasm of the mediastinum and this term is limited to tumours originating in the thymic epithelium. The distinction between benign and malignant thymoma may be difficult even from histological sections. The prognosis and therapeutic approach is frequently determined by whether the tumour has invaded the tissue beyond its capsule. CT and MRI have become the most precise modalities to detect thymomas and to evaluate their extent.

In patients with myasthenia gravis, a thymoma or thymic hyperplasia is present in 10%-20% of cases. Thymic hyperplasia is a term used by pathologists to describe numerous active lymphoid germinal centres in the medulla. The role of CT and MRI is limited in detecting this abnormality because 50% of thymic hyperplasias appear entirely normal on CT while other glands with hyperplasia typically are diffusely enlarged [10].

The spectrum of CT findings in patients with thymoma has been extensively described [11]. Noninvasive thymomas appear as round or oval, well-circumscribed masses, growing asymmetrically to one side of the anterior mediastinum. The CT density is similar to that of a normal young thymus and slightly increases with administration of contrast material. Intratumoural calcifications are seen in one third of cases and areas of cystic degeneration are common. The tumour can occur in the prevascular space but also around the base of the heart and anywhere between the lower pole of the thyroid gland and the anterior surface of the pericardium. Invasive thymomas appear on CT as irregular, ill-defined masses. They grow along pleural surfaces and extend downwards along the aorta to involve the crus of the diaphragm and the retroperitoneum. A full CT examination in these patients should extend to the upper abdomen. Pleural extension in the form of droplet spread without continuity with the primary tumour is seen in 15% of cases. Invasion of the thoracic wall, mediastinal vessels, trachea, pericardium and lung parenchyma is frequent. CT is the most precise method for detecting local and regional spread. However, caution should be used to avoid overdiagnosing invasion. Direct contact and absence of cleavage planes are not strictly reliable criteria to predict invasion. In contrast, clear delineation of fat

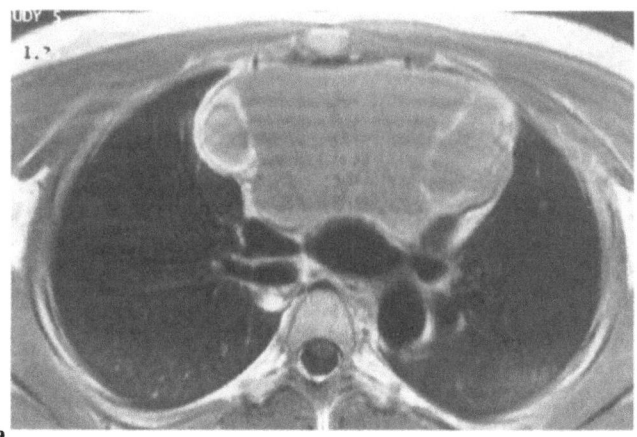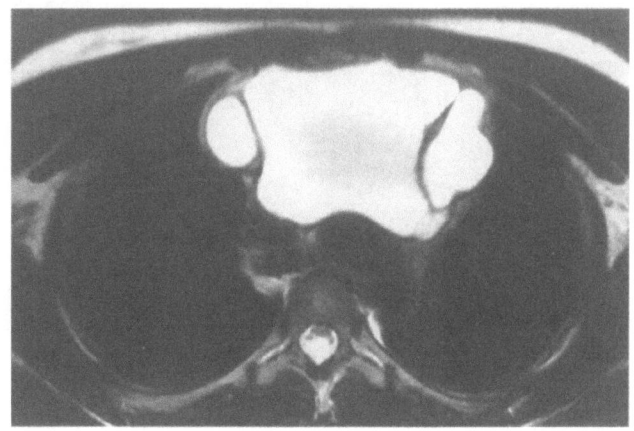

a                                                                                    b

**Fig. 3 a, b.** Benign cystic teratoma. Gadolinium enhanced T1- (**a**) and T2- (**b**) weighted magnetic resonance images show a multiloculated cystic mass with thick walls. The T1 high signal intensity of one of the loculi is related to its proteinaceous content

planes surrounding a tumour should be interpreted as indicating an absence of extensive local invasion [5, 6].

MRI has a limited role in the evaluation of thymomas. MRI signal characteristics are not useful in the clinical setting of myasthenia gravis, thymic hyperplasia and thymic mass. However, vascular and cardiac extension of invasive thymoma is well identified by MRI [12].

## Germs Cell Tumours

Germs cell tumours arise from malignant transformation of germinal elements. Sixty per cent are benign teratomas that occur with equal frequency in men and women. Malignant varieties have a strong male predominance and include teratocarcinomas, embryonic carcinomas, seminomas, endodermal sinus tumour and choriocarcinomas.

Benign teratomas are commonly found in the anterior mediastinum and typically contain a mixture of CT densities [3, 13]. Fatty and cystic components are present in half of the cases and sometimes the fat-fluid level strongly suggests the diagnosis but these features are not specific for benignancy. Cystic teratomas are differentiated from pleuropericardial cyst by the identification of a thicker wall in the latter (Fig. 3).

Malignant germ cell tumours have CT and MRI features similar to invasive thymomas. Invasion of mediastinal structures is diagnosed according to obliteration of fat planes and replacement of mediastinal fat by tumoural tissue. Confirmation of the primary nature of these tumours requires that there is no evidence of testicular or retroperitoneal tumour. The role of imaging modalities is to define disease extent and to monitor response to therapy [14].

## Lymphoma

With the advent of CT, the detection of all thoracic manifestations of lymphomas has become significantly less a diagnostic challenge. To date, CT has also played a major role in the follow-up of patients undergoing therapy. Reduction of the tumour is satisfactorily monitored with CT. However, partial size regression is often observed and in this case residual tissue has to be differentiated from active residual disease. CT is unreliable in this assessment, only being capable of monitoring the size of the lesion.

The role of MRI in the management of patients with lymphomas remains to be defined.

## Thyroid Masses

Mediastinal goiters constitute 5%-10% of all resected mediastinal masses. Most patients are asymptomatic and the abnormality is detected on a routine chest radiograph. Occasionally, symptoms of airway or esophageal compression are present. The combination of findings on CT or MRI is characteristic in most instances. In most cases thyroid masses represent direct contiguous growth of a goitre into the mediastinum almost always connected to the thyroid gland. In 80% of cases, the thyroid extends into the thyropericardiac prevascular spaces but posterior extension behind the brachiocephalic vessels along the trachea represents 20% of cases. Identification of substernal thyroid tissue is made on the following findings:
– Communication between the cervical thyroid gland and the mass by contiguous slices
– Mass of inhomogeneous density with cystic areas, calcifications of various shape and high density areas
– Marked and prolonged contrast enhancement

However, limitations in histological specificity similar to sonography have been noted with CT. The role of CT is important in the preoperative assessment of substernal goitres because the surgical approach depends on their precise anatomic location [3].

On MRI, multinodular goitres have been shown to be relatively hypointense as compared with normal tissue

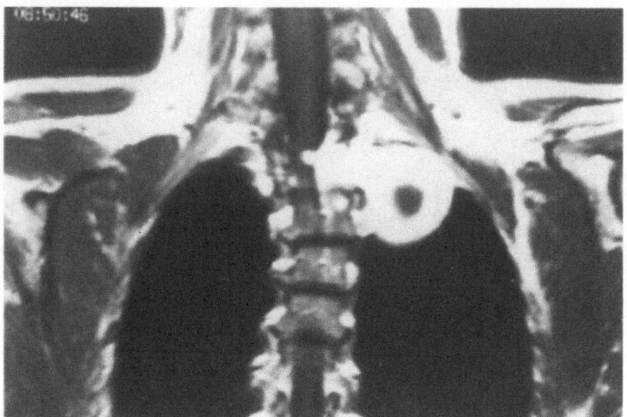

**Fig. 4.** Dumbbell neurinoma. Coronal magnetic resonance image after gadolinium injection shows a large enhancing mass with a central necrotic area of the paravertebral gutter extending into the spinal canal

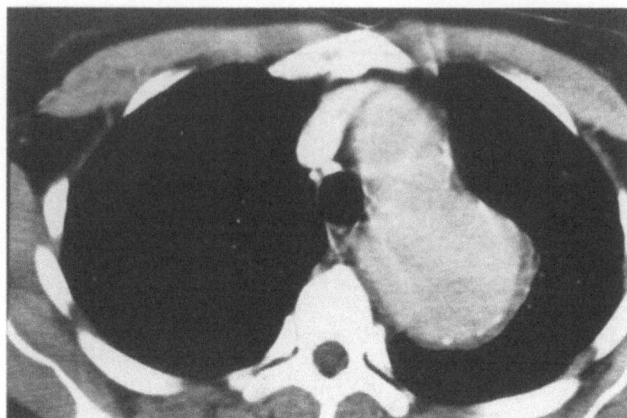

**Fig. 5.** Aneurysm of the aortic arch: large vascular mass with a calcified thrombus

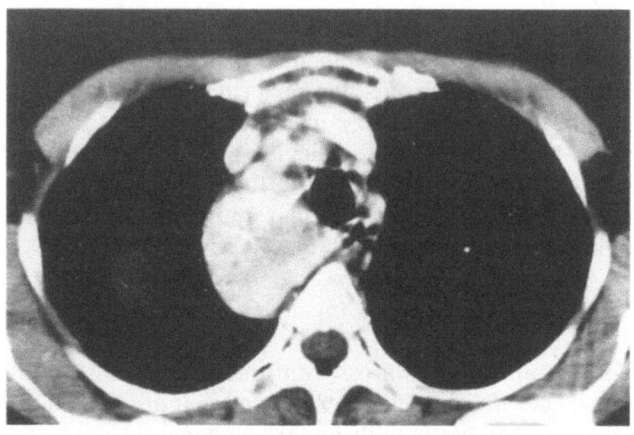

**Fig. 6.** Castelman disease. Computed tomographic scan shows a large laterotracheal mass with calcification and strong enhancement after contrast injection

on T1-weighted images, except foci of haemorrhage and cysts that may be hyperintense. T2-weighted images show a typically heterogeneous appearance with high signal intensity throughout most of the gland. MRI has not proven to be any more specific than CT histologically. Displacement of mediastinal vessels, trachea, oesophagus and relationships between the cervical and thoracic components of the goiter are exquisitely demonstrated by MRI [15].

*Neurogenic Tumour*

Neurogenic tumours are the most common posterior masses of the mediastinum, 30% of them being malignant. They can arise from peripheral nerves (schwannoma, neurofibroma and malignant tumours), symphathetic ganglia (ganlioneuroma, ganglioneuroblastoma, neuroblastoma) or from paraganglia (paranganglioma and pheochromocytoma).

Chest radiography typically shows a sharply circumscribed round or oval mass located in the paravertebral gutter. Other locations are along the course of the vagus or phrenic nerves. Rib erosion with a sclerotic border is suggestive of a benign lesion. Spreading to multiple ribs with erosion or destruction is in favour of malignancy. On CT scans, neurogenic tumours have a soft tissue attenuation but may show a low attenuation value attributed to lipid content, cystic degeneration and entrapment of peripheral neural tissue. Relationships with vertebrae, ribs and the spinal canal are essential for planning therapy. MRI can demonstrate spinal involvement without the use of intrathecal contrast material (Fig. 4). Moreover, its multiplanar capabilities help to demonstrate the longitudinal extent along the spine.

A diverse group of entities may involve the posterior mediastinum, including lipomatosis, lymphadenopa-

thies, aortic aneurysm, cystic masses and thoracic spinal inflammatory or neoplastic lesions. CT is often diagnostic but this is one of its best indications for MRI.

**Vascular Masses**

Approximately 10% of mediastinal masses are vascular in origin. Aneurysm of the aorta should be considered whenever a mass is in direct relation or cannot be separated from the course of the thoracic aorta. Dynamic CT scanning, spiral CT and/or MRI are usually diagnostic (Fig. 5). Chronic aortic dissection can also be demonstrated by dynamic CT or MRI, although transoesophageal echocardiography seems to be the procedure of choice in acute aortic dissection. Other vascular lesions can mimic mediastinal masses: aberrant right subclavian artery mediastinal varices or pulmonary artery aneurysms. A strong contrast enhancement of a solid mass as in Castelman disease rarely mimics a vascular lesion (Fig. 6).

# Conclusion

Identification of a mediastinal mass essentially remains the role of chest radiography. CT examination is the next logical step and is often sufficient to suggest a limited differential diagnosis adequate for therapeutic decisions. MRI and transthoracic needle biopsies provide additional information in selected cases.

# References

1. Davis RD, Oldham HN, Sabiston DC (1987) Primary cysts and neoplasms of the mediastinum: recent changes in clinical presentation, methods of diagnosis, management, and results. Ann Thorac Surg 44:229-237
2. Heitzman ER (ed) (1988) The mediastinum: radiologic correlations with anatomy and pathology, 2nd edn. Springer, Berlin Heidelberg New York
3. Naidich DP, Zerhouni EA, Siegelman SS (1991) Computed tomography and magnetic resonance of the thorax, 2nd edn. Raven, New York, pp 35-149
4. Herman SJ, Holub RV, Weisbrod GL, Chamberlain DW (1991) Anterior mediastinal masses: utility of transthoracic needle biopsy. Radiology 180:167-70
5. Laurent F, Drouillard J, Joullie M et al (1990) Mediastinal tumours: comparison between CT and MRI in the evaluation of nature and extension. Diagn Interven Radiol 2:201-209
6. Webb WR, Sostman HD (1992) MR imaging of thoracic disease: clinical uses. Radiology 182:621-630
7. Wernecke K, Potter R, Peters PE et al (1988) Parasternal mediastinal sonography: sensitivity in the detection of anterior mediastinal and subcarinal tumour. AJR 150:1021-1026
8. Glazer HS, Siegel MJ, Sagel SS (1989) Low-attenuation mediastinal masses on CT. AJR 152:1173-1177
9. Mendelson D, Rose J, Efremidis S et al (1983) Bronchogenic cysts with high CT numbers. AJR 140:463-465
10. Baron RL, Lee JKT, Sagel SS et al (1982) Computed tomography of the abnormal thymus. Radiology 142:127-134
11. Batra P, Herrmann C JR, Mulder D (1987) Mediastinal imaging in myasthenia gravis: correlation of chest radiography, CT, MR and surgical findings. AJR 148:515-519
12. Molina PL, Siegel MJ, Glazer HS (1990) Thymic masses on MR imaging. AJR 155:495-500
13. Levitt RG, Hesband JE, Glazer HS (1984) CT of primary germ-cell tumours of the mediastinum. AJR 142:73-78
14. Lee KS, Im JG, Han Ch et al (1989) Malignant primary germ cell tumours of the mediastinum: CT features. AJR 153:947-951
15. Noma S, Kanaoka M, Minami S et al (1988) Thyroid masses: MR imaging and pathologic correlation. Radiology 168:759-764

# Congenital Abnormalities Affecting the Respiratory System

D. Shaw

Department of Radiology, Great Ormond Street Hospital for Children, Great Ormond Street, London WC1N 3JH, UK

Among the various and multiple causes of respiratory distress in the young child, some are the result of congenital abnormalities. Of these, some may present immediately while others present as a result of complications, particularly infection. In this article, the spectrum of such abnormalities is reviewed.

## Larynx and Trachea

Respiratory distress in the young may be caused by "physiological immaturity". Laryngomalacia is a common, essentially benign condition associated with inspiratory stridor and a flaccid larynx.

More serious congenital abnormalities of the larynx include clefting, atresia, webs, cysts and tumours, particularly subglottic haemangiomas. Although there may be radiographic signs of these conditions, they are essentially evaluated by endoscopy.

Excessive narrowing of the trachea may be associated with tracheomalacia, in which the cartilaginous rings of the airways do not provide adequate support. This may be a local deficiency in the trachea or major bronchi but more importantly is associated with oesophageal atresia. Oesophageal atresia is most commonly associated with a fistula from the distal trachea to the distal segment of the oesophagus although in about 15% of cases, there are variable connections between the atretic oesophagus and the airways. Oesophageal atresia is often associated with malformations in other systems such as the kidneys, skeleton, heart and other parts of the alimentary tract. Radiological evaluation is essentially conducted using plain radiography and air or a radio-opaque tube in the upper pouch. The presence of abdominal distension is a clue to the presence of a tracheo-oesophageal fistula. Imaging is especially pertinent to the evaluation of other alimentary tract abnormalities, particularly duodenal and anorectal atresias and malformations and to the evaluation of abnormalities in other systems. It is of particular importance to define the side of the aortic arch as this is a determinant of the side of operative approach.

## Foregut Duplication Cysts

Alimentary tract duplications may occur from mouth to anus and about a fifth or so are associated with lesions in the thorax. Some of these are asymptomatic but, if large, can lead to compression and respiratory distress and feeding difficulties. Those associated with the oesophagus are often noncommunicating, round cystic structures but communication with the alimentary tract can occur. Transdiaphragmatic duplication cysts, particularly arising from the upper small gut, are well recognised and such duplications may be multiple. Plain film, alimentary contrast medium studies and ultrasonography are simple evaluative techniques which can be supplemented by computed tomography if necessary. An important plain film correlate is the presence of vertebral column anomalies. Duplication cysts may contain gastric mucosa and this can be detected following injection of radioactive technetium on nuclear medicine studies.

## Oesophageal Lung

Some very severe tracheal abnormalities occur, of which tracheal agenesis is a fatal condition, but less severe malformations can include the bronchial tree arising from the oesophagus to give oesophageal lung.

## Congenital Diaphragmatic Hernia

Congenital diaphragmatic hernia (CDH) occurs in between one and two per 5000 births. There is a female preponderance. Polyhydramnios is an important presenting feature and carries a poorer prognosis when present. Prenatal ultrasonographic diagnosis is well established and allows suitable preparations for immediate postnatal management. Although survivors of CDH do not have a particularly high incidence of associated malformations, those neonates who are stillborn and die soon after birth have a much higher incidence of major anomalies, particularly in the central nervous and cardiovascular systems.

The anatomical defect can be divided into three major types: firstly, varying degrees of agenesis of the diaphragm; secondly, septum transversum defects including Cantrell's pentalogy and the smaller Morgagni hernias; thirdly, by far the commonest posterolateral defects, (Bochdalek) hernias. The posterolateral diaphragmatic hernias are very much more common on the left.

Lung hypoplasia, particularly on the ipsilateral side, is a major association of CDH. It has been suggested that the presence of the stomach, as opposed to small bowel in the hemithorax, indicates a longer duration of the hernia in utero and a correspondingly poor prognosis.

The immediate presentation is with respiratory distress, cyanosis, tachypnoea and often a scaphoid abdomen. The diagnosis is made by plain radiography of the chest and abdomen and ultrasound can delineate the diaphragmatic defect. Occasionally, contrast media studies are indicated in the unusual case of failure to differentiate other cystic looking lesions in the lung.

Extracorporeal membrane oxygenation (ECMO) has proved helpful in the management of respiratory compromise in infants with CDH, either due to lung hypoplasia or persisting pulmonary hypertension. The role of radiology in ECMO is essentially to manage complications, which are often haemorrhagic, such as pulmonary haemorrhage, pleural bleeding and intracranial haemorrhage. Careful ultrasound monitoring of the brain is important before instituting ECMO. Anticoagulation is an integral part of this regime.

## Cystic Adenomatoid Malformation

Accounting for some 5% of congenital lung malformations, cystic adenomatoid malformations (CAM) show overgrowth of the terminal bronchiolar structures with varying sized cystic structures lined by columnar epithelium but without organised architecture. No cartilage is evident. Usually a single lobe is affected and the lower lobes more commonly so than the upper lobes, although occasionally, the entire lung may be involved.

On histological grounds, three types have been described. Type 1, the commonest, usually on the right, consists of large cystic structures and generally is of good prognosis. Type 2 shows multiple small cysts often associated with other anomalies, with preterm delivery and carrying a poor prognosis. Type 3, with cysts 5 mm or less, are typically seen in male children. The lesions are frequently diagnosed on prenatal ultrasound or on chest radiography or ultrasound postnatally. In the immediate neonatal period, the cysts may be fluid filled and show opacities in the affected lung, which over the course of a few days become aerated, giving rise to hyper-radiolucent cystic structures. There are several reports of prenatally diagnosed CAMs resolving by the time of birth. Treatment is by surgical excision and if

there are no other associated lesions or adverse medical factors, the long-term outcome is satisfactory.

## Congenital Lobar Emphysema

Congenital lobar emphysema is most usually seen in the left upper or right middle lobe, with multiple lobes occasionally being involved. The pathogenesis is probably multifactorial. Abnormalities of elastic properties of the lobar bronchus, polyalveolar lobes and variable cartilaginous abnormalities in the bronchial wall have been postulated.

Important associations are with cardiac disease, particularly persistent ductus arteriosus and absent pulmonary valve syndrome. The presentation is usually fairly soon after birth, with increasing respiratory distress, wheezing, cough and poor feeding.

Radiography reveals a hyperlucent area within the lung with compression of typically unaffected other lobes in the same lung. Radio-isotopic pulmonary ventilation and perfusion scans allow delineation of those functionally affected lobes and confirm good function in other compressed parts of the lung.

In acute and progressive respiratory compromise, resection of the affected lobe is curative and surgical treatment is usually indicated in children with associated heart lesions. In children less critically affected, conservative management has proved satisfactory in many cases, with resolution of the changes in the radiographs and with functional improvement.

## Bronchial Atresia

Bronchial atresia, a condition in which a bronchus is occluded, is associated with some peripheral development of the lung parenchyma. By far, the left upper lobe is the one most commonly involved, but other lobes, particularly the right middle and right upper lobes may be involved, too.

Although congenital in origin, this lesion may be asymptomatic or present with localised pneumonia in the affected lobe. The radiographic signs are a paradoxically overinflated lobe with, in later childhood, a bronchocoele distal to the atresia which is sometimes apparent on plain radiographs and usually identifiable on computed tomography. The overdistension is believed to be due to aeration through the collateral pathways of the pores of Kohn and canals of Lambert. Bronchography is now seldom used do evaluate this lesion.

## Bronchogenic Cysts

Bronchogenic cysts occur as anomalous developments of the branching of the tracheobronchial tree, most commonly in the region of the trachea and central bronchi. Typically they do not connect with the airways and are usually singular and unilocular. The epithelium is mucous secreting, but, if infected, the cysts may contain pus. Altrough small cysts may be asymptomatic throughout life, larger cysts present with symptoms of airway compression, often with hyperinflation of the lung distal to the obstruction. Treatment is by surgical excision, which is often curative, but if a large hilar bronchogenic cyst has compromised vascular development of the lung, some persisting abnormalities in ventilation and lung function will be present.

## Pulmonary Lymphangiectasia

Three types of abnormal dilatation of the pulmonary lymphatics are recognised: primary pulmonary lymphangiectasia with diffuse bilateral involvement of the lungs and without other abnormalities, which presents as stillbirths or hydrops fetalis, but if less severe may be found incidentally on chest radiography in adults. Generalised pulmonary lymphangiectasia is associated with cardiac abnormalities, particularly those with obstruction of pulmonary venous return. Prognosis in this group is generally poor. Thirdly, pulmonary lymphangiectasia may occur with lymphatic abnormalities in other systems, particularly gut and bone, and involvement of the lungs is often asymmetrical and variable.

## Pulmonary Arteriovenous Malformations

Arteriovenous malformations (AVMs) are an important feature of hereditary haemorrhagic telangiectasia. There may, however, be incidental findings or occasionally associated with advanced liver disease. Clinical findings result from shunting with arterial desaturation, clubbing and polycythaemia. More serious complications include paradoxical cerebral embolism and abscess and frank pulmonary haemorrhage.

The lesions may be seen as opacities associated with a sinuous vessel and digital angiography allows good delineation of the lesions and any other associated similar lesions in the lungs. Embolisation of feeding vessels is eminently feasible, but direct operative intervention occasionally is needed.

## Pulmonary Hypoplasia

Pulmonary hypoplasia may be bilateral or unilateral. Bilateral hypoplasia may occur in an idiopathic form but is frequently symptomatic. Oligohydramnios, particularly associated with renal deseases and urinary tract obstruction prenatally, myopathies and hydrops are important causes. Unilateral hypoplasia may occasionally be isolat-

ed but is often associated with pulmonary vasculature problems and cardiac abnormalities. Pulmonary artery hypoplasia and aplasia can be satisfactorily demonstrated on pulmonary V/Q isotope studies, and abnormal vessels such as those associated with sequestrations and a scimitar syndrome may be detectable with colour flow Doppler. Congenital diaphragmatic hernia is a particularly important and common cause of pulmonary hypoplasia especially on the ipsilateral side.

In the neonate, pulmonary hypoplasia is typically manifested by a small lung, deviation of the mediastinum and sparsity of the pulmonary vasculature on plain radiography. Bilateral hypoplasia is manifest as a small thorax, an additional cause of which are some skeletal dysplasias such as asphyxiating thoracic dystrophy and thanatophoric dysplasia. Minor degrees of bilateral pulmonary hypoplasia are essentially a pathological diagnosis.

## Pulmonary Sequestrations

Two forms of pulmonary sequestrations are generally recognised. Intralobar sequestrations are the most important and consist of areas of structurally disorganised lung tissue, usually cystic in origin and usually aerated but without typically normal connections with the bronchial tree. Collateral air drift and minor communications account for the aeration. The majority of these lesions occur in the lower lobes posteriorly, particularly on the left but occasionally bilateral lesions and lesions in other lobes are encountered. The vascular supply is by the systemic arteries and these may be multiple. The venous drainage is typically into the pulmonary veins, especially in those lesions occurring on the left, but some on the right may have anomalous connections into the systemic venous system.

The commonest presenting symptom is recurrent chest infections, particularly in later childhood and surgical resection is curative.

Extralobar sequestrations can be looked upon as dysplastic accessory lungs and are particularly found on the left between the left lower lobe and the diaphragm. Venous drainage is variable as in intralobar sequestrations, but those associated with extralobar sequestrations are significantly more frequently into the systemic venous system. Extralobar sequestrations are often found as incidental findings in children with multiple other malformations, sometimes coincidentally post mortem.

## Vascular Rings

Anomalies of segmentation of the aortic arch and the major intrathoracic vessels may be associated with ring compressions of the trachea and the oesophagus, either by reduplication of the vessels or the presence of a constricting ligamentum arteriousus. Some vascular anomalies, such as the aberrant right subclavian artery, are typically asymptomatic. Those anomalies which cause problems present typically with feeding difficulties and stridor. Evaluation is by plain radiography, barium swallow and ultrasound of the cardiovascular system. Computed tomography and magnetic resonance imaging can give exquisite anatomical delineation but may not be necessary.

The pulmonary artery sling is a condition in which the left pulmonary artery arises on the right and passes between the lower trachea and the oesophagus. This is often associated with right pulmonary hypoplasia but is an important cause of bilateral overdistension of the lungs. The diagnosis can be established by contrast studies and plain radiography but magnetic resonance imaging, in particular, is of great use.

A persistent ductus arteriosus may be associated with overdistension of the left upper lobe as a result of compression of the associated bronchus. Cardiac enlargement may cause collapse and consolidation in the right middle and left lower lobe, and left lower lobe consolidation is a very frequent finding following cardiac surgery for congenital malformations.

## Further Reading

1. Silverman FN, Kuhn JP (1993) Caffey's paediatric X-ray diagnosis. Mosby, St. Louis
2. Carty H et al (ed) (1994) Imaging children. Churchill Livingstone, Edinburgh
3. Loughlin GM, Eigen H (1994) Respiratory disease in children. Williams and Wilkins, Baltimore
4. Freeman et al (ed) (1994) Surgery of the newborn. Churchill Livingstone, Edinburgh

# Radiology in Chest Emergencies

L. Bonomo, M.L. Storto, C. Ciccotosto and A. Guidotti

Istituto di Radiologia, Università di Chieti, Via P.A. Valignani, 66100 Chieti, Italy

## Introduction

Thoracic trauma represents an increasingly large proportion of emergencies in chest radiology. Chest injuries, alone or in combination with other injuries, account for more than half of all traumatic deaths. The overall death rate is 2%-12% for isolated chest injuries and 35% for chest injuries associated with polytrauma [1].

In recent years, the number of immediate survivors of accidents has increased to over 50% due to prompt emergency medical treatment and rapid admission to the hospital [1]. Thus, the radiologist is increasingly likely to be faced with an urgent need for diagnostic evaluation of injured patients. Imaging studies play no role in the initial management of critically ill, unstable patients in whom the restoration and maintenance of vital cardiocirculatory function and assurance of adequate ventilation through an effective airway are the first priorities [1-3]. However, radiologic imaging is a major component of the secondary clinical treatment aimed at the identification and correction of potentially fatal injuries.

Optimum use of imaging depends on: (a) recognition of the technical advantages and limitations of various imaging modalities; (b) thorough understanding of the pathogenetic mechanism of injury; and (c) familiarity with the clinical and radiologic manifestations of chest trauma involving the lung, chest wall, mediastinum and other organs.

Plain chest radiograph is the first examination to be performed; because of the condition of these patients, most radiographs have to be obtained in the supine position using portable equipment. The radiologist should immediately scan the radiograph for evidence of life-threatening abnormalities such as tension pneumothorax, haemothorax, blurring or widening of the upper mediastinal margins suggesting injury to the aorta, and enlargement of the cardiac region consistent with haemopericardium. At this stage, the radiologist should also control the location of central lines and endotracheal and nasogastric tubes. Then the plain film should be examined a second time for the presence of rib fractures, subcutaneous emphysema, diaphragmatic abnormalities, and parenchymal densities or lucencies. Moreover, a decision for additional views or examinations should be made [3]. Computed tomography (CT) has enhanced the ability to detect those structural abnormalities associated with chest trauma. In this regard, spiral CT, which allows volumetric acquisitions in a short scanning time, may improve the evaluation of severely traumatized patients. Aortography remains the imaging procedure of choice in patients with suspected aortic injury.

## Biomechanics

Chest trauma is traditionally described as either blunt or penetrating. This distinction is based on whether the chest wall remains intact (blunt trauma) or whether the primary injury produces an open communication between the intrathoracic content and the external environment (penetrating trauma).

Blunt chest trauma is much more common than penetrating chest trauma, accounting for almost 90% of all chest injuries in civilians [2, 3]. The specific injuries associated with blunt trauma can be caused directly, by the force of impact on the chest wall and thoracic content, or indirectly, by the differential rates of deceleration that thoracic structures experience at the time of impact. The effects of a direct blow depend on the complex interaction of the characteristics of the applied force (magnitude, duration, direction, rate of application, surface area of impact) with the intrinsic properties (elasticity) and the general stress condition of the tissues. Different rates of deceleration in a tissue or organ cause damage by either producing internal collision between intrathoracic organs and the chest wall, or producing intrinsic strain that exceeds an organ's tolerance level.

Penetrating chest trauma is usually the result of the abrupt, direct application of mechanical force to a small focal area on the external surface of the chest, usually with a knife blade or a bullet. Tissue damage is produced by stretching and crushing and is confined largely to organs and tissues situated directly in the path of the projectile.

# Chest Wall Injury

The chest wall is the first line of defence against blunt thoracic trauma. The soft tissues of the chest wall may be contused, lacerated, perforated or avulsed by blunt or penetrating trauma. These injuries have a minor physiologic impact but may have radiographic significance as they can either obscure important underlying abnormalities or may simulate more significant parenchymal injuries.

## Skeletal Trauma

Rib fractures represent the most common injury in patients who have substained blunt trauma of the chest and are usually caused by chest wall compression. Up to 50% of acute rib fractures are not seen on conventional radiographs because of their position or lack of displacement [1, 3]. In most instances, failure to detect an acute rib fracture is of little importance, as no specific therapy is required. However, some fractures assume a greater significance by virtue of specific features. Fractures of the lower ribs (9th-12th) are often associated with injury to the liver, spleen or kidneys. Fractures of the first three ribs are the expression of severe trauma because these ribs are protected by the shoulder girdles and the associated musculature; the possibility of injury to the aorta and the tracheobronchial tree is therefore greater. However, the presence of fractures of the first three ribs, in the absence of other clinical or radiographic abnormalities, does not constitute an indication for angiography or bronchoscopy [1, 3, 5].

Two-point fractures of three or more contiguous ribs may result in a flail chest with paradoxical movements during respiration and potentially serious clinical consequences. On conventional radiographs, multiple rib fractures with marked angulation of the fractured segments suggest the three-point fractures of flail chest [1].

Sternal fractures occur in 8% of patients admitted for blunt chest trauma and tend to involve the sternomanubrial junction or the sternal body. Their presence indicates significant trauma, and the physician should be alert to the possibility of a deceleration injury to the aorta, the great vessel or the pericardium [3, 4]. These fractures cannot be visualized on frontal chest radiographs; lateral views and CT are the best methods for detecting sternal fractures and retrosternal haematomas [1].

Vertebral fractures may result from hyperflexion and compression injuries of the chest. On well-penetrated chest radiographs, a paraspinal haematoma may be the first sign of a vertebral fracture.

## Pleural Space

Abnormal accumulation of fluid or gas in the pleural space is common in patients with blunt or penetrating chest trauma.

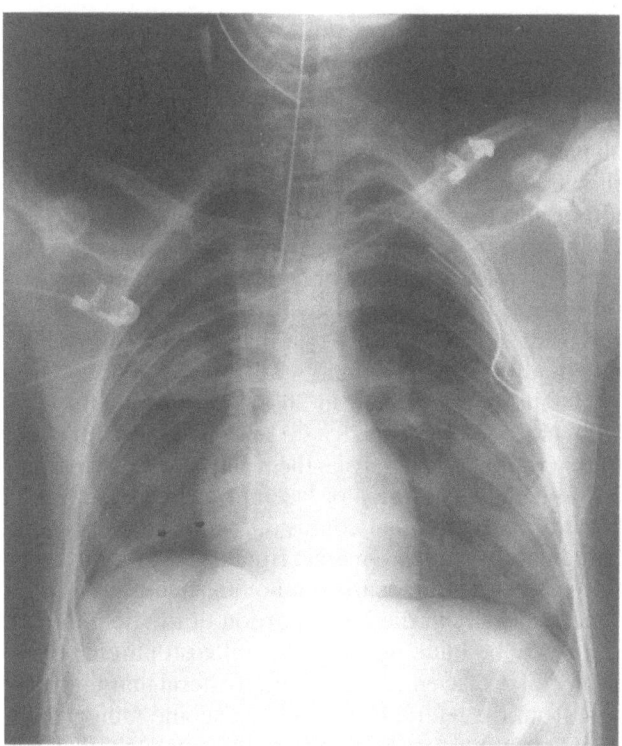

**Fig. 1.** Supine chest radiograph shows contusion of the left lower lobe and right upper lobe and bilateral pneumothorax. The right pneumothorax (*arrows*) is responsible for the basilar hyperlucency with unusual definition of the right cardiophrenic angle

Pneumothorax occurs in 15%-38% of patients with blunt trauma and 18%-19% of patients with penetrating trauma and is often associated with haemothorax [2, 3]. There are many potential causes, including alveolar compression in crushing injuries, lung laceration and tracheobronchial tears. On frontal chest radiographs obtained with the patient erect, a pneumothorax is seen as an apical lucent area, devoid of bronchovascular markings, which separates the superior and lateral margins of the lung from the chest wall. Most trauma patients are unable to stand and their films are obtained in the supine position. In the supine patient, pleural space air preferentially collects in the anterior, medial and subpulmonic pulmonary recess and may be difficult to detect on supine radiographs (Fig. 1). Subtle signs suggesting pneumothorax on supine chest radiographs include: (a) the presence of a deep costophrenic sulcus ("deep sulcus" sign); (b) double diaphragm sign – a double contour of a hemidiaphragm caused by air in the anterior costophrenic sulcus that allows the anterior attachment of the diaphragm to be visualized, in addition to the normally seen diaphragmatic dome; (c) unusually clear definition of the right cardiophrenic angle or the left cardiac apex; and (d) basilar hyperlucency [2, 3]. Additional views, such as a cross-table lateral radiograph or a lateral decubitus view of the chest with the pleural space under study uppermost can demonstrate pneumothorax in patients who cannot assume an erect position. A number of studies have shown the superiority of CT scans for detecting pneumothorax in patients with thoracic and nonthoracic trauma. For this reason, some authors recommend that all patients being scanned for head or abdominal trauma should have some CT sections through the lower thorax to rule out the presence of pneumothorax [2, 3, 6, 7]. It has also been suggested that all trauma patients have a chest CT prior to surgery or being placed on mechanical ventilation to allow the diagnosis and treatment of occult, simple pnemothorax that may develop into a life-threatening tension pneumothorax [3].

Haemothorax is seen in 20%-59% of patients with blunt chest trauma and 28%-63% of patients with penetrating trauma [3]. It may be the result of various injuries, including lung contusion or laceration, intercostal vessel laceration, mediastinal contusion, aortic tears and diaphragmatic tears [1]. On erect frontal chest radiographs, free pleural fluid appears as a homogeneous area of increased density in the lower portion of the hemithorax; there may be blunting of the lateral costophrenic angle or medial displacement of the inferolateral margin of the lung from the lateral chest wall. On supine radiographs, free pleural fluid collects in the posterior pleural space, causing a uniform increase in density in the hemithorax. There may be blunting of the diaphragmatic contours or the lateral costophrenic angle; a radiopaque apical cap and a crescent-shaped opacity between the inner margin of the ribs and the lung may form. Although lateral decubitus views may be helpful in questionable cases, an ultrasound examination represents a more sensitive method for detection of pleural effusion.

## Lung Injury

The elastic nature of the pulmonary parenchyma minimizes the amount of damage that the lungs sustain during penetrating trauma. However, the fragility of the pulmonary interstitial tissues makes the lungs susceptible to blunt trauma with a resultant contusion or laceration [3].

Pulmonary contusion may be seen underlying the point of chest wall impact or as a contrecoup lesion. It represents a focal or diffuse area of interstitial and alveolar haemorrhage and oedema in which the structural integrity of the lung is preserved [3, 8]. Alveolar capillary disruption has been implicated in the pathogenesis. The most common radiographic findings are patchy, nonsegmental, ill-defined areas of increased airspace density (Fig. 1). These abnormalities appear within 6 h of injury in 70%-85% of patients and begin to clear within 48-72 h with complete resolution in 4-5 days. However, complete radiographic clearing may take as little as 24 h or as long as 8 days. Persistence of lung opacities after 10 days suggests a complicated contusion [1]. Contusion is initially indistinguishable from other causes of consolidation such as aspiration, oedema, and pneumonia. The clinical his-

tory and the timing of the radiographic abnormalities help to differentiate these processes.

Pulmonary laceration implies the disruption of pulmonary parenchyma. The normal elastic recoil of lung converts the resultant tear into spheric or ovoid spaces. Associated tears of bronchi and blood vessels cause the space to fill with air (pneumatocoele), blood (haematoma) or both. Pneumatocoeles and haematomas may be multiple but are more commonly isolated lesions. On occasion they are large, up to 14 cm in diameter, but most are 2-5 cm. The radiographic finding classically described in haematoma is a focal, well-defined, homogeneous soft tissue density which becomes more evident when the surrounding lung contusion clears. Haematomas may take months to resolve and may be mistaken for a neoplasm or an abscess during the phase of resolution [4, 8]. The lucency of a pneumatocoele may become more apparent as the degree of surrounding lung contusion increases during the first 6-8 h after injury. Sometimes, pneumatocoeles become quite obvious when they rapidly enlarge in response to high-pressure mechanical ventilation [1].

## Mediastinal Injury

### Aortic Injury

Major decelerating trauma following high-speed motor vehicle accidents may cause shearing of the thoracic aorta. In clinical series, 90%-95% of aortic ruptures occur in the region of the isthmus, which represents a transition zone between the relatively mobile aortic arch and the tethered descending aorta; the other 5% occur in the ascending aorta [2-4, 8, 9]. In autopsy series, the incidence of ascending aorta rupture is greater, accounting for 20%-25% of all aortic injuries [2, 3]. Seventy per cent of all patients with aortic injury die at the scene of trauma from complete transection of the vessel, and 80%-90% die before treatment can be started. However, 60%-70% of those who reach the hospital alive and who receive prompt and appropriate treatment survive [2, 3, 9]. In survivors the degree of damage falls just short of complete transection and the adventitial layer preserves the integrity of the aorta, at last for a time. The risk of ultimate rupture is higher as more than 50% will rupture within 24 h and most of the remainder within the next few weeks [4, 8]. Diagnosis of impending aortic rupture is therefore vital.

A great deal has been written about the sensitivity and specificity of the plain frontal chest radiographic changes as indicators of aortic injury [3, 5]: (a) Fractures of the upper ribs or an apical "cap" have no diagnostic value; (b) a shift of the trachea to the right, deviation of a nasogastric tube to the right of the T4 spinous process, widening of the right and left paraspinal line, and depression of the left main bronchus more than 40° below the horizontal are all fairly specific (about 90%) but

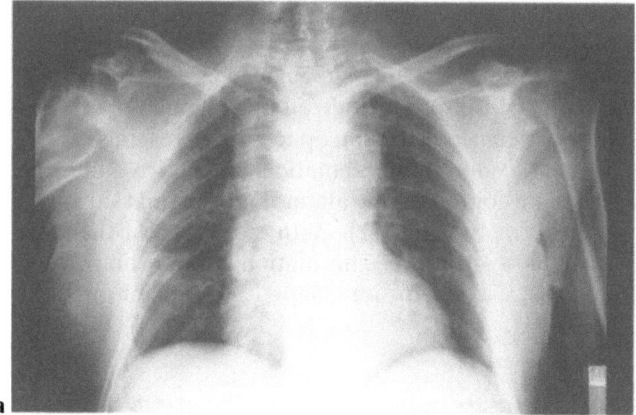

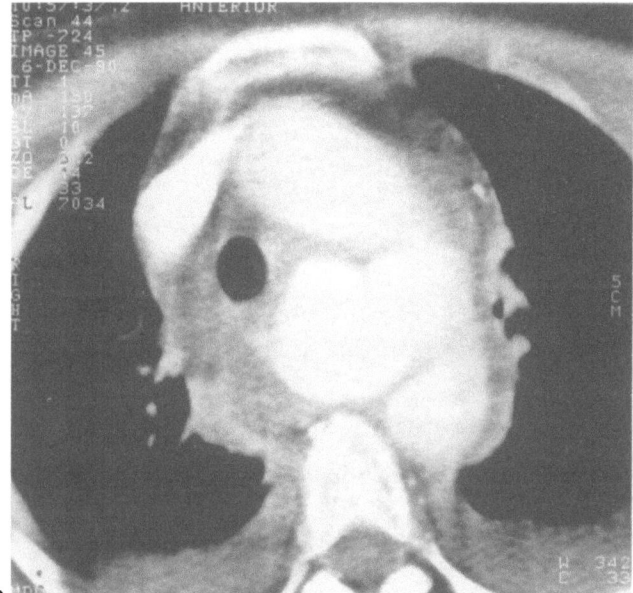

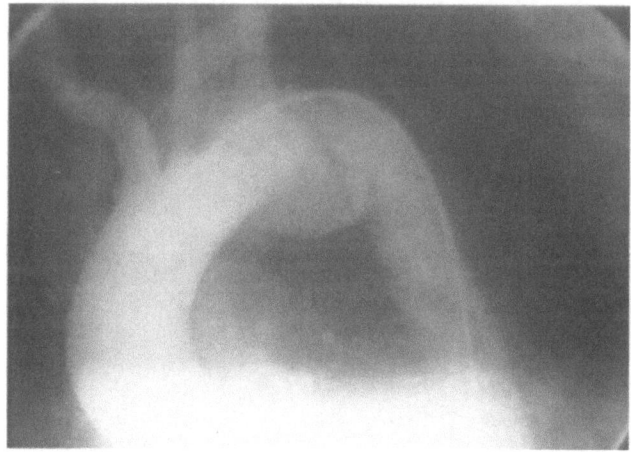

Fig. 2 a-c. Ruptured aorta following a severe blunt chest trauma. a The supine chest radiograph demonstrates widening of the superior mediastinum and loss of definition of the aortic knob with deviation of the trachea to the right. b The spiral computed tomogaphic scan shows a large pseudoaneurysm on the inferomedial aspect of the aortic arch. Massive mediastinal hematoma and bilateral hemothoraces are also present. c Aortogram shows pseudoaneurysm distal to the origin of the left subclavian artery

have poor sensitivity (12%-70%); (c) a subjective impression of widening of the mediastinum, preferably assessed on an erect frontal radiograph and an abnormal aortic arch contour are the best indicators of aortic damage; and (d) the absence of abnormalities has a greater predictive value than does their presence [2, 3]. Even under the best circumstances, the described findings on the plain chest radiograph can only suggest the diagnosis of aortic rupture; another study must be performed to confirm its presence (Fig. 2). Traditionally, the next step in the diagnostic algorithm has been aortography, the high sensitivity and specificity of which are well known [2]. Since other traumatic and nontraumatic abnormalities other than aortic injury may cause mediastinal widening, most emergency aortograms are normal [2, 3]. A sensitive, less invasive, and easily performed screening test would be desirable.

CT can easily show mediastinal haematoma and provide information about the presence of other significant intrathoracic injuries. However, it cannot be recommended as the primary means of diagnosing traumatic aortic rupture because the laceration is often transverse and parallel to the scan plane. Chest CT may be useful in stable patients with low-to-moderate risk of aortic rupture and equivocal findings on the plain film. Any direct evidence of aortic injury or mediastinal haematoma on CT is an indication for an aortogram. Using this approach, 50% of normal aortograms could be avoided [3].

Magnetic resonance imaging has assumed a major role in the diagnosis of nontraumatic disorders of the thoracic aorta; however, it has not achieved widespread acceptance in the evaluation of traumatic aortic rupture because of the difficulty to monitor the patient [2].

Transoesophageal echocardiography is well suited to examining the aortic isthmus region. Partial ruptures have been observed with transoesophageal echocardiography, but its role in trauma patients has not yet been evaluated.

**Cardiac Injury**

The exact incidence of cardiac injuries is difficult to determine because they are either clinically silent or the signs and symptoms are obscured by or attributed to other major thoracic injuries [3]. They include myocardial contusion, pericardial laceration, pericardial tamponade, coronary artery occlusion or tear, and bullet embolization. If cardiac trauma is suspected, chest radiographs should be obtained, although the information they provide is seldom diagnostic. Echocardiography may demonstrate pericardial effusion or focal areas of myocardial damage.

**Tracheobronchial Tear**

Tracheal or bronchial rupture may result from penetrating injuries or severe blunt trauma and is associated with a 30% overall mortality rate. Diagnosis is often difficult and a significant proportion of cases go undiagnosed until complications develop. Radiographic findings include: pneumomediastinum, which is most commonly seen in tracheal or proximal main stem bronchial rupture; pneumothorax, which may be large and often fail to resolve after correct positioning of a chest tube; and the "fallen lung" sign, which may be observed with complete disruption of a main stem bronchus.

### Oesophageal and Thoracic Duct Tears

Oesophageal and thoracic duct tears are usually iatrogenic. Radiographic signs of oesophageal rupture are pneumomediastinum and pneumothorax or pleural effusion, most commonly on the left side. Oesophagoscopy or a barium study will confirm the diagnosis. Mediastinitis, abscess and empyema are complications of unrecognized injuries to the oesophagus. Injury to the thoracic duct may remain unsuspected until chyle is recovered from the pleural space.

## Diaphragmatic Tear

Rupture or laceration of the diaphragm occurs in 3%-7% of patients with blunt and 6%-46% of patients with penetrating thoracoabdominal trauma [2]. The left hemidiaphragm is affected more often than the right leaflet, accounting for 70%-90% of ruptures [8, 10]. This is explained by the cushioning effect of the liver, which does not allow the propagating shock waves to impact on the right hemidiaphragm. Some authors believe that rupture of the right hemidiaphragm occurs with almost the same frequency as rupture of the left one; it is simply more often clinically "silent" and more difficult to diagnose [2].

Up to 70% of diaphragmatic tears are initially missed because they are usually not life-threatening and because the associated clinical and radiographic signs are often nonspecific and are attributed to more commonly encountered processes. Diagnosis of diaphragmatic rupture can be delayed for hours to years [10]. Complications of such a delay include strangulation with haematemesis, melena, intestinal obstruction and respiratory impairment.

Seventy-five to 95% of patients with acute diaphragmatic rupture have abnormal chest radiographs, but only 17%-40% have radiographic findings highly suggestive of rupture [2]. Diagnostic abnormalities on plain radiographs include the presence of air or contrast-containing stomach or bowel above the diaphragm and superior displacement of the nasogastric tube into the left hemithorax. Nonspecific but suggestive radiographic findings of rupture include an unexplained pleural effusion, a persistent basilar opacity that resembles atelectasis or a supradiaphragmatic mass, an irregular diaphragmatic contour, contralateral mediastinal shift, and lower rib fractures [2, 11]. With laceration of the right hemidiaphragm (Fig. 3), herniation of a portion of the liver causes a mushroom-shaped supradiaphragmatic density [11].

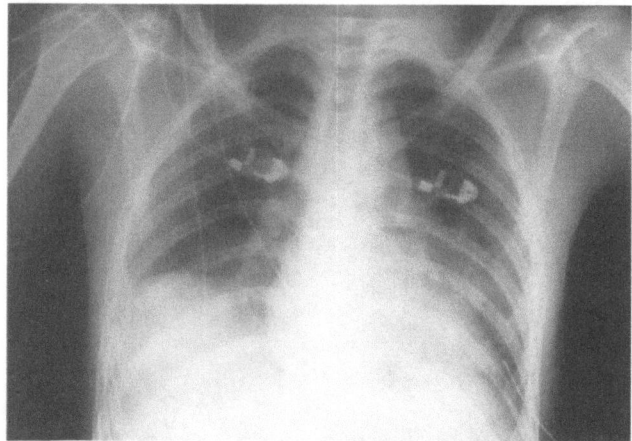

a

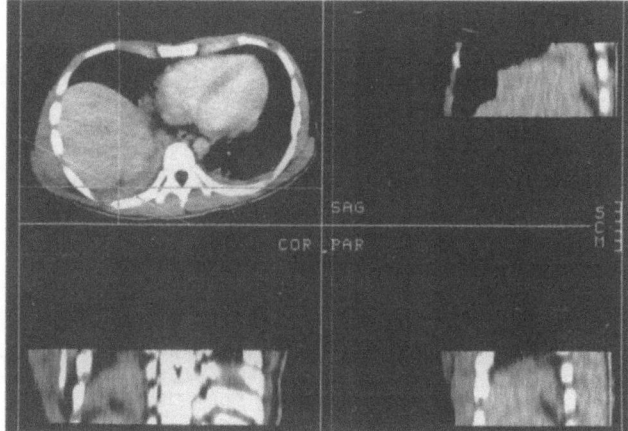

b

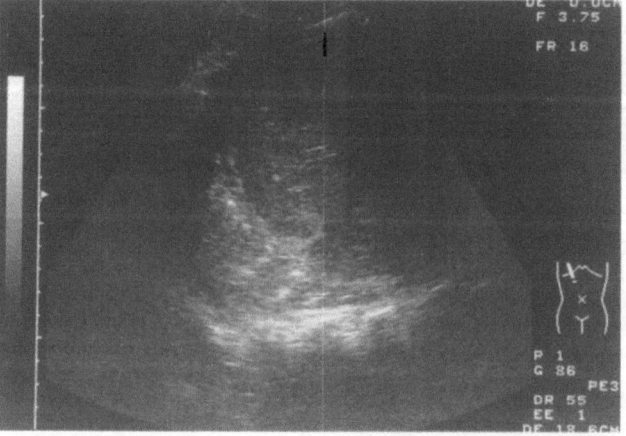

c

**Fig. 3 a-c.** Right hemidiaphragm rupture with herniation of the liver. **a** Apparent elevation of the right hemidiaphragm is visible on the supine chest radiograph. **b** The computed tomographic scan with multiplanar reconstructions shows herniation of the liver into the right hemithorax with a mushroom-like appearance. **c** Ultrasound confirms the interruption of the right hemidiaphragm and herniation of the liver

CT may explain the origin of abnormal opacities in the thorax and can also demonstrate the interrupted diaphragm. The relationship of abdominal organs to the hemidiaphragm can be determined: abdominal viscera are normally located centrally on axial CT images of the thoracoabdominal junction. A ruptured diaphragm will allow the abdominal viscera to occupy part of the outer ring, lateral to the diaphragm [10].

Ultrasound can be used to visualize the diaphragm directly and can demonstrate actual disruption. It is particularly useful for evaluating patients with suspected rupture of the right hemidiaphragm, since the liver offers an excellent acoustic window (Fig. 3).

## Indirect Effects of Trauma to the Lungs

Severe trauma can have indirect effects on the lungs that may severely complicate the clinical and radiographic diagnosis. Three main processes require consideration: fat embolism, adult respiratory distress syndrome and neurogenic pulmonary oedema.

## Conclusions

The radiologist's role in the evaluation and management of chest trauma is complex and multifaceted. The radiologist must be able to quickly and efficiently extract all information from what are often technically limited studies and recognize what additional information and supplementary studies are needed to ensure optimal patient care. The radiologist's most important responsibility, however, is to communicate with members of the clinical team caring for the patient.

## References

1. Greene R (1992) Blunt thoracic trauma. In: Greene R (ed) Syllabus: a categorial course in diagnostic radiology. Chest radiology. RSNA, Oak Brook, pp 297-309
2. Groskin SA (1992) Selected topics in chest trauma. Radiology 183:605-617
3. Groskin S, Maresca M, Heitzman ER (1990) Thoracic trauma. In: McCort JJ (ed) Trauma radiology. Churchill Livingstone, New York, pp 75-127
4. Dee P (1995) Chest trauma. In: Armstrong P (ed) Imaging diseases of the chest. Mosby, St. Louis, pp 869-893
5. Woodring JH, Fried AM, Hatfield DR, Stevens RK, Todd EP (1992) Fractures of first and second ribs: predictive value for arterial and bronchial injury. AJR 138:211-215
6. Tocino IM, Miller MH, Frederick PR, Bahr AL, Thomas F (1984) CT detection of occult pneumothorax in head trauma. AJR 143:987-990
7. Wall SD, Federle MP, Jeffrey RB, Brent CM (1983) CT diagnosis of unsuspected pneumothorax after blunt abdominal trauma. AJR 141:919-921
8. Dee P (1992) The radiology of chest trauma. Radiol Clin North Am 30:291-306
9. Cowley RA, Turney SZ, Hankins JR, Rodriguez A, Attar S, Shankar BS (1990) Rupture of thoracic aorta caused by blunt trauma: a fifteen year experience. J Thorac Cardiovasc Surg 100:652-660
10. Stark P (1993) Radiology of thoracic trauma. Andover, Boston
11. Mindelzun RE (1990) Diaphragmatic trauma. In: McCort JJ (ed) Trauma radiology. Churchill Livingstone, New York, pp 129-133

# Interventional Radiology of the Chest: Percutaneous Procedures

R.F. Dondelinger and B. Ghaye

Department of Medical Imaging, University Hospital Sart Tilman, 4000 Liege 1, Belgium

## Percutaneous Transthoracic Biopsy

Percutaneous lung biopsy was first performed in 1883 by Leyden to establish the infectious nature of lung disease. Actually, percutaneous tissue sampling of a pulmonary, pleural or mediastinal lesion is indicated when histological diagnosis will further influence diagnostic strategy and therapeutic options or modify tumour stage and the sequence of oncologic therapy. Cost efficiency due to a shortened hospital stay and reduced hospital bills has been demonstrated.

### Indications

The main indications for percutaneous fine-needle thoracic biopsy can be summarized as follows [1]: pulmonary nodule(s) without specific diagnostic criteria on computed tomography (CT) ascertaining benignity: pulmonary nodule(s) or mass suggesting malignancy when surgery is to be postponed after chemotherapy and/or radiotherapy or replaced by these treatments. A patient who refuses invasive diagnostic procedures and therapy may change his mind when irrefutable proof of malignancy is established by percutaneous biopsy; pulmonary nodule(s) with a history of extrapulmonary primary malignancy, with the patient in clinical remission or presenting with several primary malignancies; a residual nonregressive lesion following radiotherapy or chemotherapy; tissue sampling for therapeutic sensitivity tests, measurements of tumour markers, hormone dependence, DNA analysis, etc.; chronic diffuse pulmonary infiltrate in selected cases; pleural nodule or mass of indeterminate origin; and mediastinal mass or adenopathies.

Percutaneous puncture is also indicated in a few other conditions: intracavitary injection of therapeutic agents for treatment of secondary aspergillomas [2]; insertion of a harpoon or injection of methylene blue or black carbon as a tracer prior to pleuroscopic resection of lung nodules [3].

### Contraindications

Vascular structures, hydatid cyst, a mediastinal meningocoele and a pheochromocytoma are absolute contraindications for percutaneous thoracic needle biopsy. The following are relative contraindications: puncture of both lungs on the same day, puncture of only one functional lung, chronic respiratory insufficiency, pulmonary arterial hypertension, cardiac insufficiency, recent myocardial infarct, angina, severe emphysema and bullae situated in the vicinity of the pulmonary lesion. A coagulation defect should be recognized and corrected temporarily before percutaneous biopsy is performed. Persistent cough, severe dyspnoea and reduced patient compliance are other limiting factors. Mechanical ventilation is not a contraindication for percutaneous lung biopsy.

### Technique

Percutaneous biopsy of thoracic lesions is preferentially performed with uni- or biplanar fluoroscopy control. CT is particularly useful for lesions that are situated at the apex and the base of the lung, in the posterior sulcus or at the pulmonary hilum. Mediastinal and hilar vascular structures surrounding a lesion are recognized with contrast-enhanced CT. In complex situations, CT reveals a tumour obscured by atelectasis, obstructive pneumonia or pleural effusion. Central tumour necrosis is recognized on the basis of central low densities after i.v. contrast injection. The biopsy needle should be directed to the viable tumour component situated at the periphery of the lesion. Percutaneous puncture performed at the side of pneumonectomy to disclose local cancer recurrence is best monitored with CT. Spiral scanning has not been proven to be superior to conventional CT in monitoring percutaneous lung biopsy in our experience, based upon a prospective comparative study. A large number of cutting and aspiration biopsy needles with a calibre of less than 1 mm and a variable needle tip design are currently used. They give similar rates of results and complications.

## Results

Percutaneous biopsy of pulmonary nodules has an accuracy greater than 90% in the confirmation of malignancy [4]. Inadequate cytologic smears were noted in up to 17% and allowed no interpretation in 9% in large series [5]. Additional false-negative diagnoses are obtained in about 5% and are due to wrong sampling, tumour necrosis, crushed cells or errors in sampling reading. The negative predictive value of percutaneous pulmonary biopsy is 84%-96% and false-positive results have been noted in 2%-4% [6]. The following criteria should be fulfilled to ascertain that a lung nodule is benign: biopsy should be technically successful; adequate material has to be sampled that is not normal lung; no suspicion of cancer should be raised on the aspirated cells and bronchoscopy should be normal. If a specific diagnosis of benignity can be reached by percutaneous biopsy, no further exploration is required. More often, a nonspecific and nonmalignant inflammatory process is found on the cytologic smears. These lesions should be followed up for 2 years. If the sampled material is inadequate or insufficient or if there is strong cytological or clinical suspicion of malignancy, biopsy should be repeated. A specific diagnosis of begnignity is demonstrated in less than 1:4 patients (Table 1). Most mediastinal lesions biopsied percutaneously are of metastatic or lymphomatous origin. The results are similar to those of lung biopsy when metastatic adenopathies are considered [7].

## Complications

Pneumothorax is the most frequent potential complication following percutaneous transthoracic puncture. The incidence is 7%-15% [5]. Less than 5% of patients have persistent clinical symptoms and need aspiration or drainage. A clinically significant pneumothorax is prevented by the roll-over technique, which consists in turning the patient following biopsy for 15-30 min to the side which has been punctured. When a large or

symptomatic pneumothorax persists, a Heimlich valve is inserted under fluoroscopic control. The pneumothorax is aspirated with a syringe, the valve is connected and its function is checked before the patient is discharged. Small bore 7-Fr to 10-Fr drainage catheters are successful in 75%-97% of iatrogenic penumothorax.

Haemoptysis is encountered in less than 10% of percutaneous lung biopsies. Other complications, such as mediastinal emphysema, thoracic wall haematoma, haemothorax, empyema, air embolism and sudden death are extremely rarely reported following transthoracic fine needle biopsy.

## Percutaneous Aspiration and Drainage of Thoracic Fluid Collections

Thoracic fluid collections can be aspirated or drained percutaneously with imaging guidance techniques. Percutaneous therapy is an important refinement compared to blind bedside technique and surgery. Diagnostic fluid aspiration includes cytological, bacteriological and chemical analyses. The presence of malignant cells, exudative fluid, blood, lymph, bile, amylase, clear fluid or gross pus provides aetiological indications.

### Guidance Modalities

*Fluoroscopy*

With fluoroscopy a pleural effusion can be recognized when the volume is sufficient to obliterate the posterior and lateral pleural sulcus. The location of encapsulated fluid pockets remains unchanged when the patient is moved. Large amounts of pleural fluid can be drained with the patient in a sitting or a posterior oblique position with the involved side up. A free pneumothorax is drained by a cephalad anterolateral approach, the patient being in an upright position. When a catheter is inserted in a peripheral pulmonary or a pleural collection with ultrasound (US) or CT control, definitive adjustment of the tip of the catheter is easily achieved with fluoroscopic control. Biplanar fluoroscopy is always helpful.

*Ultrasonography*

US is particularly useful in guiding percutaneous aspiration and catheter drainage of pericardial and pleural fuid, even when of reduced amounts. Pulmonary abscesses that are in a subpleural location can also be included. Shifting of free pleural and pericardial fluid during respiratory movements and changes of patient position are easily observed with US. The percutaneous approach is performed in the position that optimally shows the fluid collection.

**Table 1.** Benign lung nodules: specific diagnosis of benignity obtained by percutaneous biopsy

| Author and year | Benign lesions biopsied (n) | Specific benign diagnosis (n) | (%) |
|---|---|---|---|
| Flower CDR (1979) | 75 | 18 | 24 |
| Johnston WW (1984) | - | - | 11.7 |
| Horrigan TP (1984) | 8 | 2 | 25 |
| Khouri NF (1985) | 137 | 93 | 67.8 |
| Greene RE (1985) | 27 | 12 | 44 |
| Winning AJ (1986) | 43 | 7 | 16 |
| Calhoun P (1986) | 132 | 16 | 12 |
| Perlmutt LM (1989) | - | - | 12 |
| Charing MJ (1991) | - | - | 5 |

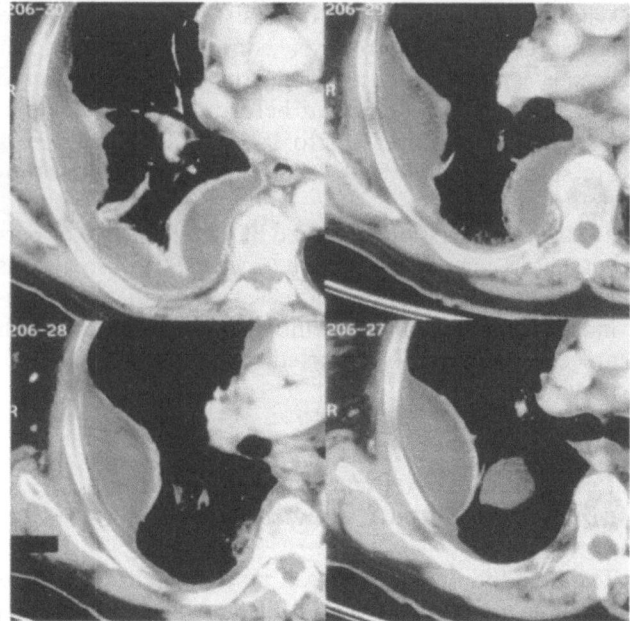

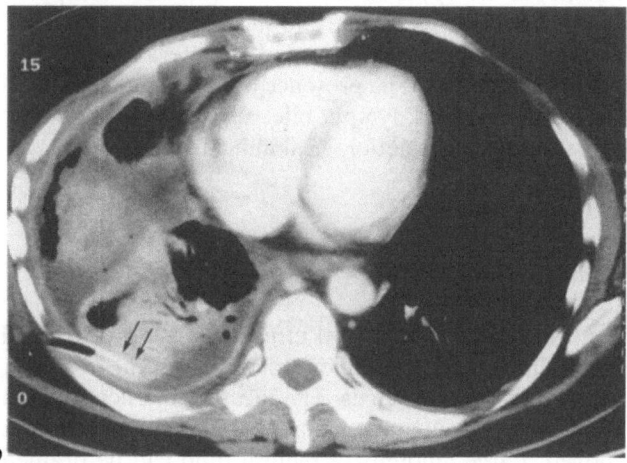

**Fig. 1 a, b.** Multiloculated right pleural empyema. Percutaneous insertion of a 20-Fr drainage catheter (→) under computed tomographic control

## Computed Tomography

CT offers precise anatomical display of all thoracic structures and allows percutaneous access to the pleura, lung and mediastinum with equal ease. However, it is not always possible to distinguish a pulmonary abscess from a pleural empyema, a distinction that often remains academic. Most catheters can be inserted with the patient remaining in the same supine position which he will adopt in bed after the drainage procedure.

CT is the optimal modality to confirm pneumothorax or pneumomediastinum following a percutaneous procedure.

## Drainage Techniques

The number and diameter of percutaneous drainage catheters should be adapted to the number and extent of collections and to the viscosity of the fluid to be drained. Small flexible 7-Fr catheters are well tolerated and sufficient for short-term drainage of water-like fluid. The trocar technique is the most expeditive. It can be used in combination with the tandem technique (a trocar is inserted parallel to a 18 – or 22 – gauge needle placed in the collection).

The angiographic catheter exchange technique is only rarely used in the thorax and is suitable for percutaneous access to deep mediastinal collections or for drainage of small or encapsulated pleural pockets that are located in the paramediastinal pleural space.

Percutaneous access through a thickened pleura can be extremely difficult, even when using regular chest tubes, and requires stiff guide wires and dilators. Chest drainage catheters are connected to a continuous negative waterseal suction.

A small drainage catheter can be left in place for pleural instillation of anticancer drugs, fibrin glue, tetracycline, bleomycin, etc. for treatment of recurrent malignant effusions.

Traumatic haemothorax should be drained in combination with lavage to prevent pleural adhesions. Larger chest tubes are usually required.

### Pleural Empyema

Imaging-guided percutaneous drainage avoids failure of blind chest tubes, which can occur in about one third of patients due to inadequate positioning of the tube or to satellite pleural pockets. Treatment of pleural empyema is most rewarding (Figs. 1, 2).

Empyemas develop secondarily to pre-existing pulmonary, mediastinal or thoracic wall infection, spread of cervical or abdominal infection, trauma, surgical or other invasive thoracic procedures, lung abscess and haematogenous spread of infection. Of the patients with pleural empyema, 50% have co-existing pneumonia. For an efficient drainage, multiple catheters are required in 23%-92% of empyemas.

Indications for drainage depend on the evolutionary stage of empyema. The main characteristics of the aspirated fluid according to stage are listed in Table 2. The diameter of the catheter has to be adapted to the viscos-

**Table 2.** Evolutionary stages of pleural empyemas

| Stage | I | IIa | IIb | III |
|---|---|---|---|---|
| Nature of fluid | Exudate | Fibrinoid | Purulent | Purulent |
| Fluid characteristics | Clear | Fibrin Strands | Pus | Pus |
| Number of cells | Few | < 25 000/ml | > 25 000/ml | |
| pH | > 7.2 | 7 > pH > 7.2 | pH < 7 | |
| Glucose (mg/dl) | > 60 | 40 - 60 | < 40 | |
| Gram staining | Negative | Positive | Positive | |

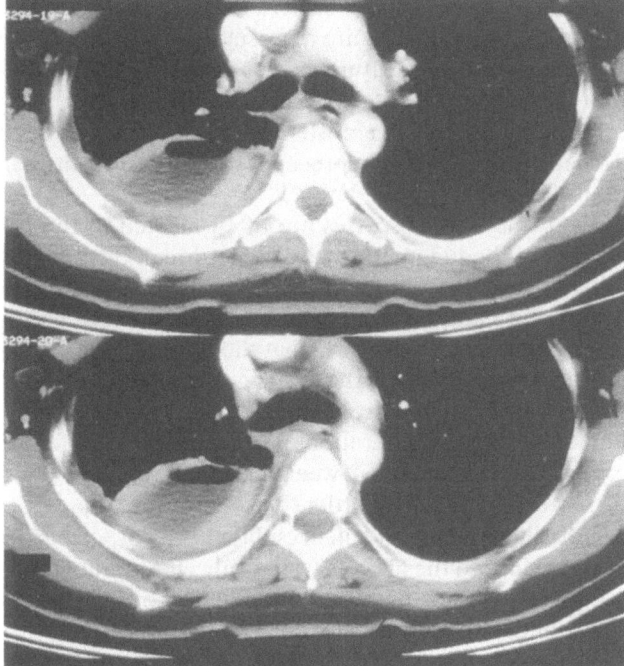

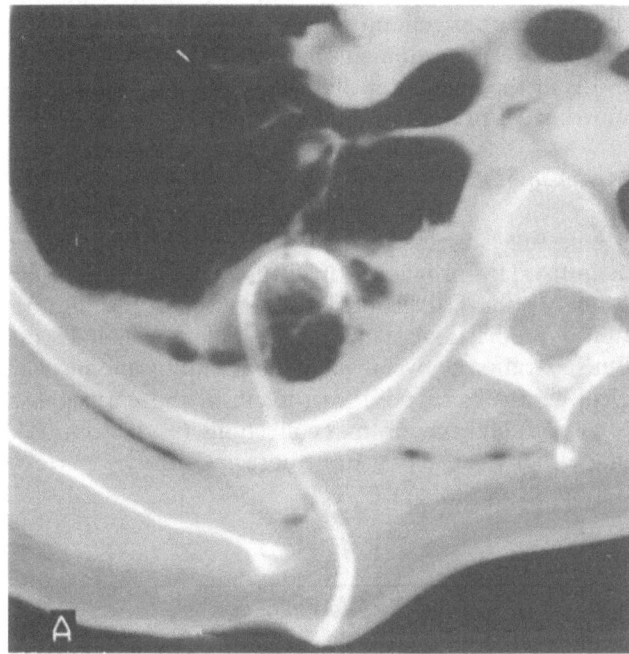

**Fig. 2 a, b.** Encapsulated empyema in the greater fissure of the right lung. Regression after percutaneous drainage with an 8-Fr pigtail catheter. Notice residual pleural peels

**Table 3.** Percutaneous drainage of pleural empyema in a first intent

| Author and year | Patients (n) | Guidance modality (%) | Clinical success (%) |
|---|---|---|---|
| Van Sonnenberg (1984) | 17 | CT : 59 US : 41 | 88 |
| Westcott (1985) | 12 | Fluoroscopy | 83 |
| O'Moore (1987) | 17 | US | 88 |
| Vasile (1987) | 11 | CT | 73 |
| Sherman (1987) | 43 | US : 70 CT : 18 Fluoroscopy : 12 | 72 |
| Merriam (1988) | 16 | CT | 75 |
| Hunnam (1988) | 20 | Fluoroscopy : 5 CT : 25, US : 40 or combination : 30 | 80 |
| Reinhold (1988) | 42 | US : 72 CT : 20 Fluoroscopy : 8 | 80 |
| Moulton (1989) | 13 | Fluoroscopy CT | 100 |
| Neff (1990) | 12 | US : 80 CT : 20 | 83 |
| Cumming (1991) | 13 | US | 85 |
| Lee (1991) | 10 | Fluoroscopy | 100 |
| Lambiase (1992) | 27 | CT or US or Fluoroscopy | 70 |
| Dondelinger (1994) | 22 | CT | 82 |

CT, computed tomography; US, ultrasound.

ity of the fluid to be drained and varies from 7 Fr to 30 Fr.

Irrigation and lavage are performed when blood or viscous material is present. Intrapleural injection of 200 - 400 000 IU of urokinase has proven to be efficient in the prevention of fibrin deposit and secondary loculation of the empyema.

Technical success of closed catheter drainage is ob-tained in almost all cases. Clinical success is achieved in 72%-89% of patients (Table 3) and depends on the stage of the disease. During stage III, with a history of illness in excess of 1 month before drainage, the procedure may fail in spite of insertion of multiple catheters. The dura-tion of percutaneous drainage is usually about 1 week. A one-session catheter treatment has been described: a large catheter is inserted in the pleural cavity and orien-tated in several directions. A negative pressure of 100 mmHg is applied until the entire pleural pus is aspirated [8]. Failure of percutaneous drainage varies from 12% to 18%. Failure of the pleural cavitiy to collapse and oblit-erate can occur in 5%-12% of patients. Massive bron-chopleural fistulae are an indication for surgery.

Even thick pleural peels often resolve spontaneously and regression can be followed by serial CT examina-tions. Pleural decortication should only be considered if pleural thickening persists after 3-4 months of follow-up.

Despite the good results obtained by closed percu-taneous drainage techniques, some pneumatologists and thoracic surgeons still advocate surgical thoracostomy and pleural decortication in stage III and also in stage IIb empyemas in a first intent. However, the results ob-tained demonstrate that radiologically guided drainage procedures are as efficient in patients in whom previous

**Table 4.** Percutaneous drainage of pleural empyema in a second intent

| Author and year | Failure of thoracostomy tube (n) | Radiologically placed catheter: successful drainage | |
|---|---|---|---|
| | | (n) | (%) |
| Van Sonnenberg (1984) | 13 | 12 | (92) |
| Westcott (1985) | 4 | 4 | (100) |
| Silverman (1988) | 3 | 3 | (100) |
| Merriam (1988) | 7 | 4 | (57) |
| Moulton (1989) | 5 | 5 | (100) |
| Lambiase (1992) | 8 | 4 | (50) |
| Total | 40 | 32 | (80) |

surgical tubes have failed as in patients treated in a first intent (Table 4).

### Malignant Pleural Effusions

Recurrent malignant pleurisies are usually drained with soft straight or 8-Fr pigtail catheters. Sclerosing drugs (tetracycline, etc.) that limit mesothelial cell secretion are injected daily through the catheter when output volume has decreased to 100 ml or less per day. Complete regression of the pleural effusion is obtained in 61%-71%.

### Post-traumatic Haemothorax

Massive haemothorax should be drained to reduce compression of the underlying lung parenchyma and prevent encapsulation and adherences. Large-bore catheters are mandatory. A pleural lavage can be useful.

### Pulmonary Abscess

Pyogenic pulmonary abscesses occur less frequently, due to progress in antibiotic treatment and more efficient eradication of the causes. Pulmonary abscesses which resist medical treatment and postural and bronchoscopic drainage require a percutaneous approach. In the past, surgical treatment of a lung abscess was required in about one fifth of patients.

A percutaneous diagnostic aspiration with an 18- to 22- gauge needle can precede catheter insertion in doubtful cases.

Pyogenic lung abscesses are often located in the periphery of the lung but usually do not break through the lobar fissure. Pleural symphyses are rapidly established. The broad pleural contact allows a percutaneous access to be planned in such a way that the normal lung parenchyma is not crossed by the drainage catheter. Generally, 7- to 14-Fr catheters are adequate for drainage of most lung abscesses. The duration of drainage is variable; the cavity closes after 1 or 2 weeks. Decompression should be performed slowly in order to avoid rupture of a vessel or a Rasmussen pseudoaneurysm that is incorporated or located close to the abscess wall. Daily chest radiographs are imperative for monitoring regression of the abscess cavity and early detection of complications.

Cure of the abscess is obtained in 73%-100% of cases, but the overall mortality is usually high in these patients due to the poor general condition or underlying disease (Table 5). Surgery remains indicated when extensive necrosis of the lung parenchyma and life-threatening haemorrhage is present.

### Mediastinal Abscess

Mediastinal abscesses result from circumscribed mediastinitis. The prognosis of diffuse mediastinitis is extremely poor. CT distinguishes between diffuse infiltration of mediastinal planes and a circumscribed abscess, but separation between acute mediastinitis and postsurgical changes can pose a problem in the early phase. Most purulent mediastinal collections result from trauma, either penetrating transthoracic injury or perforation of the oesophagus.

**Table 5.** Percutaneous drainage of pulmonary abscess

| Author and year | Patients (n) | Guidance modality | Calibre of drainage catheter | Duration of drainage (days) | Clinical success (%) |
|---|---|---|---|---|---|
| Vainrub (1978) | 3 | Fluoroscopy | 16 - 18 Fr | | 100 |
| Lorenzo (1985) | 5 | Fluoroscopy | 18 G Teflon sheathed needle | Aspiration | 100 |
| Rami Porta (1985) | 13 | - | Repeat aspiration 5 - 30 Fr | 15 | 100 |
| Yellin (1985) | 7 | Fluoroscopy | - | 15 | 100 |
| Parker (1987) | 6 | Fluoroscopy | 10 Fr | - | 100 |
| Rice (1987) | 11 | Fluoroscopy | - | - | 73 |
| Dondelinger (1990) | 7 | CT | 8 - 14 Fr | 12 | 43[a] |
| Van Sonnenberg (1991) | 19 | CT | 9 - 20 Fr | 10 | 84 |

CT, computed tomography

[a] Four of seven patients died from underlying disease after successful drainage.

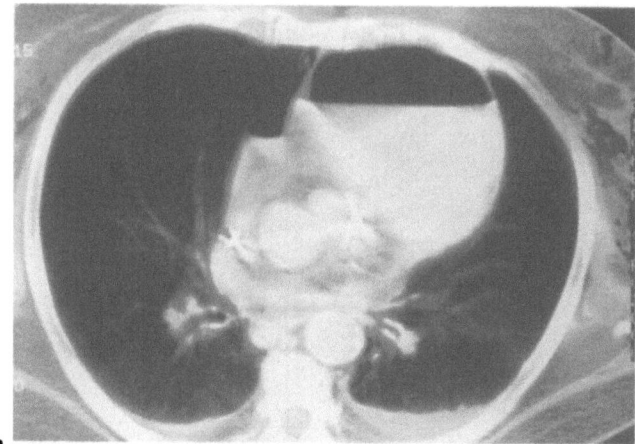

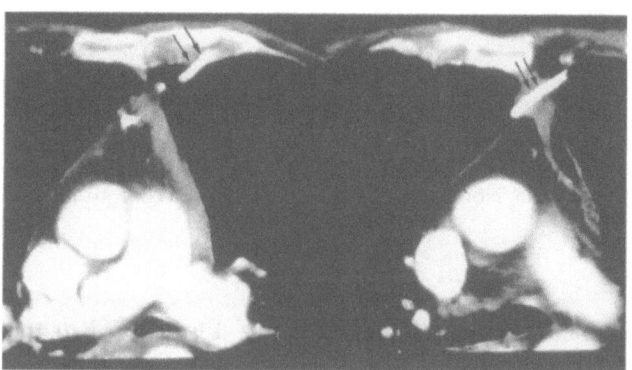

**Fig. 3 a, b.** Large, infected mediastinal haematoma after mediastinoscopy. Regression after percutaneous drainage with an 8-Fr catheter (→)

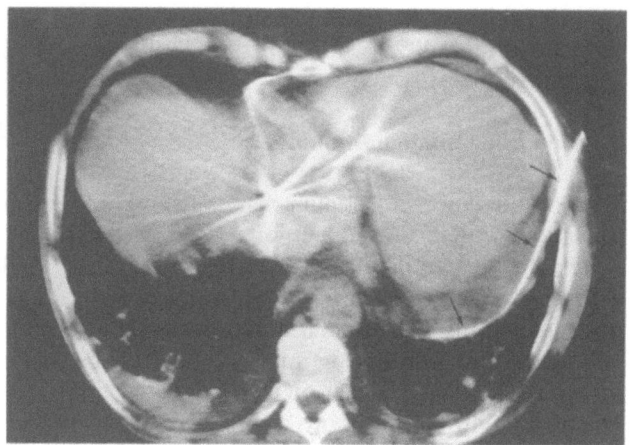

**Fig. 4.** Percutaneous drainage of a pericardial effusion by a left anterolateral approach with a 5-Fr pigtail catheter (→)

servative treatment is commonly applied to oesophageal perforation. An endo-oesophageal catheter can be inserted through an oesophageal tear or in combination with a percutaneous drainage catheter placed at the site of perforation. Only a limited number of patients with percutaneous drainage have been reported on (Table 6). Cure can be obtained in 83%-100% of patients according to the radiological literature, which does not consider the 30-day mortality rate.

*Pericardial Fluid Collection*

Pericardial effusion is suspected on the basis of clinical signs and electrocardiography. The diagnosis is confirmed with imaging techniques, mainly with transthoracic or endo-oesophageal US.

Percutaneous aspiration of pericardial fluid is indicated for diagnosis; percutaneous drainage prevents cardiac tamponade. Large amounts of pericardial fluid can be drained under CT control, sometimes with an atypical left anterolateral puncture, but most effusions are evacuated under US guidance, by a subcostal or a subxiphoid approach (Fig. 4). A 5-Fr to 7-Fr pigtail catheter is placed in the pericardial space. Technical success of the procedure and decompression of the

Abscesses that are located in the anterior mediastinum are drained by a parasternal approach, avoiding the internal mammary vessels which are well demonstrated with contrast-enhanced CT (Fig. 3). Abscesses that are located in the middle and posterior mediastinal compartment are treated by a paravertebral and extrapleural approach. It is also possible to drain the mediastinal compartments by a percutaneous cervical descending approach following the pathway of the infection.

Multiple catheters are often necessary and are placed either at both sides of the thoracic spine or the sternum or in the upper and lower part of the mediastinum. Con-

**Table 6.** Percutaneous drainage of mediastinal abscess

| Author and year | Patients (n) | Guidance modality | Calibre of drainage catheter (Fr) | Duration of drainage | Clinical success (%) |
|---|---|---|---|---|---|
| Gobien (1984) | 6 | CT and fluoroscopy | 8.3 - 12 | 5 - 91 days (mean 35) | 83 |
| Meranze (1987) | 8 | Fluoroscopy | 8.3 - 12 | 2 - 4 weeks | 88 |
| Carrol (1987) | 5 | CT | - | - | 100 |
| Ball (1989) | 5 | Fluoroscopy, US, CT | 8 - 12 | Mean 28 days | 100 |

CT, computed tomography; US, ultrasound.

heart is achieved in almost all cases, when there is a sufficient amount of effusion. Duration of drainage is short, several days only.

## Tension Pneumomediastinum

Tension pneumomediastinum results from barotrauma in patients with increased pulmonary resistance who are mechanically ventilated, with an elevated PAP and PEEP. Alveolar rupture results in interstitial emphysema that migrates to the mediastinum along the bronchovascular sheaths. When the mediastinal air fails to escape due to adhesions, tension pneumomediastinum develops. Compromised venous return, cardiac and respiratory insufficiency and anuria require rapid decompression. A left-sided pneumothorax is usually associated.

A soft 12-Fr or 14-Fr drainage tube can be inserted into the mediastinum behind the sternum under CT guidance by a left anterolateral percutaneous approach. When a left pneumothorax is also present, the mediastinal catheter should be inserted before exsufflation of the pleural air collection. We have successfully treated four patients with tension pneumomediastinum.

## Complications of Percutaneous Catheter Drainage

Complications resulting from percutaneous drainage of thoracic fluid collections guided by imaging techniques occur in 5% of patients and are mainly due to inadequate technique during percutaneous insertion of the catheter. Life-threatening haemorrhage is rare, but can be observed following rupture of the wall of a pulmonary abscess, erosion of a branch of the pulmonary artery or transfixation of the internal mammary or mediastinal vessels by the catheter.

Pericardial drainage is prone to most of clinically significant complications, such as haemopericardium with tamponade, dysrhythmia, pneumopericardium or superinfection.

A thoracic catheter can be introduced erroneously into the subdiaphragmatic space, the liver or spleen when cross-sectional imaging is not used properly. When the catheter creates a communication between a pulmonary abscess and the pleural space, a secondary empyema or a bronchopleural fistula can be established.

When the normal lung is crossed with a large-bore catheter using the trocar technique, pulmonary infarction can result. Pneumothorax is a potentially frequent complication, but can be avoided during percutaneous drainage of most pleural collections and pulmonary abscesses, provided that there is pleural contact. During pleural drainage under fluoroscopic guidance, a rate of pneumothorax of 6% has been noted; under US guidance a rate of 25% has occurred. When fluoroscopy is used predominantly as a guidance modality for thoracic drainage procedures, the overall complication rate is as high as 20%, most being minor problems.

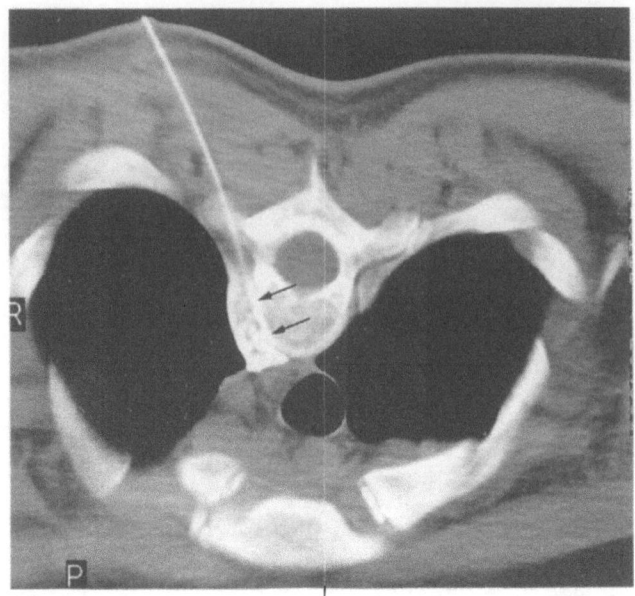

**Fig. 5.** Percutaneous phenol blockage of the left thoracic sympathetic chain. Note local diffusion of phenol and contrast medium (→)

## Percutaneous Block of the Upper Thoracic Sympathetic Chain

CT-guided percutaneous phenol block of the upper sympathetic chain was described and performed on an outpatient basis without premedication (Fig. 5) [9]. The neurolytic effect is obtained by injection of 5-15 ml of a solution of phenol 400 mg, glycerin 2.5 g and water to 5 ml at the level of T3 by a posterior paravertebral approach. Injection of phenol is stopped when optimal dryness and heat of the hand is reached.

The best results following percutaneous CT-guided phenol lysis of the upper thoracic sympathetic chain are obtained with palmar and axillary hyperhidrosis. A complete and durable cessation of sweating is noted in 82% of patients with the percutaneous procedure and in 94% following surgery. Primary Raynaud disease tends to recur after several months or 1-2 years after treatment. In case of failure, the percutaneous procedure can also be repeated. With surgical resection of the upper thoracic sympathetic ganglia (T2-T4), good results are noted in 22%-56% of patients with vasomotor syndromes.

Among the complications that may result from percutaneous CT-guided phenol block, a temporary or definitive incomplete Horner syndrome is most likely, but can be avoided by a careful technique. It has been noted in 23% of patients. Neuralgia of the upper limb and compensatory sweating are unpredictable side effects and are observed in 8% and 16% of the patients, respectively [10].

# References

1. Dondelinger RF (1993) Interventional radiology of the chest: percutaneous procedures. In: Imaging of the chest (Syllabus). ECR, Vienna CC-1001, pp 165-175
2. Giron JM, Poey CG, Fajadet PP, Balagner GB, Assoun JA, Richardi GR, Haddad JH, Caceres JC (1993) Inoperable pulmonary aspergilloma: percutaneous CT-guided injection with glycerin and Amphotericin B paste in 15 cases. Radiology 188:825-827
3. Plunkett MB, Peterson MS, Landerneau RJ, Ferson PF, Posner MC (1992) Peripheral pulmonary nodules: preoperative percutaneous needle localization with CT guidance. Radiology 185:274-276
4. Westcott JL (1980) Direct percutaneous needle aspiration of localized pulmonary lesions: results in 422 patients. Radiology 137:31-35
5. Sinner WN (1975) Wert und Bedeutung der perkutanen transthorakalen Nadelbiopsie für die Diagnose intrathorakalen Krankheitsprozesse. ROFO 123:197-202
6. Dahlgren S, Nordenstrom B (eds) (1966) Transthoracic needle biopsy. Almquist and Wiksell, Stockholm
7. Rosenberger A, Adler O (1978) Fine needle aspiration in the diagnosis of mediastinal lesions. AJR 131:239-242
8. Moulton JS, Moore PT, Mencini RA (1989) Treatment of loculated pleural effusions with transcatheter intracavitary urokinase. AJR 153:941-945
9. Dondelinger RF, Kurdziel JC (1987) Percutaneous phenol block of the upper thoracic sympathetic chain with computed tomography guidance. Acta Radiol 28:511-515
10. Adler O, Engel A, Rosenberger A, Dondelinger R (1990) Palmar hyperhidrosis CT guided chemical percutaneous thoracic sympathectomy. ROFO 153:400-403

# SKELETAL RADIOLOGY

# Digital Skeletal Radiography

H. Pettersson

Department of Radiology, University Hospital, S-221 85 Lund, Sweden

Digital radiography may be defined as an imaging system in which conventional X-rays are used, but in which conventional film-screen combinations are replaced by radiation detectors connected to computer systems to produce the image. Today, digital radiography for examination of the musculoskeletal system is routine in many departments. The systems used most for such digital radiography are based on imaging plates, using phosphor storage screens, but there are also several other systems developed or under development in which the imaging plate is no longer needed.

The image obtained may be evaluated either on a monitor or on hard copies. If hard copies are used, it is common that two differently processed images are obtained from each exposure. One image is preprogrammed to simulate the characteristics of a conventional film, while the other has a low global contrast and increased unsharped masking (Fig. 1).

## Potential Advantages and Disadvantages

The advantages and disadvantages of digital radiography are well known today. The advantages are: the broad exposure range, the free choice of data processing and the possibility of image evaluation and reporting at

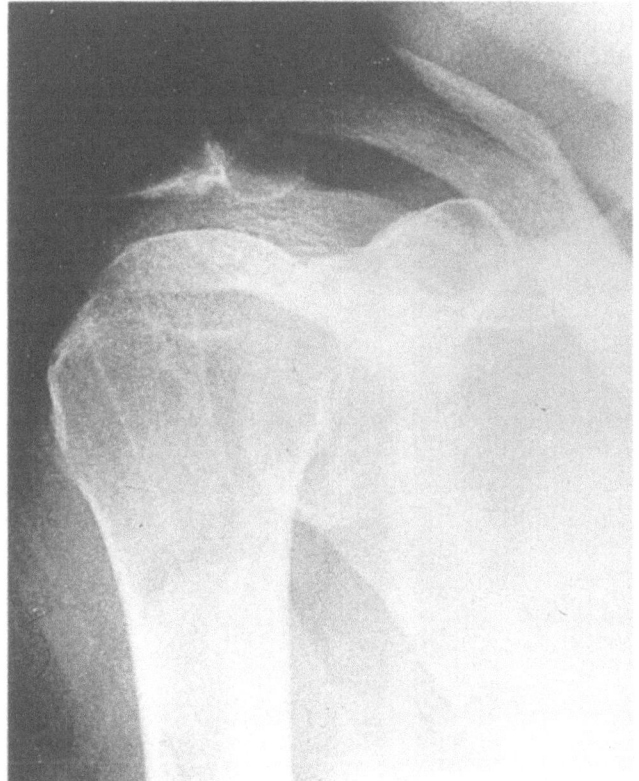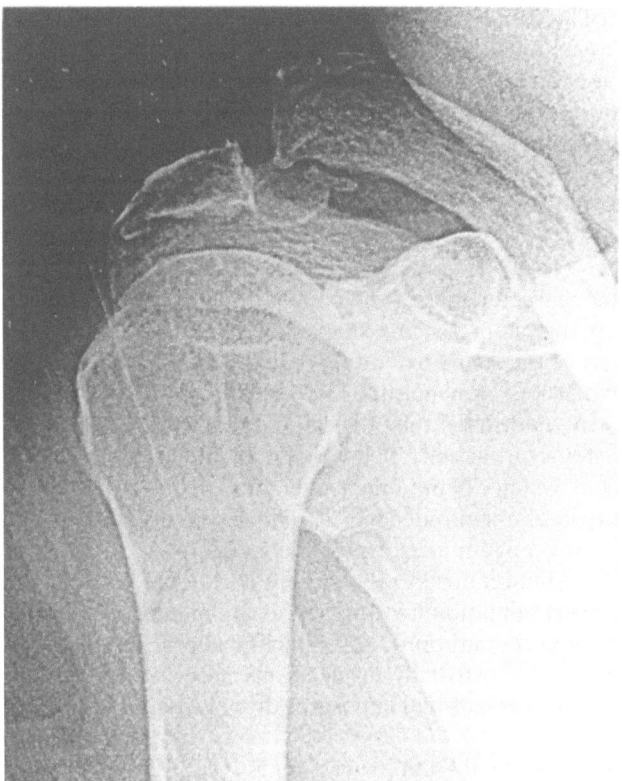

**Fig. 1 a, b.** Digital radiology, routine hard-copy processing. Commonly, each exposure is processed in two ways: one simulates a conventional film (**a**); the other enhances contrast edges (**b**)

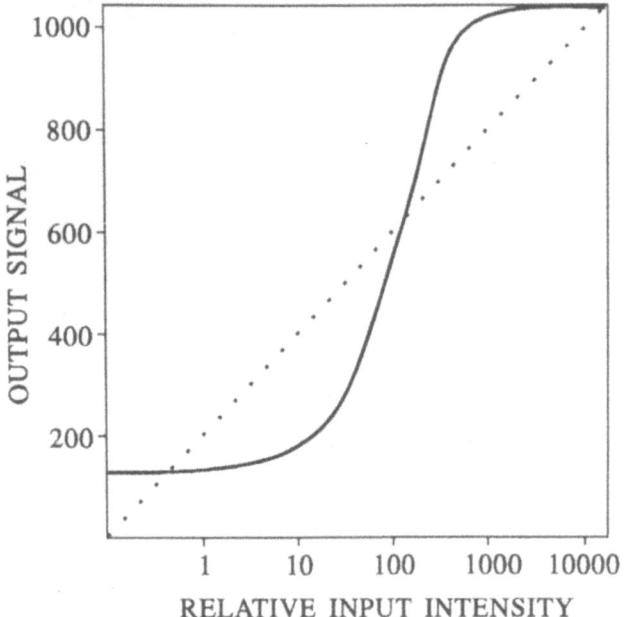

**Fig. 2.** A dose-response curve for a modern film-screen system (sigma-shaped), and for a digital radiography system (*dotted line*). The linear part of the curve for the film-screen system extends only over about two orders of magnitude, while the digital system is linear over four or five orders of magnitude

work stations, facilitating picture archiving and communication systems (PACS) solutions [1, 2].

The disadvantages may be efficiently controlled today and are therefore of clinically less importance than they were only a few years ago: the limited spatial resolution, the limited possibility to evaluate bone density, and contrast artefacts [1, 2].

## Broad Exposure Range

The typcal dose-response curve describing the characteristics of the conventional film-screen system is sigma-shaped, with a linear part of the sigma extending only over about two orders of magnitude [3].

In contrast, the digital radiographic systems principally behave almost like an ideal system, being linear over four or five orders of magnitude (Fig. 2). This broad exposure range makes it possible to decrease the radiation dose to the patient and hence to the population (A. Jónsson et al., manuscript in preparation). Also, in clinical practice there is virtually no need anymore for re-exposures, as bad exposures do not exist.

## Free Choice of Data Processing

Free choice of data processing means that from one and the same exposure, virtually an unlimited number of different images may be processed, with different combinations of grey scale, latitude, contrast steps, density, noise, etc. This obviously implies the possibility of getting additional information out of one and the same exposure, as compared with the traditional film-screen imaging.

## Evaluation and Reporting at the Monitor

If reporting of examinations at the monitor is made routine, and if monitors are also available in demonstration rooms, at the doctors' offices, on wards, etc., there is no need anymore for the hard copy. When the PACS system is fully developed in a department, there is no longer a need for films. In the long run this will diminish the costs for handling of images and it will also change the working situation both within the radiological department, and the means of communication between the radiologist and the referring clinicians.

## Limited Spatial Resolution

The limited spatial resolution inherent in early versions of digital radiography systems was a definite limitation for its use in skeletal radiology. However, with increasing spatial resolution in new systems, the pixel size today in most systems is about 0.1 mm, or even less, and the work station often operates at a matrix of 2000 x 2000. This will correspond to about five line pairs/mm, using conventional film-screen systems, and is thus still below the spatial resolution obtained with high-resolution film-screen combinations. However, the difference in resolution seems to be of negligible importance for the diagnostic accuracy, even for evaluation of subtle changes in bone texture [4-6] (Fig. 3).

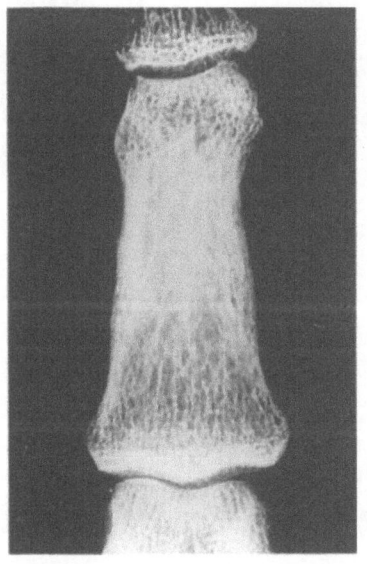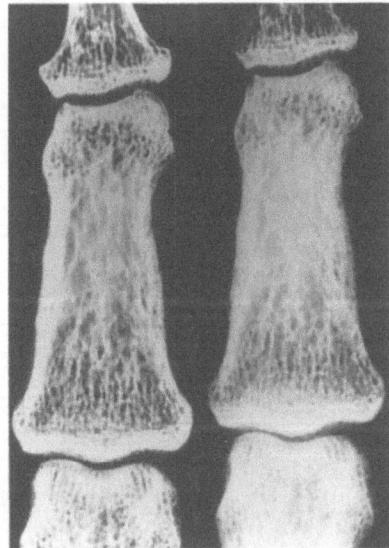

**Fig. 3 a, b.** Spatial resolution. A patient with hyperparathyroidism, examined with (**a**) a conventional film-screen system, and (**b**) digital radiography. Subtle subperiosteal changes can be seen with both systems

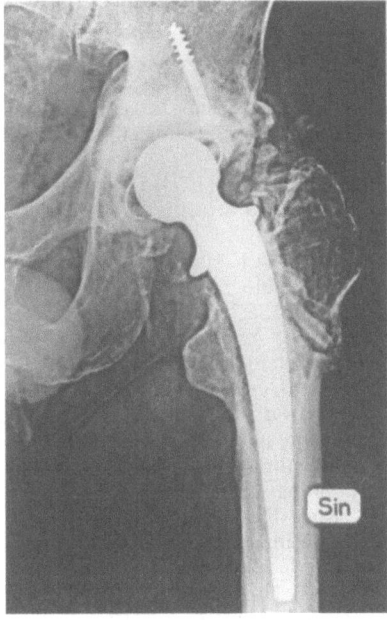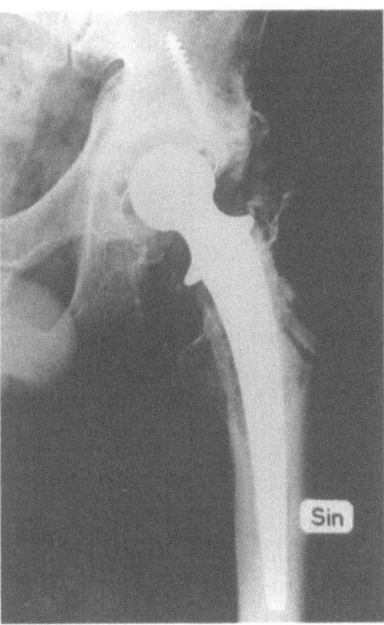

**Fig. 4 a, b.** Contrast artefacts. Hip prosthesis, digital radiography. **a** The image is processed with enhanced contrast edges, and there is a halo effect that may simulate radiolucent zones. **b** The image is processed to simulate a conventional film, and the halo effect is no longer visible

### Decreased Possibility for Evaluation of Bone Density

The apparent bone density in an image processed in a digital radiographic system depends totally on how the imaging parameters are set. Therefore, osteopenia may be suggested even if it is not present. However, if this is kept in mind when dealing with, for instance, patients with arthritis, metabolic disturbances and bone tumours, the problem can be kept under control.

### Contrast Artefacts

Again, if the imaging parameters are inadequately set, a contrast step artefact may appear in regions where there are high contrast steps, such as at the interface between a metal prosthesis and the bone or soft tissue (Fig. 4a). However, knowing the problem, and adjusting for the contrast steps, the artefacts may be avoided (Fig. 4b).

## Clinical Experience

Digital radiography has now been in use worldwide for several years, and considerable experience as to the clinical feasibility and the diagnostic accuracy has accumulated. There is a general experience that the digital systems facilitate the daily work in the emergency rooms and intensive care units, as the need for retakes is almost nil. In the same way, the system is highly appreciated for its ability to give adequate information in anatomical regions that are notoriously difficult to visualize because of

exposure problems using conventional film-screen systems, such as the transition region between the cervical and thoracic spine, in the thoracic spine/lumbar spine at the level of the diaphragm [7, 8], etc. Also, for visualization of skeletal detail and soft tissue structures, the digital systems are ideal (Fig. 5).

## Accuracy

For a solid evaluation of the diagnostic accuracy, scientifically planned investigations are mandatory. Several reports from such investigations are on record. Most of these investigations have used Receiver Operating Characteristic (ROC) studies as an instrument for comparison between the digital systems and the conventional film-screen combinations [9-11].

Generally, it may be said that digital systems, as evaluated on hard copies, have at least the same diagnostic accuracy as the film-screen combinations. This is also valid for pathologic conditions in which the changes may be subtle, such as in rheumatoid arthritis, hyperparathyroidism and scaphoid fractures. However, some investigators have found that when the accuracy using digital systems evaluated at a monitor is compared with the film-screen combinations, the film-screen combinations may be more reliable [12].

Generally, given the clinical experience gained in several large departments around the world, and the results of scientific investigations on record, it could be said that modern digital radiographic systems may well be used for all types of examinations in musculoskeletal radiology.

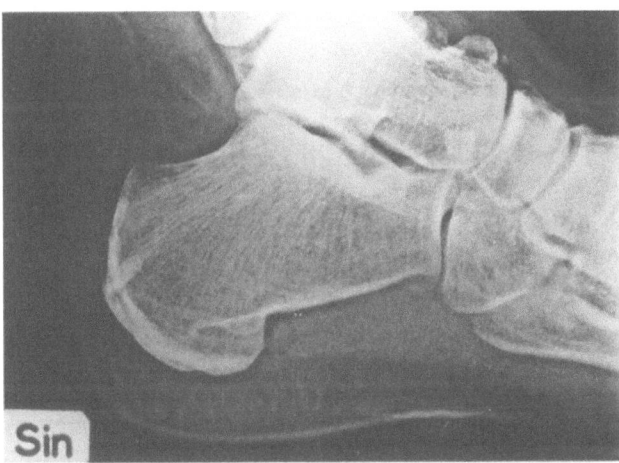

**Fig. 5.** Digital radiography is ideal for visualization of skeletal detail and soft tissue structures in one and the same image

## Computed Diagnosis

The storage of all diagnostic information in digitized form opens up possibilities for computed diagnosis, using some type of artificial intelligence. Around the world, several research groups are involved in these questions. Several approaches have been tried, for instance using chaos mathematics and fractal geometry or neural networks. This research is still in its infancy, but no doubt, the results from this will change the possibilities for X-ray diagnosis in skeletal radiology in the long run.

## Conclusion

Digital radiography has proven to be a safe and accurate technique for examinations of the musculoskeletal system. The diagnostic accuracy is high, and in the future will probably be even higher than conventional film-screen combinations. The cost for the system is still relatively high, but with increased use, very probably it will prove not only to be superior from a diagnostic point of view, but also more cost effective.

## References

1. Pettersson H (1992) Digital skeletal radiography. In: Resnick D, Pettersson H (eds) Skeletal radiology. Merit Communications, London, pp 1-8 (NICER series on diagnostic imaging)
2. Schmidt Ch, Deininger HK (1990) Die digitale Bildverstärkerradiographie: Ein neues Konzept für die traumatologische Röntgendiagnostik. ROFO 152:51-55
3. Pettersson H, Aspelin P, Boijsen E, Herrlin K, Egund N (1988) Digital radiography of the spine, large bones and joints using stimulable phosphos. Early clinical experience. Acta Radiol 29:267-271
4. Jónsson Á, Borg A, Hannesson P et al (1994) Film-screen vs. digital radiography in rheumatoid arthritis of the hand: a ROC analysis. Acta Radiol 35:311-318
5. Jónsson, Á, Hannesson P, Herrlin K et al (1995) Computed vs. film-screen magnification radiography of fingers in hyperparathyroidism. Acta Radiol 36:290-294
6. Scott WW Jr, Rosenbaum JE, Ackerman SJ et al (1993) Subtle orthopedic fractures: teleradiology workstation versus film interpretation. Radiology 187:811-815
7. Wilson AJ, Mann FA, West OC, McEnery KW, Murphy WA Jr (1994) Evaluation of the injured cervical spine: comparison of conventional and storage phosphor radiography with a hybrid cassette. Radiology 193:419-422
8. Kreipke DL, Silver DI, Tarer RD, Braunstein EM (1990) Readability of cervical spine imaging: digital versus film/screen radiographs. Comput Med Imaging Graph 14:119-125
9. Hanley JA, McNeil BJ (1982) The meaning and use of the area under a receiver operating characteristic (ROC) curve. Radiology 143:29-36
10. Prokop M, Galanski M, Oestmann JW et al (1990) Storage phosphor versus screen-film radiography: effect of varying of exposure parameters and unsharp mask filtering on the detectability of cortical bone defects. Radiology 177:109-113
11. Wegryn SA, Piraino DW, Richmond BJ et al (1990) Comparison of digital and conventional musculoskeletal radiography: an observer performance study. Radiology 175:225-228
12. Wilson AJ, Hodge JC (1995) Digitized radiography in skeletal trauma: performance comparison between a digital workstation and the original film images. Radiology 196:565-568

# Surface Lesions of Bone

A.M. Davies

Royal Orthopaedic Hospital, The Woodlands, Bristol Road South, Birmingham B31 2AP, UK

## Introduction

There are a large variety of neoplasms and tumour-like lesions that arise from the surface of bone. To the unwary observer these lesions produce a bewildering spectrum of radiographic appearances that can lead to misinterpretation and suboptimal management. The purpose of this review is to describe the differential diagnosis and highlight the value of imaging in identifying the correct diagnosis.

Surface lesions of bone may be categorized either by site of origin (e.g. subperiosteal, parosteal etc.) or by aetiology (e.g. neoplastic, post-traumatic etc.). A number of lesions of similar nature (e.g. osteosarcoma) may arise in several sites on the surface of bone (e.g. periosteal and parosteal). It is simpler, therefore, to classify the lesions by aetiology rather than site of origin. It is important, however, to note the site of origin as this will obviously influence the radiographic appearance. Two broad groups exist: tumour-like lesions and true neoplasms.

Difficulties in understanding this subject are undoubtedly aggravated by the confusion in use of terminology [1]. Many texts use a variety of different terms, some of which are interchangeable. If one considers that the surface of bone comprises three structures, the cortex, the periosteum and adjacent soft tissues, then the term juxtacortical is nonspecific and refers to all surface lesions of extracortical origin.

Subperiosteal lesions lift the periosteum from the cortex, whereas periosteal lesions arise in the deep layer of the periosteum. The former are typically non-neoplastic and the latter neoplastic. Parosteal lesions arise within the fibrous outer layer of the periosteum. Cortical lesions are only included in the differential diagnosis because the subperiosteal space may be involved secondarily and thereby mimic a surface or juxtacortical lesion.

## Tumour-like Conditions

The group of tumour-like conditions includes all the metabolic, systemic and hormonal disorders which may elevate the periosteum from the cortex and result in periosteal new bone formation. The conventional radiograph is the optimum imaging technique for the demonstration of periosteal new bone formation although it is only visible when sufficient mineralization has occurred. The speed of mineralization is faster in younger patients.

The underlying cause of a periosteal reaction may be determined by analysing a number of factors. These include the age of the patient, the nature of the periosteal reaction (e.g. lamellated or spiculated), the distribution (e.g. bilaterally symmetrical or asymmetrical) and, finally, associated abnormalities such as an arthropathy. For example, a bilaterally symmetrical periosteal reaction in an adult is likely to be hypertrophic osteoarthropathy or diffuse idiopathic skeletal hyperostosis. A bilaterally asymmetrical periosteal reaction in an adult will include the arthritides such as Reiter's syndrome and psoriatic arthropathy.

The remaining juxtacortical lesions which may mimic tumours are largely post-traumatic in origin. Again, the literature is confusing, with a large number of different names being employed. However, the subject can be significantly simplified by acknowledging that the lesions represent a spectrum of post-traumatic disorders, whereby histological and radiographic variation can be accounted for by the maturation of the lesion, the anatomical location and the age of the patient. The following entities are discussed.

### Periostitis Ossificans

Sometimes known as florid reactive periostitis or periosteal fasciitis, periostitis ossificans is typified by the presence of a subperiosteal haematoma which matures in 6-8 weeks. It is important to recognize the zoning pattern of ossification with radiodensity at the periphery and a

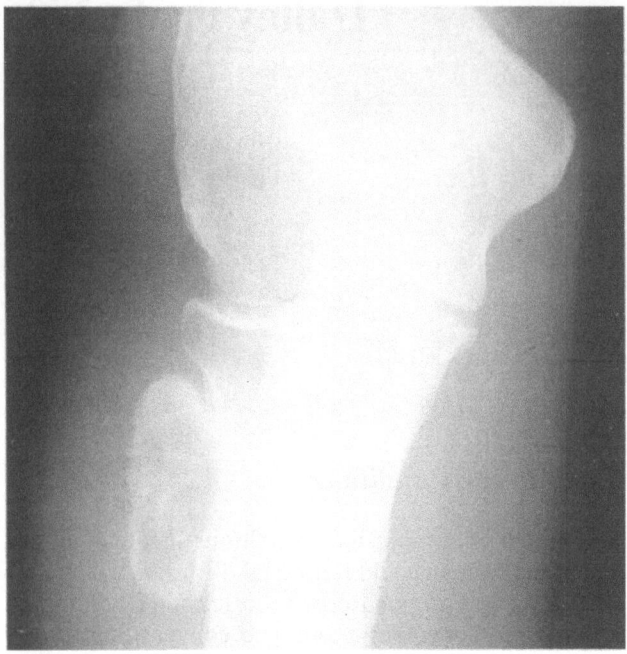

**Fig. 1.** Periostitis ossificans of the proximal radius adherent to the outer cortex, with peripheral mineralization

lucent centre (Fig. 1). This feature helps to differentiate the lesion from juxtacortial malignancies such as parosteal osteosarcoma. The soft tissue counterpart of periostitis ossificans is myositis ossificans which arises within skeletal muscle. Again, the zoning phenomenon visible on radiographs, computed tomography (CT) and magnetic resonance imaging (MRI) is typical. It is important to identify the diagnosis radiographically as histologically it may easily be mistaken for an osteosarcoma.

## Bizarre Parosteal Osteochondromatous Proliferation

A relatively rare benign condition is bizarre parosteal osteochondromatous proliferation, frequently known by the acronym BPOP [2]. Although there is rarely a definite history of antecedent trauma it is generally thought to belong to the spectrum of post-traumatic reparative conditions. It arises from the long bones of the hands and feet and is identified radiographically as a bony "exostosis" with a pedicle attached directly to the outer cortical surface with no communication with the medullary cavity. This distinguishes BPOP from an osteochondroma. In many respects BPOP may resemble a parosteal osteosarcoma but this malignancy is virtually unknown in the hands and feet. An interesting feature to note for management is the high tendency to local recurrence.

## Subungual Exostosis

Subungual exostosis is an easily recognizable lesion on radiographs most commonly reported in the great toe. It is seen as a benign exostosis, either subungual or para-

ungual. The aetiology is unknown although trauma is considered a contributory factor.

## Stress Fracture

The clinical and radiographic features of fatigue type stress fractures can frequently mimic a malignant tumour. Strictly speaking, the fracture involves the cortex and is only included in surface lesions as the fracture line may be occult and the periosteal reaction predominate. Although textbooks claim the clinical picture is usually typical, personal experience indicates that the history of unusual, strenuous physical activity is frequently absent. The diagnosis should be established from the radiographs as more advanced imaging, such as bone scintigraphy and MRI, will reveal an extensive abnormality which may be misinterpreted as neoplastic infiltration.

## Avulsion Injuries

The mechanism of avulsion injuries is either a single, violent contraction or repeated contraction of a muscle or group of muscles transmitted to the bone through their

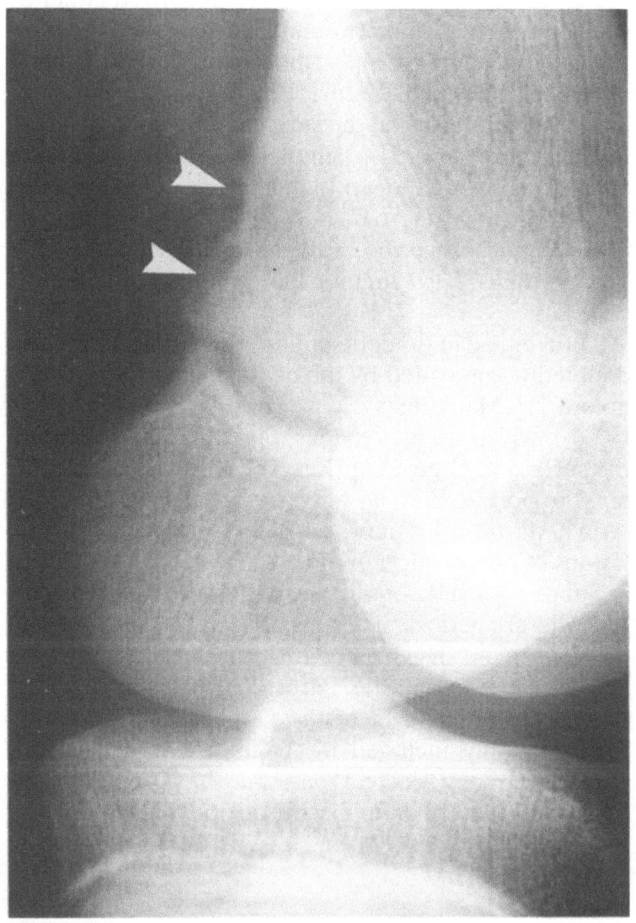

**Fig. 2.** Avulsive cortical irregularity of the posteromedial aspect of the distal femoral metaphysis (*arrowheads*)

tendons. In all these injuries, the soft tissue component remains intact, but the skeletal element is disrupted, either by fracture separation or physeal separation. These are particularly common in the pelvis where there may be involvement of the iliac crest, anterior superior and inferior iliac spines, the ischial tuberosity and the lesser trochanter. The acute injuries rarely cause problems in diagnosis and are easily identified on the radiographs. Problems may arise with an acute apophyseal avulsion where the fragment continues to grow to produce a large osseous body in the soft tissues. Chronic avulsion injuries, frequently seen in the adolescent age group, typically show subperiosteal and cortical irregularity without frank bone destruction or a soft tissue mass at the site of origin/insertion of a muscle group. One lesion that merits particular mention is the cortical irregularity seen along the posteromedial aspect of the distal femoral condyle in adolescents (Fig. 2) [3, 4]. Known in the American literature as a *periosteal desmoid*, this lesion frequently mimics a sarcoma. Usually an incidental finding, the aetiology is attributed to traction at the insertion of the adductor muscles. One factor against the suggestion of a traumatic origin is the absence of increased activity on bone scintigraphy.

## Tumours

Juxtacortical neoplasms may be both benign or malignant and can be further subdivided by their principal tissue of origin (Table 1).

### Bone-Forming Tumours

*Periosteal Osteoid Osteoma/Osteoblastoma*

The majority of osteoid osteomas arise within the cortex but on occasion may develop within the medulla or on the surface of bone. The nidus elevates the periosteum to produce reactive bone locally. CT is excellent in demonstrating the nidus. Scintigraphy and MRI reveal the

**Table 1.** Classification of tumours of juxtacortical origin

**Bone-forming**
  Periosteal osteoid osteoma/osteblastoma
  Parosteal osteoma
  Parosteal osteosarcoma
  Periosteal osteosarcoma
  High-grade surface osteosarcoma

**Cartilage-forming**
  Osteochondroma
  Periosteal chondroma
  Periosteal chondrosarcoma

**Miscellaneous**
  Parosteal lipoma
  Periosteal Ewing's sarcoma

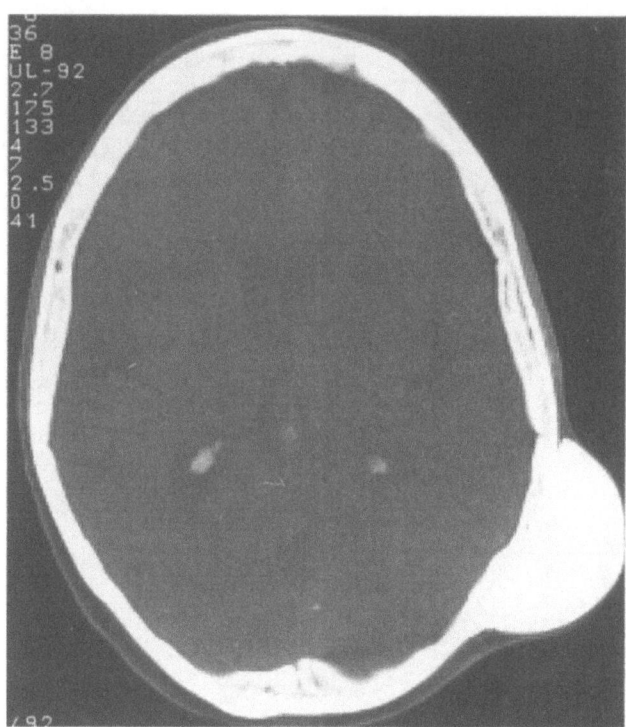

**Fig. 3.** Computed tomography of parosteal osteoma of the skull vault

extent of the surrounding inflammatory process in bone and the adjacent soft tissues.

*Parosteal Osteoma*

Parosteal osteoma is a benign, compact, bone forming lesion, usually asymptomatic, which presents as a dense, slow growing tumour. Typical sites include the skull vault (Fig. 3) and the mandible. There is a well recognized association between mandibular osteomas and Gardner's syndrome. Radiographs and CT demonstrate a dense mass, with no soft tissue component, closely adherent to the cortex with no plane of cleavage. The osteoma appears uniformly dark on all MRI sequences due to the relative lack of mobile protons.

*Parosteal Osteosarcoma*

Parosteal osteosarcoma is the commonest of the surface osteosarcomas and is associated with the best prognosis [5]. The posterior aspect of the distal femur is the most common site (Fig. 4), followed by the tibia and the humerus. Radiographically the tumour is densely ossified at the centre and relatively lucent at the periphery, distinguishing it from myositis ossificans. The tumour has a tendency to wrap around the underlying bone and, in part, there will appear to be a plane of cleavage from the underlying cortex. Although the cortex may be invaded, the trabeculae of the medulla are not continuous with

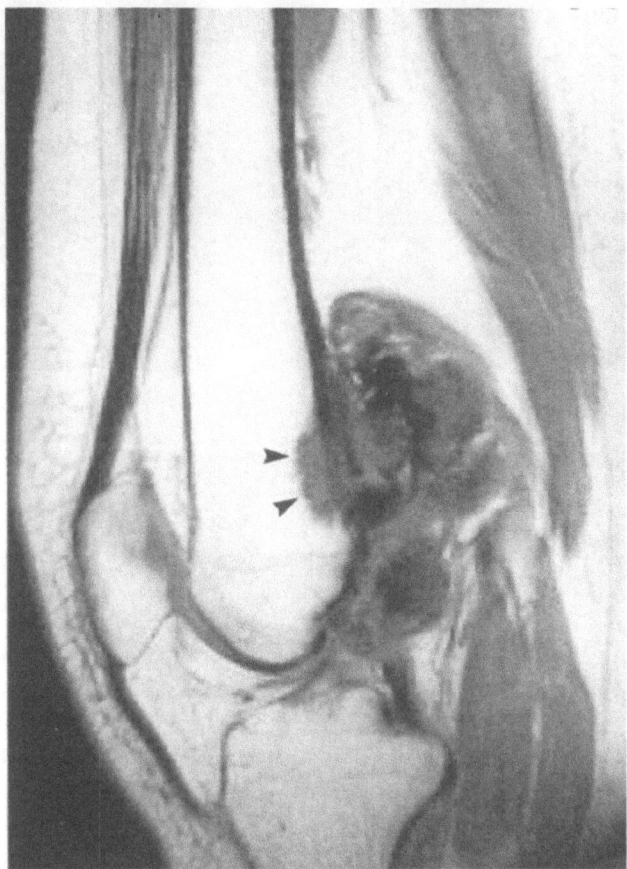

**Fig. 4.** Sagittal T1-weighted image of a parosteal osteosarcoma arising from the posterior femoral metaphysis. There is early invasion of the underlying medulla (*arrowheads*) and the posterior knee joint

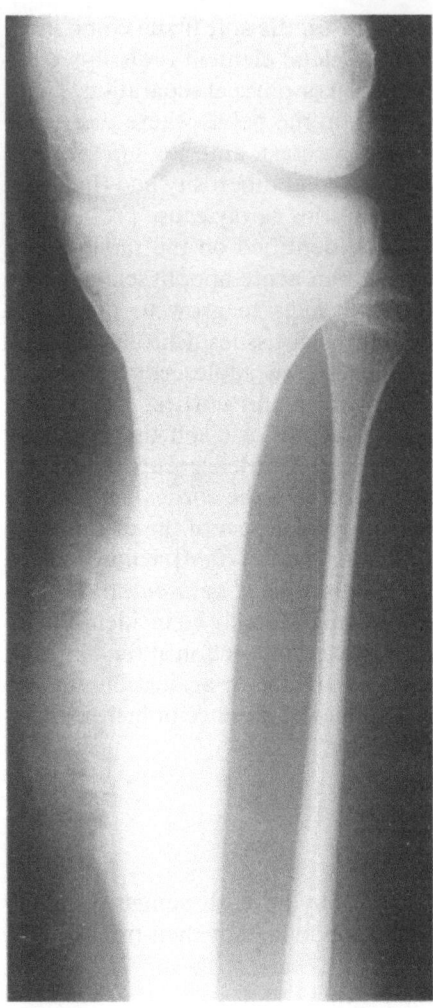

**Fig. 5.** Periosteal osteosarcoma of the tibia. Typical site and appearance with a spiculated periosteal reaction

the tumour, allowing for distinction from an osteochondroma. CT elegantly demonstrates the relationship of the tumour to the underlying bone but MRI gives a more accurate depiction of cortical breaching. Approximately 20% of parosteal osteosarcomas dedifferentiate, which may be suspected by the presence of increasing radiolucency within the tumour [6].

### Periosteal Osteosarcoma

First described in 1976, this tumour classically arises in the proximal tibial metaphysis (Fig. 5) [7]. Typical features are the fusiform soft tissue mass with a spiculated periosteal reaction firmly adherent to the underlying cortex with no evidence of a plane of cleavage. This is a low grade malignancy with a predominantely chondroblastic histology.

### High-Grade Surface Osteosarcoma

High-grade surface osteosarcoma is a rare tumour first reported just over a decade ago [8]. Radiographically it may mimic a periosteal osteosarcoma although MRI

frequently reveals underlying medullary invasion. It is associated with a poorer prognosis than the periosteal variant and is similar to that of conventional osteosarcoma.

### Cartilage-Forming Tumours

#### Osteochondroma

Strictly speaking, osteochondromas present an extension of bone with a cartilage cap and are, therefore, not truly a surface lesion. Nevertheless, it is important to include them in the differential diagnosis of surface lesions as they may be mistaken for a parosteal osteosarcoma, or more significantly, vice versa. The cartilage cap may be easily measured with CT, MRI or ultrasound. A thickness in excess of 3 cm in an adult is suspicious of malignant degeneration into a peripheral chondrosarcoma.

#### Periosteal Chondroma

Arising within or under the periosteum this benign tu-

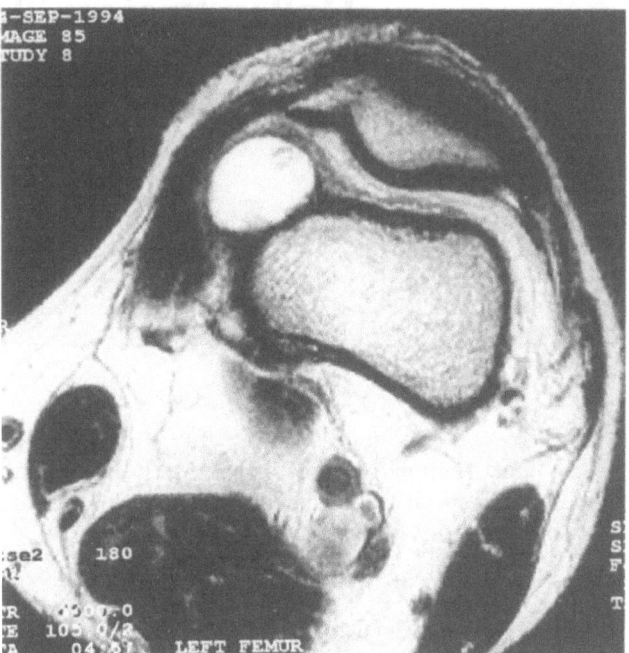

**Fig. 6.** Axial T2-weighted image of a periosteal chondroma arising from the cortex of the distal femoral metaphysis

mour produces cortical erosion (Fig. 6) [9, 10]. There is underlying saucerization of the cortex with buttress formation peripherally and minor marginal calcification. The relationship of the tumour to the cortex can be well demonstrated with either CT or MRI.

*Periosteal Chondrosarcoma*

The malignant counterpart of the periosteal chondroma, this rare, low grade tumour arises in an older age group [11]. Typically there is a large soft tissue mass containing punctate cartilage calcification. The underlying cortex is usually not breached.

**Miscellaneous Tumours**

*Parosteal Lipoma*

Parosteal lipoma is a rare benign tumour of adipose tissue. The soft tissue component exhibits typical fat density on both radiographs and CT [12]. Frequently there are reactive bone changes, including periosteal reaction, cortical erosion and bony excrescences.

*Periosteal Ewing's Sarcoma*

Small, round-cell tumours arising within the medulla of

bone or at an extraskeletal site are well recognized. Primary periosteal Ewing's sarcoma is extremely rare [13]. The tumour presents as a large, ill-defined, fusiform, soft tissue mass lying on bone. The underlying cortex appears permeated and there is usually a complex periosteal reaction.

## Conclusion

A large spectrum of tumours and tumour-like lesions may arise from the surface of bone. Excluding metabolic, hormonal and systemic disorders, the majority of tumour-like juxtacortical lesions are post-traumatic in origin. Close attention to the history, typical site of occurrence and the conventional radiographic features will allow for accurate diagnosis in the majority of cases.

The remaining surface lesions are likely to be neoplastic. As with all bone tumours, it is the conventional radiographs which reveal the most diagnostic information with regard to periosteal reaction, mineralization and pattern of bone destruction. CT and MRI have less of a role in diagnosis but are of value in demonstrating the integrity of the cortex and, depending on availability, one or the other technique is required in the staging of suspected malignant surface lesions of bone.

## References

1. Kenan S et al (1993) Lesions of juxtacortical origin (surface lesions of bone). Skeletal Radiol 22:337
2. Nora FE et al (1983) Bizarre parosteal osteochondromatous proliferations of the hands and feet. Am J Surg Pathol 7:245
3. Bufkin WJ (1974) The avulsive cortical irregularity. AJR 112:180
4. Dunham WK et al (1980) Developmental defects of the distal femoral metaphysis. J Bone Joint Surg 62A:801
5. Ahuja SE et al (1977) Juxtacortical (parosteal) osteosarcoma histological grading and prognosis. J Bone Joint Surg 59A:632
6. Wold L et al (1984) Dedifferentiated parosteal osteosarcoma. J Bone Joint Surg 66A:53
7. Unni KK et al (1976) Periosteal osteogenic osteosarcoma. Cancer 37:2476
8. Wold L et al (1984) High grade surface osteosarcoma. Am J Surg Pathol 8:181
9. Lewis MM et al (1990) Periosteal chondroma: a report of 10 cases and review of the literature. Clin Orthop 256:185
10. Desantos LA, Spjut HJ (1981) Periosteal chondrosarcoma: a radiographic spectrum. Skeletal Radiol 6:15
11. Schajowicz F (1977) Juxtacortical chondrosarcoma. J Bone Joint Surg 59B:473
12. Fleming RJ et al (1962) Parosteal lipoma. AJR 87:1075
13. Bator SM et al (1986) Periosteal Ewing's sarcoma. Cancer 58:1781

# Advances in Joint Imaging

I. Watt

Directorate of Clinical Radiology, Bristol Royal Infirmary, Bristol BS2 8HW, UK

## Introduction

The mainstay of radiological rheumatological diagnosis remains the plain X-ray. Films should be of high quality and always relevant to answer a clinical management problem. Examinations must be performed with clear objectives in mind. What do we want to know? Will the information affect patient management? Is the treatment that will be offered useful? As in all radiological situations it is vital to co-ordinate the imaging 'orchestra' for the best and most efficacious use. Obviously the best person to do that is a radiologist, preferably one skilled in musculoskeletal diseases. The major roles of the various imaging modalities are discussed in this paper.

## Plain Radiographs

The plain film offers much benefit even though soft tissue changes can only be seen in those areas that have suitable fat planes next to them, and bony changes take at least 10-14 days to develop. However, plain films are readily available, (relatively) inexpensive and carry a reasonable radiation dose. Their main uses include:
- Initial diagnosis.
- They are often sufficient to monitor disease and for preoperative assessment (for example to show the load line and the degree of varus / valgus instability).
- Follow-up of disease and therapy, including after surgical intervention.
- Detection of complications, for example a single lateral film of the cervical spine in flexion is sufficient to detect atlantoaxial instability in rheumatoid disease.
- With the use of contrast medium to delineate synovial masses, joint rupture and so on.
- Microfocal techniques are enjoying a resurgence. They allow very acute delineation of fine-detail lesions, proving helpful in the assessment of patients on treatment regimens [1]. As fine trabecular detail can be seen, texture analysis methods can be applied, including fractal signature analysis. These show differences between normal bone, juxta-articular osteoporosis and rheumatoid erosion. Similarly insights are being gained on trabecular organisation, and failure, in osteoarthritis (OA) [2].

## Ultrasound

Ultrasound is inexpensive, hazard free, undervalued and widely available. Disadvantages include the operator dependence of the method. However, with the benefit of colour flow or power Doppler useful information is available, including:
- Detection of ganglia, joint cysts, rupture and synovial masses and soft tissue "tumours" in general.
- Screening for extra-articular complications of the inflammatory rheumatic diseases, for example venous thrombosis.
- Detecting and staging tendon lesions, from the peroneal sheath to the rotator cuff.
- Some data suggest that cartilage thickness may be measurable, where access is possible without overlying bone. Transducers applied directly to the surface of cartilage at arthroscopy allow exact measurement of cartilage thickness and quality.
- Early work suggests that colour flow Doppler may be used to monitor therapeutic responses to intra-articular therapy in rheumatoid disease of the knee [3].

## Radionuclide Scintigraphy

The $^{99m}$ technetium skeletal scintigram is of considerable value for:
- The initial evaluation, following plain films, for occult causes of bone pain, including soft tissue lesions. For example, tendon or ligamentous disease is shown when plain X-rays are normal [4].
- With emphasis on the blood pool phase, detect and show the effect of treatment on acute inflammatory lesions, for example synovitis or septic arthritis.
- Assess the painful joint replacement. The blood pool phase of the scintigram is crucial as it reflects in-

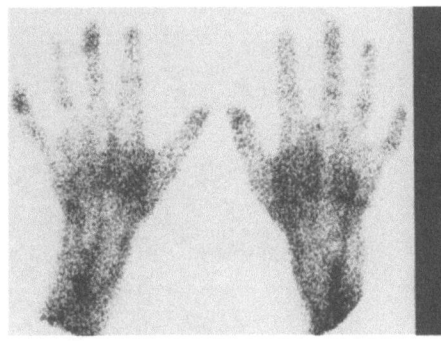
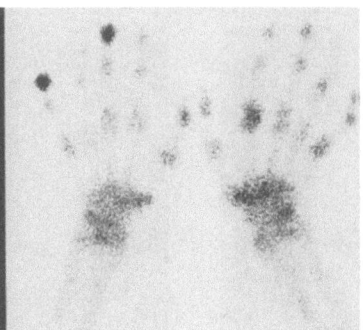
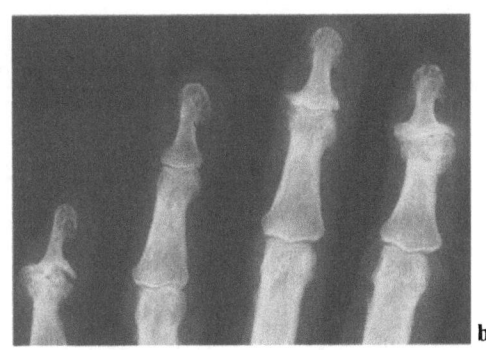

a                                                                  b

**Fig. 1 a, b.** Scintigraphy in the assessment of osteoarthritis (OA). **a** The scintigram using $^{99m}$Tc-labelled diphosphonate on the blood pool and delayed images demonstrates three abnormal active joints. **b** The X-ray, however, shows three. The implication is that a time lag exists between the pathophysiological processes shown by the scintigram and the X-ray, and that the radiographic changes may be perceived as biologically inert or 'healed'

creased vascularity and is cheaper and more readily available than a labelled white cell or $^{67}$gallium scan. The late phase appearances alone are sensitive to prosthetic problems, but may not be discriminatory in their own right. Ultrasound may confirm the presence of a joint effusion and allow real-time visualisation for joint aspiration.

– Detect and confirm the presence of arthritis, for example rheumatoid disease, even when an X-ray is normal and a joint is asymptomatic. A disparity may occur between scintigraphic and radiographic features in OA (Fig. 1 a, b). Scintigraphy will predict eventual joint failure in OA of the hand or knee [5, 6]. Data show that those joints which are scintigraphically active have a substantially greater chance of failing and requiring surgery than those which are normal on the scan. Skeletal scintigraphy shows four types of abnormality in knee OA, each with possibly a different prognostic significance [7].

– Demonstrate incidental, nonrheumatogical causes of bone and joint pain, including metastasis and insufficiency or osteomalacic fractures.

The radionuclide $^{99m}$technetium may label other pharmaceuticals, including nanocolloid or liposomes, to distinguish between the inflammatory component of synovitis and the secondary bone changes in rheumatoid disease (Fig. 2a-d). Similarly $^{99m}$technetium may be used with human immunoglobulin [8].

## Computed Tomography

In many ways computed tomography (CT) has been superseded by magnetic resonance imaging (MRI). CT has had a number of important uses in joint disease, including:

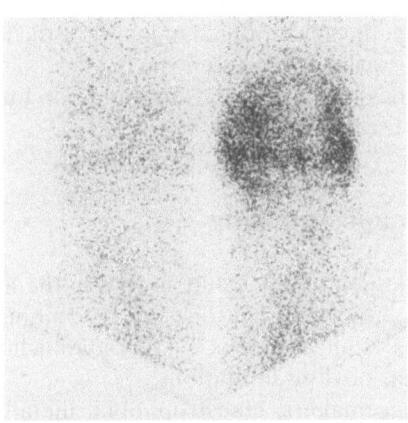

a

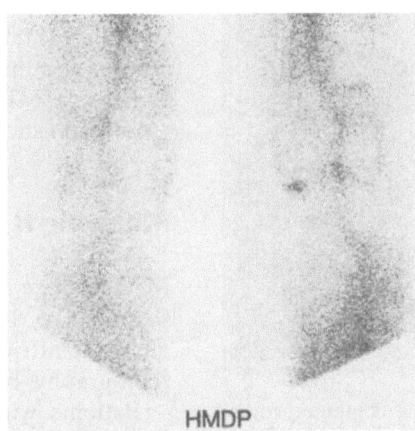
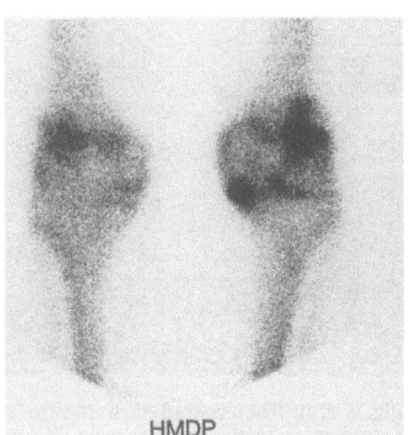

b                                           c                                          d

**Fig. 2 a-d.** In rheumatoid arthritis the different processes within the knee joint are shown by the use of two radiopharmaceuticals. **a, b** $^{99m}$Tc-labelled nanocolloid reflects the blood pool changes around the knee as well as reflecting synovial activity. **c, d** $^{99m}$Tc-labelled diphosphonate shows similar appearances on the blood pool phase, but the late phase shows features of secondary bone response

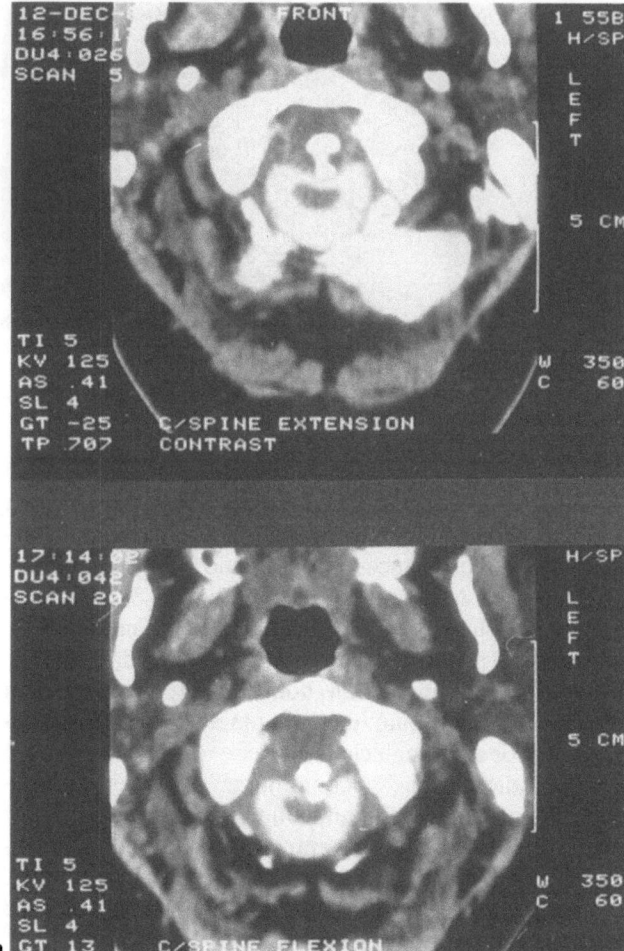

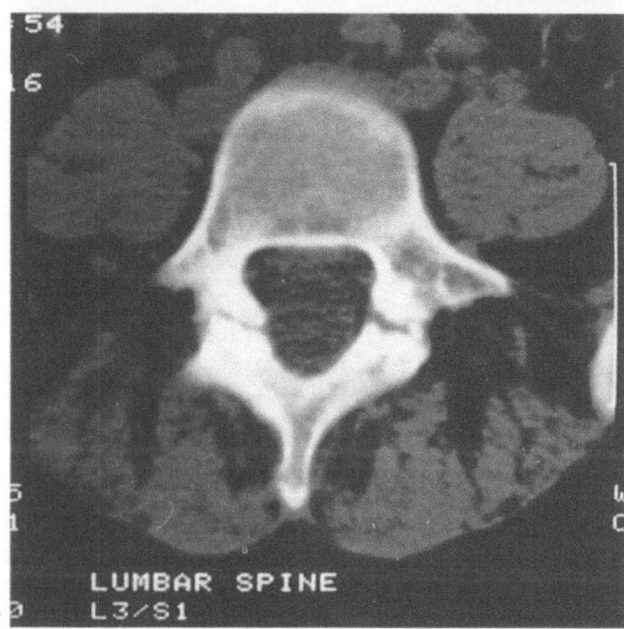

Fig. 3 a, b. Rheumatoid neck disease. a The computed tomographic scan in flexion and extension with intrathecal contrast medium shows obvious cord indentation (especially on flexion) and odontoid peg erosion. b T2-weighted magnetic resonance imaging shows all this to better advantage with much less patient discomfort and potential hazard

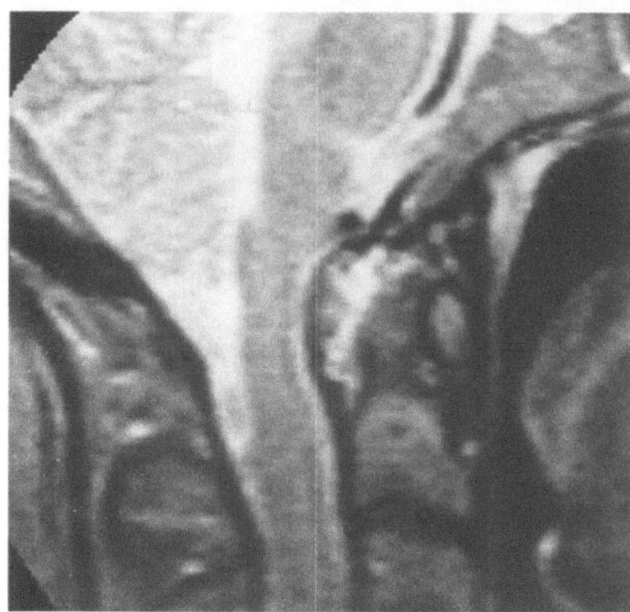

Fig. 4. Spondylolysis shown by computed tomography (CT). The exact anatomy is clearly shown, although to show disc morphology magnetic resonance imaging would be better. CT carries far less overall radiation burden for two or three scans than multiple oblique lumbar spine X-rays

- Lumbar spine degenerative disc disease, facet joint OA, spondylolysis and spinal stenosis.
- Evaluation of the lung parenchyma in rheumatic disorders. [67]Gallium citrate indicates how much active inflammatory infiltrate is present, as opposed to fibrosis. So does MRI.
- Atlantoaxial subluxation in rheumatoid disease, but to distinguish the cord adequately, intra-thecal contrast medium may be needed. As this is invasive, MRI is preferable (Fig. 3 a, b).
- The evaluation of spondylolysis. Plain oblique films carry a high radiation burden and are often repeated before the 'right' projection is obtained. Two or three CT scans through the appropriate lamina show the lesion and any associated local stenosis or disc bulge (Fig. 4). MRI does this too, carries no radiation burden and shows discal anatomy as well.

## Magnetic Resonance Imaging

MRI has become an extremely valuable tool in the assessment of rheumatological joint disease. It combines all of the attributes of ultrasound, CT and radionuclide scintigraphy, but has obvious limitations:
- Patients with pacemakers, claustrophobia, metallic implants and other metallic foreign bodies cannot be scanned.
- Cost and relative inaccessibility compared with other imaging modalities.

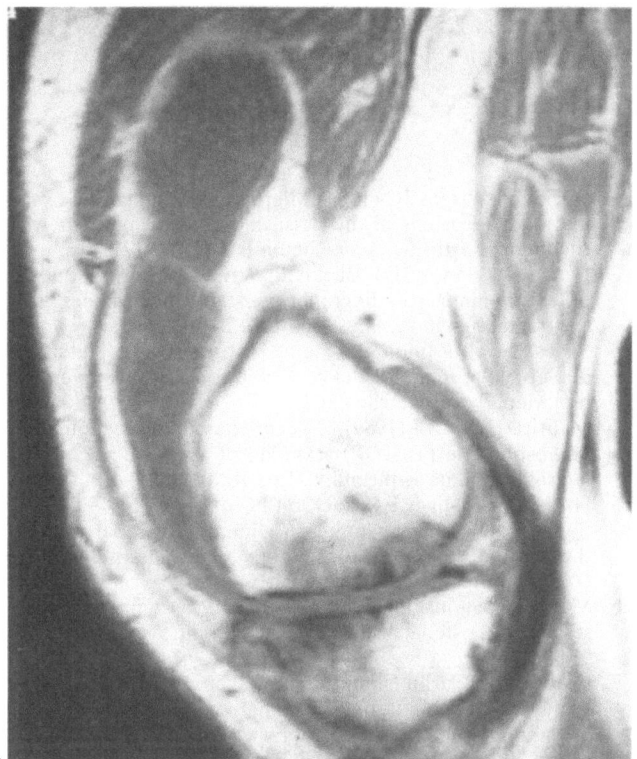
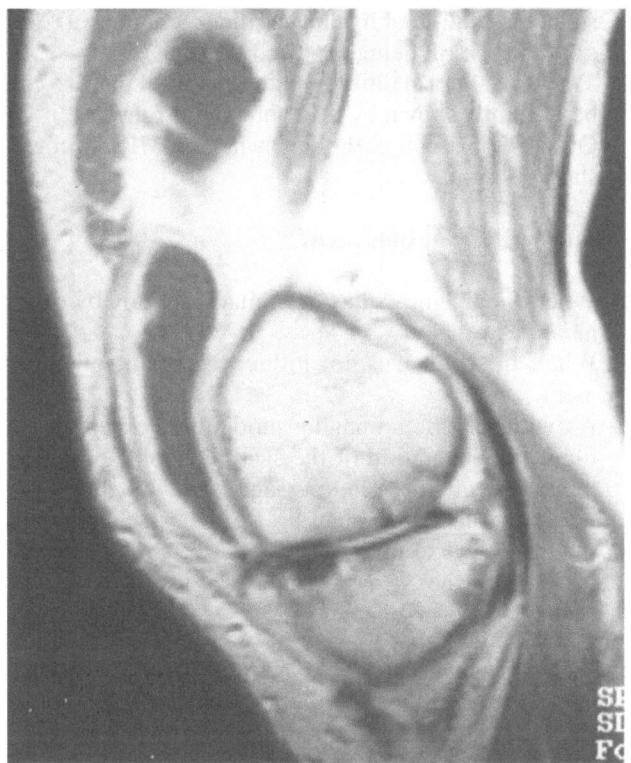

**Fig. 5 a, b.** Rheumatoid disease. **a** Synovitis is difficult to assess with plain, T1-weighted magnetic resonance image. **b** However, following intravenous gadolinium chelate excellent delineation of the enhancing active synovitis is demonstrated

MRI can be used in all the investigations listed above, but good housekeeping would suggest that it is kept as a backup procedure in many instances. For example, it is easier and more economical to use ultrasound to assess the Achilles tendon, whereas MRI is the investigation of choice in demonstrating fully craniocervical problems in rheumatoid disease.

### Where Is MRI the Investigation of Choice?

- The assessment of craniocervical instability, when needed, after plain films.
- The investigation of other spinal symptoms and signs. CT of the lumbar spine may be preferable in possible spinal stenosis since bony structures are easier to see on CT.
- The evaluation of possible soft tissue tumours or synovial masses if ultrasound assessment is inconclusive.
- Demonstration of internal joint derangement, particularly the knee and ankle.
- The demonstration of active synovitis (Fig. 5 a, b) [9] and cartilage disease (Fig. 6).

### Where Is MRI Still Being Evaluated?

- Assessment of therapy regimes for synovitis [10]. Careful study of the hand changes in rheumatoid disease shows that distinct subsets occur [11]. Response

to treatment may be shown by changes in synovial contrast medium enhancement. MRI may differentiate types of seronegative arthritis [12].
Whilst good demonstration of hyaline cartilage is pos-

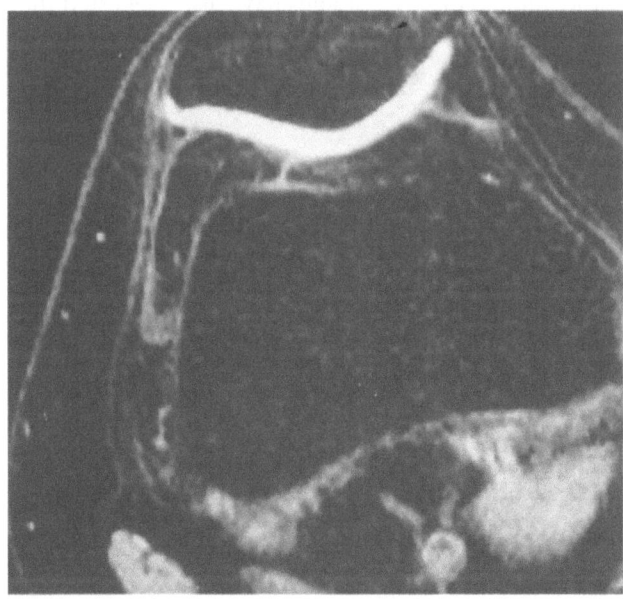

**Fig. 6.** Hyaline cartilage in a normal knee. The FLASH sequence demonstrates superb detail. Such techniques are readily available on most commercial scanners, without the need for sophisticated software

sible, calculation of hyaline cartilage volumes in osteoarthritis is still being explored [13].
- Tracking abnormalities in patellofemoral disease can be elegantly shown by MRI, but is this relevant?
- Obscure or occult pathology, when an MRI scan can show a lesion.

## When Is MRI Not Indicated?

- When the diagnosis has been made already by other means!
- When the scan will not influence patient management.
- As with all other imaging modalities, except plain films, the evaluation of the sacroiliac joints in ankylosing spondylitis. The message is always the same: when symptoms and signs are equivocal, chances are that radiological investigation will be too! Treat the patient, not the X-rays remains a good adage.

## Dual Energy X-Ray Absorptiometry Scanning for Bone Density Studies

The use of bone absorptiometry has been linked traditionally to the assessment of bone loss in postmenopausal osteoporosis. However, a number of other important roles are emerging:
- Detection and early therapy in algodystrophy.
- Quantification of bone loss in the hands in rheumatoid disease.
- Demonstration of early changes in the knee between density levels in normal people and those with OA or rheumatoid disease. Studies have also suggested that repair processes in OA may vary and be monitored by dual energy X-ray absorptiometry.

## Conclusion

Radiological investigations increasingly give valuable insight into disease processes and staging of rheumatological diseases. The role of the radiologist is increasing, too, as available investigations become more complex. Clear guidelines for the use of investigations are needed if unnecessary cost is to be avoided, both in terms of patient discomfort and hazard and financially.

## References

1. Buckland-Wright JC (1984) Microfocal radiographic examination of erosions in the wrist and hand of patients with rheumatoid arthritis. Ann Rheum Dis 43:160-171
2. Lynch JA, Hawkes DJ, Buckland-Wright JC (1991) Analysis of texture in macroradiographs of osteoarthritic knees using the fractal signature. Phys Med Biol 36:709-722
3. Silvestri E, Martinoli C, Onetto F et al (1994) Valutazione dell'artrite reumatoide del ginocchio con color Doppler. Radiol Med (Torino) 88:364-367
4. Maurice H, Watt I (1989) $^{99m}$Technetium hydroxymethylene diphosphonate (TcHDP) scanning of acute injuries to the lateral ligaments of the ankle. Br J Radiol 62:31-34
5. Hutton CW, Higgs ER, Jackson PC et al (1986) $^{99m}$Technetium HMDP bone scanning in generalised nodal osteoarthritis - the 4 hour bone scan image predicts radiographic change Ann Rheum Dis 45:622-626
6. McCrae F, Shouls J, Dieppe PA et al (1992) Scintigraphic assessment of osteoarthritis of the knee joint. Ann Rheum Dis 51:938-942
7. Dieppe PA, Cushnaghan J, Young P et al (1993) Prediction of the progression of joint space narrowing in osteoarthritis of the knee by bone scintigraphy. Ann Rheum Dis 52:557-563
8. De Bois MHW, Arndt JW, Van der Velde EA et al (1994) Joint scintigraphy for quantification of synovitis with $^{99m}$Tc-labelled human immunoglobulin G compared with late phase scintigraphy with $^{99m}$Tc-labelled diphosphonate. Br J Rheumatol 33:67-73
9. König H, Sieper J, Wolf K-J (1990) Rheumatoid arthritis: evaluation of hypervascular and fibrous pannus with dynamic MR imaging enhanced with Gd-DTPA. Radiology 176:473-477
10. Creamer P, Keen M, Zananiri F et al (1996) MRI of the knee: a method of monitoring efficacy of intra-articular therapies. Br J Rheumatol (in press)
11. Jevtic V, Watt I, Rozman B et al (1993) Pre contrast and post contrast (Gd-DTPA) magnetic resonance imaging (MRI) of hand joints in patients with rheumatoid arthritis. Clin Radiol 48:176-181
12. Jevtic V, Watt I, Rozman B et al (1995) Distinctive radiological features of small hand joints in rheumatoid arthritis and seronegative spondyloarthritis demonstrated by contrast enhanced (Gd-DTPA) magnetic resonance imaging. Skeletal Radiol 24:351-356
13. Peterfy C, F van Dijke C, Janzen D L et al (1994) Quantification of articular cartilage in the knee with pulsed saturation transfer subtraction and fat - suppressed MR imaging: optimisation and validation. Radiology 192:485-491

# Radiological Assessment of Pain in the Knee

C. Masciocchi and M.V. Maffey

Cattedra di Radiologia, Università degli Studi, Ospedale Collemaggio, 67100 L'Aquila, Italy

## Introduction

Pain in the knee is a clinical condition due to several aetiopathogenetic mechanisms, primarily trauma and degenerative joint disease. Physical injury to bone and soft tissue represents the most common indication for radiological examination of the musculoskeletal system. However, radiography is not most important in the evaluation of trauma and should be never considered a substitute for the history and physical examination: serious injuries commonly exist in the absence of radiographic findings.

The imaging assessment of injury may require information obtained from methods other than radiographs, such as computed tomography (CT), magnetic resonance imaging (MRI) or bone scintigraphy, which commonly demonstrate the extent of the injury within the soft tissue or bone marrow.

Intra-articular blood effusion and painful contracture adversely affect clinical evaluation of the traumatized knee [1]. CT can visualize various pathological conditions because of its capability to recognize all articular formations and their anatomical relationships using high-resolution technique, while the non-invasive nature of MRI has facilited evaluation of even acutely traumatized patients.

## Techniques

In studying the knee joint with CT, the patient is positioned supine with only the leg under examination in the gantry tunnel, immobilized on a wooden support and in semiflexed position (8°-10°) in order to have the scanning plane parallel to the articular surface of the tibia. To align the patient correctly, two digital radiograms, anteroposterior and lateral, are obtained first and on the second one the distal scanning level is centred a few millimetres caudal to the head of the tibia with the gantry angled: starting from this first slice, 12-14 contiguous scans (20-25 scans if the patellofemoral joint must be studied) with a slice thickness of 2 mm are taken, moving cranially until the proximal insertion of the cruciate ligaments is reached.

The standard MRI examination [2] is performed with the affected knee in semiflexed position (about 10°) to have good visualization of the anterior cruciate ligament (ACL) and femoropatellar joint. Spin echo, sagittal, T1-weighted and transverse scan planes are used, while gradient echo T2*-weighted sequences are performed on coronal scan planes: in all cases the slice thickness is 4 or 5 mm. Spin echo, T2-weighted sequences are used in selected cases. Higher spatial and contrast resolution made possible by new technical improvements in MRI account for the growing accuracy of this diagnostic technique in the study of bone and joint disease, such as using a "dedicated" system [3]. In fact, the comfortable position of the patient and the low level of noise allows examination of claustrophobic patients who normally would refuse examination with a whole body unit. Besides, the field of view of 11-16 cm allows a complete and detailed evaluation of the knee joint, recognizing all articular structures and their anatomical relationships.

## Normal CT and MRI Findings

On CT scans meniscal structures have both homogeneous fibrocartilaginous density (70 to 90 HU) and, on the planes of the intercondylar eminence and intercondylar spines, demostrate a characteristic C shape for the medial meniscus and an incomplete O for the lateral one. The middle part of the medial meniscus is connected with the medial collateral ligament (MCL), the posterior part with the Hughston ligament and posterior joint capsule. The lateral meniscus is connected with the popliteus muscle tendon and the fibular collateral ligament at its middle and posterior parts, while the posterior horn is connected with the meniscofemoral ligaments.

On sagittal MRI scans, the medial meniscus appears as a homogeneous dark band and the posterior horn is larger than the anterior one. The lateral meniscus appears as two triangles for two to three 5-mm sections and is separated from the lateral collateral ligament (LCL), which is extracapsular. In contrast to the medial meniscus, which is firmly attached to the joint capsule throughout, the popliteal tendon violates the meniscocapsular junction of the lateral meniscus, creating two fascicles that function as the peripheral meniscal attachments. The vascular supply to the meniscus is derived from the genicular arteries, which provide an arborizing network of perimeniscal capillary vessels that supply the peripheral border of the meniscus throughout its attachment to the joint capsule [4].

Considering the capsuloligamentous structures, the ligamentous system is composed of the extra-articular ligaments, tibial and fibular collateral ligaments, as well as the intra-articular ACL and posterior cruciate ligament (PCL). On CT, the ACL has an average density value between 50 and 70 HU and appears in the distal section with well-demarcated points of attachment, in the middle section as a characteristic "horseshoe" and in the proximal insertion with a ribbon-like form.

The PCL (average density 80 - 100 HU) has an oval shape at the distal insertion and is triangular in the middle section and in the proximal insertion. The MCL and the LCL have a ribbon- and a cord-like appearance, respectively. They are both homogeneous, with a density between 50 and 70 HU.

On MRI examination, the ACL consists of two major fibre bundles (anteromedial and posterolateral band), each composed of a collection of individual fascicles; it appears as a single, dark, continuous band or as two- to three separated fibre bundles extending from the medial aspect of the lateral femoral condyle to the anterior tibial plateau. The normal PCL is generally the structure within the knee most easily depicted using MRI and it appears as a smooth, mildly convex posterior curve of uniform low-signal intensity band, sometimes associated with the meniscofemoral ligament.

The tibial collateral ligament is seen as a thin, dark band extending from the medial femoral epicondyle to the medial tibia on T1-weighted coronal images and frequently is separated from the joint capsule and meniscus by an intraligamentous bursa that can be seen on MRI. The iliotibial band, fibular collateral ligament, biceps femoris tendon, popliteal muscle and tendon, lateral patellar retinaculum, lateral capsular ligament, arcuate ligament, and fabellofibular ligament all provide lateral support. The normal iliotibial band is seen on coronal MRI as a thin, dark, vertically oriented line, coursing distally in the bright subcutaneous fat of the lateral thigh to insert on the lateral tibia just below the plateau. The fibular collateral ligament and its common insertion with the biceps femoris tendon on the fibula are seen on coronal images and on extremely lateral sagittal views. The normal lateral ligaments produce no signal at most imaging parameters.

## Pathological CT and MRI Findings

Lesions of the menisci are among the most frequent causes of knee pain and disability. Isolated meniscal injuries are more commonly associated with torsional forces rather than the violence of external contact. Clinically, the pain is only in the articular line and, at this level, the digital pressure accentuates it. On CT, meniscal tears are characterized by hypodense, multiple and irregular streaks or gaps in longitudinal or, less frequently, transverse or oblique direction, while overlap of a meniscal flap onto the remnant structures produces a hyperdense lesion [5]. The meniscal detachments may or may not be associated with a lesion of the capsular ligament structures of the internal compartment. On CT, they have the appearance of a hypodense, longitudinal area separating the meniscal structures from the capsular ligament, which normally adhere to the posterior horn. Medial meniscal cysts are found in rare cases. They are quite small and monolocular and may or may not be associated with a complete longitudinal lesion of the meniscus.

A characteristic hyperdense "knot" is seen at the anterior meniscal horn when a "bucket-handle" tear is present, with the inner fragment dislocated into the intercondylar fossa. It should not be confused with the ACL [6]. CT can also show discoid meniscus and complications, such as lesions or cystic degenerations, which more often affect the lateral meniscus. The most common indication for MRI of the knee is to assess the menisci. A common injury is the horizontal meniscal tear which separates the meniscus in two halves and more often occurs in older individuals as a degenerative lesion, in contrast to vertical tears which are associated with acute trauma (bucket-handle tear). Peripheral tears occur through the outer third of the meniscus or at the meniscosynovial junction and represent an important subgroup of meniscal injuries as a consequence of their ability to heal or be repaired. The radial or transverse tears occur across the body of the meniscus and extend from the inner edge to the periphery; these tears may be complete or incomplete and are most common in the posterior horn and body of the lateral meniscus. The oblique tear is produced by sudden straightening of the medial meniscus and represents a full-thickness tear through its body. Flap tears occur in a degenerated meniscus and may involve either the superior or inferior half of the meniscus. Meniscal tears are considered complex when there are several tears, each in a different place, such as a flap tear, horizontal tear etc. and these usually occur in the degenerated meniscus. Meniscal cysts demonstrate increased signal intensity on T2-weighted sequences because of the fluid that accumulates in the parameniscal region of either meniscus, more commonly in the lateral one, where it remains confined to the joint line, while medially it can expand if it has occurred posterior to the MCL [7].

In acute injuries rapid assessment of the full extent of ligament damage is extremely important for correct management of knee trauma.

Rupture of the ACL is much more frequent than rupture of the PCL. The ACL is one of the most important stabilizers of the knee and, most of the time, its isolated disruption is the result of an internal rotation of the femur on the tibia with the leg extended. Pain cannot be localized precisely by palpation and sometimes the various clinical test results are normal.

On CT, in the case of acute lesions, both the ACL and PCL appear nonhomogeneous, hypodense and enlarged while in the case of complete laceration there may be an absence of the ligament on some of the scanning planes, indicated by a "black area", or detachment of its insertion, with a persistent reduction in volume of the ligament [8].

Evaluation of damage to the ACL is more difficult because of its anatomical proximity to structures of higher density and the presence of the surrounding synovial sheath.

MRI may demonstrate the several types of cruciate ligament lesions. Acute partial or complete lesions appear with an increase of signal intensity due to oedema and serous-sanguinous change and inflammatory reaction [9]. The acute lesion of the collateral ligament is characterized on CT by different degrees of nonhomogeneity, hypodensity and enlargement of the ligament, depending on the severity of the lesion. In contrast, an old lesion presents thickening, hyperdensity and, sometimes, calcifications. Use of MRI is particularly suitable for the assessment of the collateral ligaments, especially the MCL, which is typically affected in severe torsional valgus stress injures. Acute tears of this ligament are always combined with intra-articular haemorrhage and haemarthrosis, and the surrounding fat tissues are infiltrated by oedema and blood. MRI shows interruption of the ligamentous contours and can demonstrate lesions of the superficial and deep portion of the ligament. In chronic lesions, the collateral ligaments appear thickened and buckled. In 80% of traumatic events involving the knee, the medial meniscus and ACL are injured [10], although osteochondral lesions, bone contusion in the intramedullary area or small subchondral or subcortical bone impactions can also be present.

CT scan cannot detect small intraosseous lesions. Arthroscopy can only indicate associated meniscal or capsuloligamentous lesions of a clinically suspected occult fracture.

Radionuclide bone imaging provides the earliest sign of an osseous lesion and may easily depict other sites of increased uptake. MRI yields specific diagnostic information not only about the bones but also about soft tissue and endoarticular structures; it also provides excellent anatomical details and, above all, more specific information about associated soft tissue lesions. Obviously, a conservative therapeutic approach is completely modified by the evidence of a meniscal or capsuloligamentous lesion.

Impaction, avulsion or shearing forces on the bone's surface can cause combined lesions of bone and cartilage, which initially are often incorrectly diagnosed. The prognosis of an osteochondral fracture depends on its mechanical stability. Trauma can occur anywhere in the knee, but most often the lateral femoral condyle and medial patellar facet are affected as the result of impaction due to dislocation and reduction or combined torsional and compression forces on the flexed knee in twisting injuries. The symptoms may mimic meniscal tears or, more rarely, ligamentous injuries. On MRI scans the articular cartilage and a thin segment of the underlying subchondral bone are sheared off and partially displaced, as can be well depicted on three-dimensional images. Partial attachment of the osteochondral fragment can be confirmed, and loose bodies are identified in the joint fluid or sometimes in para-articular recesses. MRI easily identifies the subchondral bone area of low signal on T1 - and T2-weighted images surrounded by a larger zone of oedema with a higher signal, while the overlying cartilage presents irregularities of contour and signal depending on the importance of the fracture. The MRI technique surpasses arthrography and arthroscopy, which can only visualize the superficial joint structures [11].

## Conclusion

In conclusion, the widespread availability of new equipment together with the technological improvement in the diagnostic application of procedures such as CT, and particularly MRI, have brought about significant changes in the diagnostic approach to pathological conditions of the knee, offering important diagnostic advantages over conventional procedures. In particular, MRI has changed the diagnostic imaging approach to traumatic and degenerative knee lesions. It has largely replaced arthrography and CT and can obviate the need for arthroscopy as a diagnostic test in many situations. An early, accurate diagnosis of pain in the knee is often of paramount importance for the full recovery of knee joint function.

## References

1. Passariello R, Masciocchi C, Barile A, Aytan E (1992) Computed tomography and magnetic resonance imaging of the knee. Acta Radiol Port 4 (15):117-119
2. Gallimore GW, Harms SE (1986) Knee injuries: high resolution MR imaging. Radiology 160:457-461
3. Barile A, Masciocchi C, Mastantuono M, Passariello R, Satragno L (1995) The use of a "dedicated" MRI system in the evaluation of knee joint diseases. Clin Magn Reson Imaging 5 (2)

4. Arnoczky SP, Warren RF (1982) Microvasculature of the human meniscus. Am J Sports Med 10:90-95
5. Steinbach LS, Helms CA, Sims RE, Gillespy T, Genant HK (1987) High resolution computed tomography of knee menisci. Skeletal Radiol 16:11-16
6. Manco LG, Berlow ME, Czajka J, Alfred R (1988) Bucket-handle tears of the meniscus: appearance at CT. Radiology 168:709-712
7. Stoller DW, Martin C, Crues JV, Kaplan L, Mink J (1987) MR imaging-pathological correlation of meniscal tears. Radiology 163:731-735
8. Passariello R, Trecco F, de Paulis F, Masciocchi C, Bonanni G, Beomonte Zobel B (1986) CT demonstration of capsulo-ligamentous lesions of the knee joint. J Comput Assist Tomogr 40/450-456
9. Li DKB, Adams ME, Mcconkey JP (1986) Magnetic resonance imaging of the ligaments and menisci of the knee. J Comput Assist Tomogr 8:1147-1154
10. Reicher MA, Hartzman S, Basset LW, Mandelbaum B, Duckwiler G, Gold RH (1987) Magnetic resonance imaging of the knee joint. Clinical update I: injuries to menisci, patellar tendon and cruciate ligaments. Radiology 162:547-552
11. Fischer S, Fox J, Del Pizzo W et al (1991) Accuracy of diagnoses from magnetic resonance of the knee. A multicenter analysis of one thousand and fourteen patients. J Bone Joint Surg [AM] 73A:2-10

# Radiological Assessment of Pain in the Foot

K. Jonsson

Department of Radiology, University Hospital, S-221 85, Lund, Sweden

Generalized diseases, such as metabolic diseases and arthritis, manifest themselves everywhere in the body, but not least in the feet. The weight-bearing situation often makes such manifestations more disabling and painful in the feet than in non-weight-bearing limbs. Trauma and fractures in the feet are common, and sequelae after foot trauma may be painful and disabling.

There are a number of diseases or conditions that are specific to the feet, and several of these may be difficult to diagnose clinically or with plain-film radiography. It is my intention to present different painful conditions of the feet, excluding acute trauma and systemic arthritis.

The basic modality in radiological diagnosis in the feet is plain-film examination. With this we clarify the basic anatomy, joint congruity, the general condition of bone mineralization and bone destruction. To clarify suspected incongruity of joints or alignment of bones, computed tomography (CT) in axial and coronal projection of the foot is most helpful. CT and magnetic resonance imaging (MRI) are of great value for mapping suspected bone destruction and to evaluate possible soft tissue extension of a malignant tumour. Also, inflammatory conditions that are not seen on plain-film radiography may be diagnosed by means of MRI.

Bone scintigraphy may be of great value as a screening procedure in patients with foot pain, in order to pinpoint a location for further, more sophisticated evaluation.

## Stress Reactions

Stress fractures within the foot skeleton are common [1]. The so-called march fractures of the metatarsals are the most common type. Initially these stress fractures are difficult to see on plain-film radiographs, but are later seen as a periosteal reaction around the fracture that often is not seen as a defect of the cortical bone. Stress fractures of the calcaneus are also relatively common and those are also seen as an irregular, dense band through the calcaneus.

Stress fractures of the navicular bone are probably common in the sporting community. However, these stress fractures are often missed and go undiagnosed [2]. The reason for this is that, initially, stress fractures of the navicular bone are incomplete fractures running longitudinally through the dorsal aspect of the bone and, because of this, they are not seen on plain-film radiographs. CT scanning, however, reveals this type of fracture (Fig. 1). If the patient continues his training activities in spite of the pain, the incomplete fracture may develop in to a longitudinal, complete fracture and is then seen on plain-film radiographs.

If CT scanning is not available, common tomography may also reveal incomplete stress fractures of the navicular bone.

As a rule of thumb, pain

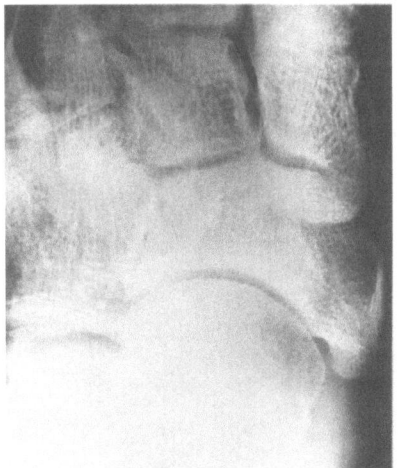

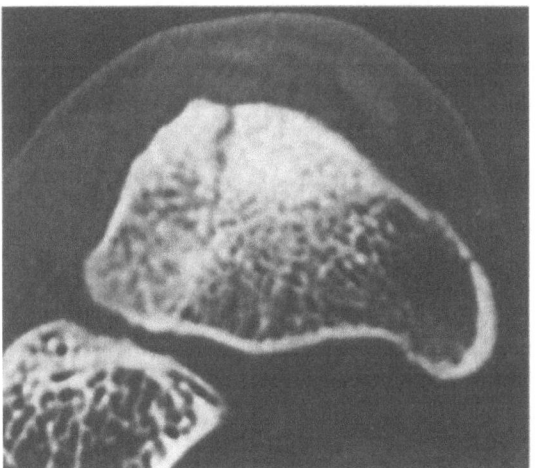

**Fig. 1 a, b.** A 22-year-old athlete with longstanding pain over the right foot. **a** Plain-film radiography reveals no fracture. **b** Computed tomography shows a stress fracture of the navicular bone

a

b

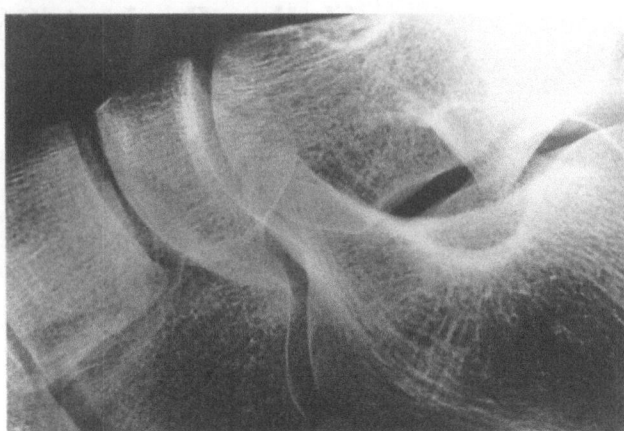

**Fig. 2.** Typical appearance of coalitio between calcaneus and the navicular bone

in the foot after hard or unusual activity should lead to the suspicion of stress fracture and a bone scan is of value for localization and, in fact, diagnosis of a stress fracture.

Pain over common normal variations, such as os trigonum, dorsal to talus or os tibiale externum on the medial aspect of the navicular bone may be related to a stress reaction [3]. The key to correct diagnosis is bone scintigraphy, which shows increased activity, although the plain-film finding is just this normal variation.

Another normal variation that may be painful for the patient is coalitio of the tarsal bones. The most common coalitio is between the calcaneus and the navicular bone (Fig. 2) and between the talus and the calcaneus. This coalitio may be bony or fibrous. The net effect is the same, i.e. the patient is unable to supinate the foot. The diagnosis is relatively easy on plain-film radiography concerning coalitio between the calcaneus and the navicular bone, but between the calcaneus and the talus it may be difficult and require special views or CT examination.

## Post-traumatic Changes

After fracture of the talus or calcaneus, regardless of whether the patient is operated upon or not, the joint surfaces are usually destroyed or irregular, causing subtalar degenerative disease.

Instability after fracture dislocation of the tarsometatarsal joints (Lisfranc's joint) are common if not treated initially. Even small evulsed fragments indicate instability of these joints. Many times such instability is an indication for arthrodesis.

Patients with neuropathy due to alcoholism or diabetes or other causes can face foot problems [4, 5]. Because of the neuropathy small traumas are repeated and, due to this major fracture-dislocations may occur. The patient is relatively free of pain although the foot is

massively deranged. This kind of Charcot joint development is not uncommon in patients with diabetes. Any joint of the foot can collapse but the Lisfranc's joint is most commonly affected.

Another painful post-traumatic condition that may occur in the hands or feet is sympathetic reflex dystrophy, also called Sudec atrophy. There is a rapid local demineralization seen on radiographs, and with bone scintigraphy there is an increased uptake locally.

Hallux valgus may be the result of repetitive trauma when pointed shoes are worn for long periods. The head of the first metatarsal is usually prominent where an inflamed bunion in the soft tissue is seen. A number of operative procedures to correct the hallux valgus are described. We used to measure different angles pre- and postoperatively in order to correlate the results of surgery. It has been proven that such angle measurements vary greatly between observers and there is also a large intraobserver variance [6]. The measured angles do not correlate to the clinical results of surgery, and, fortunately, we have now stopped conducting these measurements.

## Infectious and Inflammatory Disease

Patients with diabetes may suffer not only from neuropathy but also from the increased risk of foot infections. These infections may involve only the soft tissues but may also cause osteomyelitis. Osteomyelitis may be evident on plain-film radiography, but in the early stages MRI is the method of choice for diagnosis. On plain-film radiography a tract filled with gas is seen leading to the deep, osseous structures which may show irregular cortical outline or destruction (Fig. 3).

**Fig. 3.** Patient with diabetes and infection of the heel pad. Infectious tract in the soft tissues and distraction/osteitis of the plantar part of the calcaneus

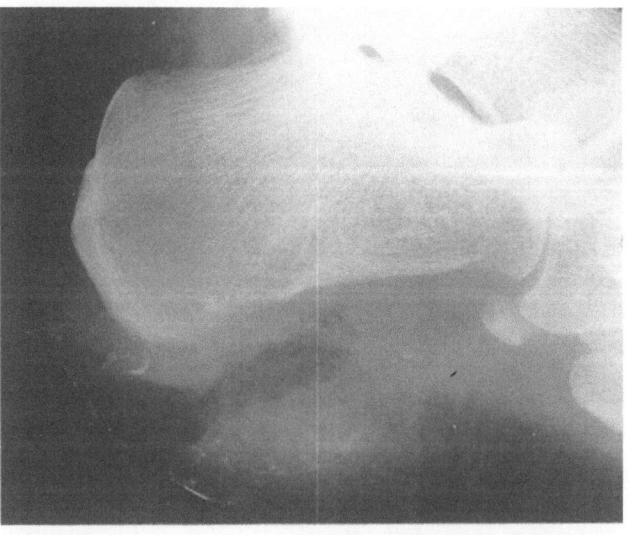

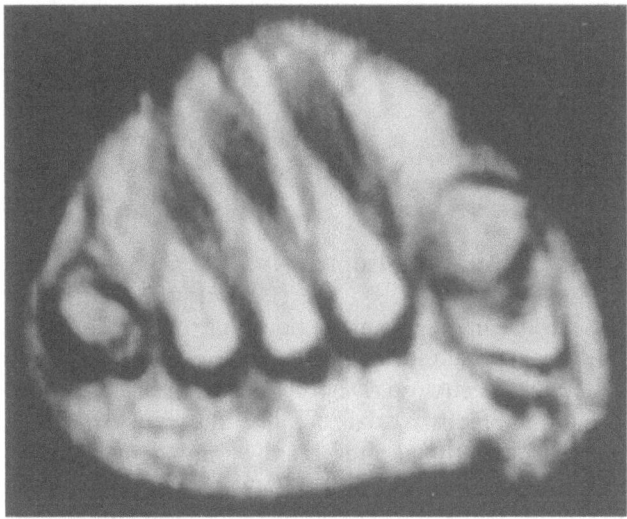

**Fig. 4.** Magnetic resonance imaging of Morton's neuroma plantar to the interspace between the third and fourth metatarsal heads

Inflammation of the tendons around the ankle may cause foot problems, not only as local swelling and pain. Inflammation of the posterior tibial tendon may lead to rupture of the tendon, causing a painful flat foot, because the valve of the foot lacks support. Tendinitis or rupture around the ankle are best seen with MRI but may also be diagnosed with ultrasound.

## Tumours

Any kind of tumour may affect the soft tissues or bones of the foot, but malignant tumours are relatively uncommon. An almost pathognomonic type of tumour of the foot is intraosseous lipoma of the calcaneus. In this condition, the tumour is lytic, with a small calcification in the middle. Evaluation of a tumour of the foot, either of the soft tissue or bone, is the same as for any other tumour. MRI is the method of choice, but CT is also of value. A specific type of tumour of the foot is Morton's neuroma. There is a neuroma formation of the digital nerves, most commonly in the space between the third and fourth interdigital space. These patients usually have longstanding pain and, if these tumours are not taken into account, they may remain undiagnosed for a long period of time [7]. MRI is the radiological method of choice for diagnosis (Fig. 4). T1-weighted images are usually diagnostic, but sometimes an interdigital bursa may be inflamed and filled with fluid, mimicking a neuroma. This is best seen on T2-weighted images.

Diseases of the feet are often disabling. Plain-film radiography and bone scintigraphy are the basic tools for localization and diagnosis. Complementary examinations with CT and MRI are often necessary to establish the diagnosis.

## References

1. Savoca CJ (1971) Stress fractures. A classification of the earliest radiographic signs. Radiology 100:519-524
2. Pavlov H, Torg JS, Freiberger RH (1983) Tarsal navicular stress fractures: radiographic evaluation. Radiology 148:641-645
3. Lawson JP (1994) Not-so-normal variants. Emerg Radiol 1:37-46
4. Björkengren AG, Weisman M, Pathria MN, Zlatkin MB, Pate D, Resnick D (1988) Neuroarthropathy associated with chronic alcoholism. AJR 151:743-745
5. Clouse ME, Gramm HF, Legg M, Flood T (1974) Diabetic osteoarthropathy. Clinical and roentgenographic observations in 90 cases. AJR 121:22-34
6. Resch S, Ryd L, Stenström A, Jonsson K, Reynisson K (1995) Measuring hallux valgus: a comparison of conventional radiography and clinical parameters with regard to measurement accuracy. Foot Ankle 16:267
7. Resch S, Stenström A, Jónsson A, Jonsson K (1994) The diagnostic efficacy of magnetic resonance imaging and ultrasonography in Morton's neuroma: a radiological-surgical correlation. Foot Ankle 15:88-92

# Bone Marrow Imaging

M.F. Reiser, A. Stäbler, A. Baur and M. Steinborn

Institut für Radiologische Diagnostik, Ludwig Maximilians Universität, Marchioninistrasse 15, 81377 Münich, Germany

The bone marrow plays an important role in many physiological processes, such as haematopoiesis, immunological response and metabolism. Various diseases, such as leukaemia, multiple myeloma, malignant lymphoma and sickle-cell anaemia manifest first within the bone marrow. Conventional radiography and bone scanning have severe limitations in sensitivity for the detection of bone marrow disorders, when cancellous and cortical bone are not involved. Magnetic resonance imaging (MRI) gives new insights into normal anatomy and physiological changes of the bone marrow. In addition, it has proved to be highly sensitive in the detection of bone marrow abnormalities. Its specificity, however, is also limited. Spin echo, opposed phase gradient echo and spectral fat-saturated pulse sequences as well as STIR (short TI inversion recovery sequences) are useful in MRI of the bone marrow [1].

## Conventional Radiography

Lesions originating from the bone marrow are visualized on conventional radiography when cancellous and cortical bone is destroyed. Destructions of the cortical bone are more readily visualized than those of cancellous bone. Conventional radiography only poorly detects bone destruction and depends on technical factors as well as the preexisting condition of the bone: In osteopenia, for example, it is more difficult to detect bony destruction than in bones with normal mineral content.

However, in various bone marrow disorders, characteristic radiographic findings may be present. In leukaemia, metaphyseal lucencies, diffuse osteopenia, bone destruction and periosteal reactions may be found (Figs. 1, 2). Skeletal metastases manifest as osteolytic, osteoblastic and combined osteolytic and osteoblastic lesions. In

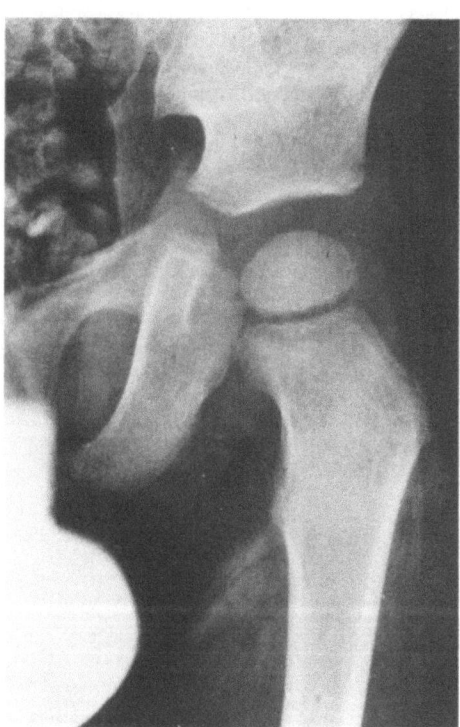

**Fig. 1.** A 2-year-old boy with acute lymphocytic leukaemia. In the metaphysis of the femur, a hyperlucent band is seen close to the epiphyseal plate

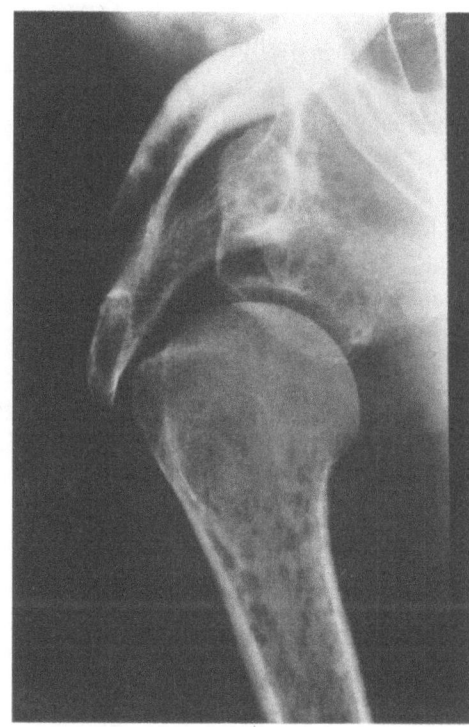

**Fig. 2.** A 58-year-old man with chronic lymphocytic leukaemia. Within the scapula and proximal humerus, ovoid destructions of trabecular and compact bone can be seen

multiple myeloma, diffuse osteopenia is the most frequent finding. Multiple destruction can also be indicative of multiple myeloma. Erlenmeyer's deformity of the long bones is typical for Gaucher's disease. Haemolytic disorders, such as thalassaemia, result in expansion of the marrow cavities with osseous expansion, coarse reticular pattern of the cancellous bone and extramedullary haematopoiesis. A diffuse increase of bone density is found in osteomyelosclerosis.

## Scintigraphic Methods

Technetium 99m ($^{99m}$Tc)-labelled methylene diphosphonate scintigraphy serves as a measure of osteoblastic activity and local blood flow. $^{99m}$Tc-labelled nanocolloid scintigraphy reflects the activity of the reticuloendothelial system [2]. However, scintigraphic methods do not provide a detailed morphological assessment of the marrow compartment due to their low spatial resolution.

## Computed Tomography

With computed tomography (CT), the trabecular and compact bone are displayed without superimposition and with high contrast resolution. Due to its fatty components, the bone marrow of the diaphysis of the long bones exhibits negative absorption values. In the metaphysis and epiphysis, however, positive HU values are found (haematopoietic bone marrow, higher concentration of trabecular bone).

Pathological alterations of the bone marrow, such as metastases, inflammation, leukaemia and multiple myeloma frequently result in an increase in density of the bone marrow, which is detected with higher sensitivity in the yellow than in the red marrow.

Moreover, CT detects minor destruction of trabecular bone which cannot be discerned on conventional radiograms.

## Magnetic Resonance Imaging

MRI has given new insight into the physiological changes and pathological alterations of the bone marrow. This is due to the inherent, high contrast resolution of MRI, its multiplanar capabilities and the large field of view.

The three major tissue constituents of the bone marrow are fat, water and bone. Fatty tissue demonstrates high signal intensity with T1 weighting and intermediate to high signal intensity with T2 weighting. Water has long T1 and T2 relaxation times and high signal intensity on T2- and low signal intensity on T1-weighted images.

Fatty marrow contains 15% water, 80% fat and 5% protein. Haematopoietic marrow is composed of 40% water, 40% fat and 20% protein. As a result of the greater water content, red marrow has longer T1 relaxation times and therefore lower signal intensity on T1-weighted images. Most pathological conditions of bone marrow produce an increase in free water with a resultant high signal intensity on T2 weighting.

At the time of birth, the bone marrow is fully responsible for red blood cell production, and all bone marrow cavities are actively engaged in haematopoiesis. Conversion from red to yellow marrow begins in the terminal phalanges of the feet. The conversion from haematopoietic to fatty marrow is a steady, gradual process that progresses from distal to proximal [3]. An adult pattern of marrow distribution is reached by the age of 25 years and red marrow is found in the vertebrae, sternum, ribs, pelvis, skull, and proximal shafts of the femura and humeri.

Myeloid depletion is seen in patients with previous radiation therapy, chemotherapy and aplastic anaemia and the fatty marrow expands in these conditions. Consequently, high signal intensity is found on the T1-weighted images. Following radiation therapy, high signal intensity is sharply defined to the radiation ports. In aplastic anaemia, high signal intensity is found throughout the entire skeleton. Scattered, small areas of intermediate signal intensity represent nests of haematopoietic marrow.

Malignant bone marrow infiltration is found in leukaemia, lymphoma, multiple myeloma and metastatic disease. Differentiation between malignant infiltration of the marrow and haematopoietic marrow may be impossible. Diffuse bone marrow infiltration in multiple myeloma is difficult to diagnose using conventional radiography and bone scintigraphy. Homogeneous and multifocal signal alterations are found in MRI (low signal intensity on T1-weighted spin echo, high signal intensity on T2-weighted spin echo and STIR sequences).

For the detection of bone marrow manifestations of malignant lymphoma and metastases, MRI is superior to any other imaging modality (Fig. 3). In patients with small-cell cancer of the lung, MRI visualized significantly more bony metastases than scintigraphy and bilateral iliac crest biopsy and no metastases could be visualized with these methods which were not found in MRI. Therefore, MRI allowed for a more precise staging.

Microscopic infiltration by tumour cells, in contrast, are better detected using bone marrow biopsy. Hoane et al. [4] evaluated 109 patients with lymphoma by MRI and iliac crest biopsy. Low-grade microscopic involvement in ten patients was negative on MRI, while MRI detected marrow involvement in 33% of patients in locations distant from the iliac crest. Similar results were reported by Gückel et al. [5, 6] (Fig. 4).

Nuclear scintigraphy has a higher sensitivity in detecting metastatic bone disease than conventional radiography. Moreover, total body imaging is possible with bone scanning.

When using phased-array spine coils and/or body coils, large areas of the axial skeleton can be evaluated. The advantages of MRI over nuclear bone scanning in

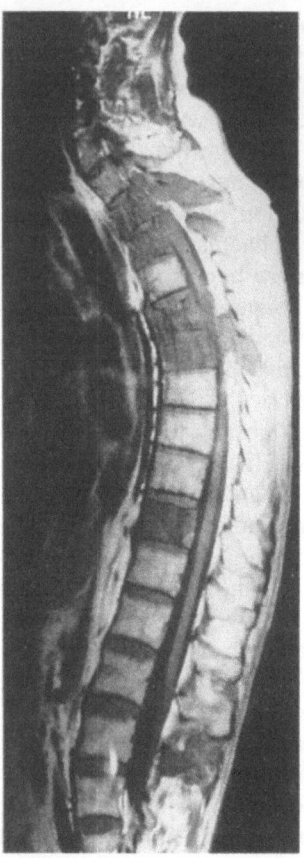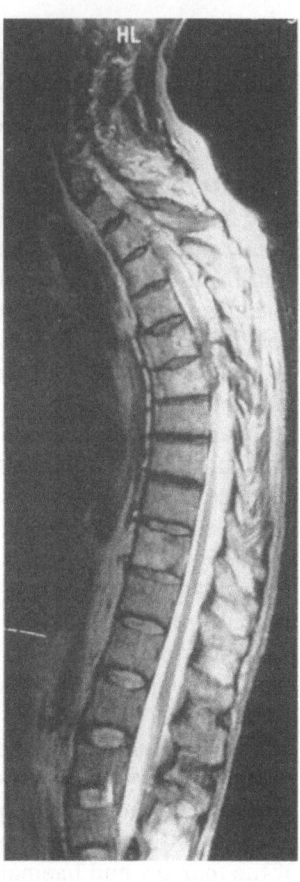

**Fig. 3 a, b.** A 63-year-old man with metastases from prostatic carcinoma. **a** T1-weighted spin echo image using the phased-array coil shows multiple metastases of the lumbal and thoracic vertebrae as well as involvement of the spinous processes. The tumour tissue is visualized with low signal intensity (*dark*) whereas the normal bone marrow has a high signal intensity in this pulse sequence. **b** T2-weighted spin echo sequence: the contrast of the neoplastic tissue versus normal bone marrow and fat tissue is greatly reduced. However, with this technique, a myelographic effect is obtained and encroachment of the spinal canal by intraspinal infiltration can be clearly assessed

imaging metastatic disease include greater sensitivity in detecting lesions and improved specificity in differentiating metastases from other pathological conditions, such as degenerative spine lesions.

The sensitivity of MRI is significantly superior to bone scintigraphy in the detection of bone metastases [7, 8]. MRI also offers important information for the differential diagnosis of bone metastases. In the spine, metastases have to be differentiated from osteochondroses, spondylitis and osteoporotic compression fractures. Convex anterior and posterior contours of the compressed vertebrae and complete and homogeneous replacement of the normal marrow are features that favour pathological fractures. Chronic benign compression fractures have a normal bone marrow signal. In acute fractures, in contrast, extensive bone marrow edema can be present. The signal alterations follow closely the distribution of the fractures. These features frequently allow differentiation from pathological fractures. If not, follow-up examinations after 2-3 months show normalization of the bone marrow signal in osteoporotic fractures.

In leukaemia, the T1 relaxation times of the bone marrow are significantly prolonged, whereas T2 relaxation times are not significantly altered [9]. The degree of marrow involvement in various types of leukaemia can be assessed with MRI. According to the classification of Olson et al. [10] five types can be differentiated, from normal to completely infiltrated bone marrow. The yellow marrow in the femoral head and the major trochanter is only involved when extensive bone marrow infiltration is present (Fig. 5).

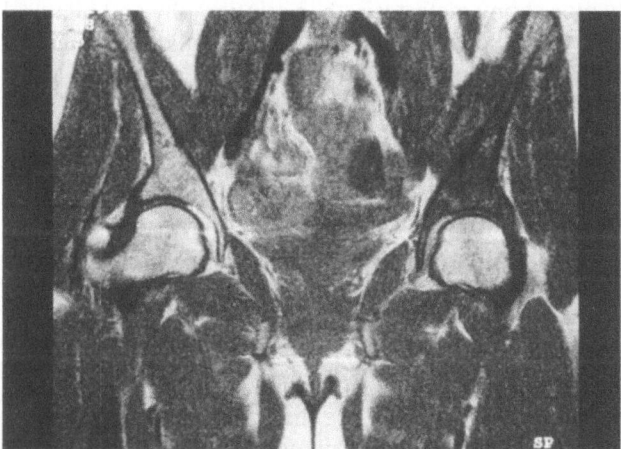

**Fig. 4.** A 48-year-old woman with stage IV Hodgkin's lymphoma. Infiltration of the left iliac bone, which exhibits low signal intensity. The iliac crest, however, shows a normal bone marrow signal

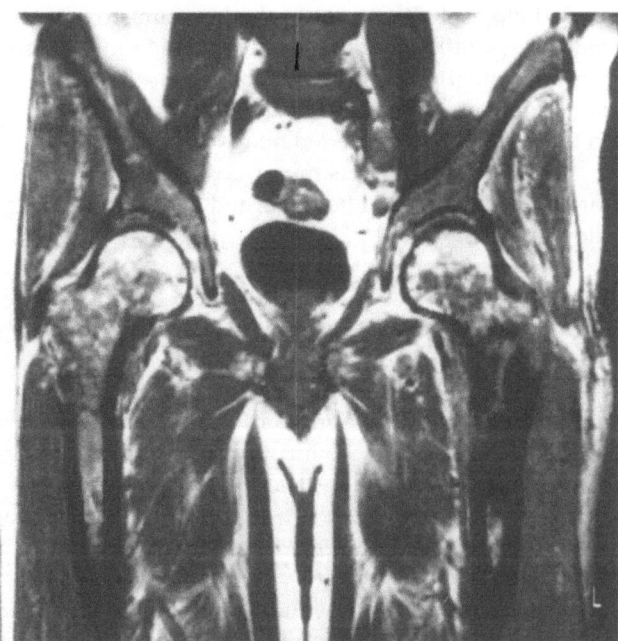

**Fig. 5.** A 60-year-old man with chronic myelogenous leukaemia. The signal intensity of the pelvis and the femoral shafts and necks is definitely reduced. In the femoral heads, high signal intensity areas are preserved

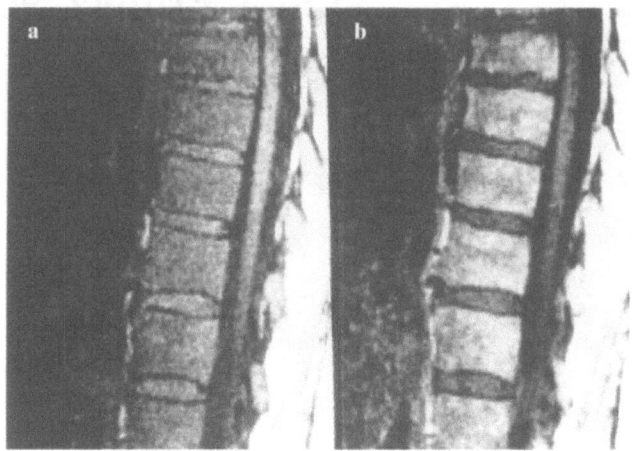

**Fig. 6 a, b.** A 72-year-old man with multiple myeloma. **a** T1-weighted spin echo sequence with diffuse signal decrease of the bone marrow within the vertebral bodies. **b** T1-weighted spin echo sequence following intravenous injection of gadolinium-DTPA. Increase of signal intensity in all vertebral bodies. These signs are found in diffuse infiltration of the bone marrow in multiple myeloma

In multiple myeloma, various types of bone marrow involvement could be differentiated and correlation of clinical stage and MRI was assessed. Nodular, diffuse and mixed marrow infiltration can be detected with MRI. As pointed out by Daffner et al. [11], MRI is far superior to bone scanning and radiography for the detection of manifestations of multiple myeloma in the spine (Fig. 6).

## Bone Marrow Edema

Various skeletal injuries and diseases are associated with bone marrow oedema and it may even be the main pathological finding in transient osteoporosis, osteonecrosis, reflex sympathetic dystrophy, bone contusion and occult fractures, osteomyelitis and tumours. Increase of extracellular fluid, hypervascularity and hyperperfusion may contribute to this "edema pattern" of the bone marrow. Even if bone marrow edema is visualized on T1- and T2-weighted spin echo sequences, STIR and fat-saturated sequences are most sensitive for the assessment of bone marrow edema.

Transient osteoporosis of the hip or knee is clearly visualized on MRI. Usually, signal intensities become normal within 6-12 months. In several reports, progression of bone marrow edema to osteonecrosis of the fe-

moral head was mentioned. Traumatic and stress fractures as well as bone contusions produce signal patterns consistent with bone marrow edema.

## Conclusion

While conventional radiography enables the indirect evaluation of the bone marrow, CT and MRI not only delineate the trabecular bone, but also allow for direct visualization of the bone marrow. With MRI, conversion of red to yellow bone marrow and a large variety of pathological disorders of the bone marrow can be detected. The sensitive assessment of alterations within the bone marrow has greatly contributed to the increased use of MRI in musculoskeletal radiology.

## References

1. Lang P, Fritz R, Vahlensieck M et al (1992) Residual and reconverted hematopoietic bone marrow in the distal femur. Spin-echo and opposed-phase gradient-echo MRI. ROFO 156:89-95
2. Cartia GL, Giambellotti E, Coda C (1991) Bone marrow scintigraphy with ⁹⁹ᵐTc-nanocolloid. A complement to bone scintigraphy with ⁹⁹ᵐTc-MDP in oncologic diagnosis. Minerva Med 82:715-721
3. Dooms GC, Fisher MR, Hricak H et al (1985) Bone marrow imaging: magnetic resonance studies related to age and sex. Radiology 155:429-432
4. Hoane BR, Shields AF, Porter BA, Shulman HM (1991) Detection of lymphomatous bone marrow involvement with magnetic resonance imaging. Blood 78:728-738
5. Gückel F, Semmler W, Dohner H et al (1989) NMR tomographic imaging of bone marrow infiltrates in malignant lymphoma. ROFO 150:26-31
6. Gückel F, Semmler W, Brix G, Bachert BP et al (1989) Bone marrow changes in Hodgkin's disease: MR tomography and chemical shift imaging. ROFO 150:670-673
7. Algra PR, Bloem JL, Tissing H et al (1991) Detection of vertebral metastases: comparison between MR imaging and bone scintigraphy. Radiographics 11:219-232
8. Avrahami E, Tadmor R, Dally O, Hadar H (1989) Early MR demonstration of spinal metastases in patients with normal radiographs and CT and radionuclide bone scans. J Comput Assist Tomogr 13:598-602
9. Moore SG, Gooding CA, Brasch RC et al (1986) Bone marrow in children with acute lymphocytic leukemia: MR relaxation times. Radiology 160:237-240
10. Olson DO, Shields AF, Scheurich CJ et al (1986) Magnetic resonance imaging of the bone marrow in patients with leukemia, aplastic anemia, and lymphoma. Invest Radiol 21:540
11. Daffner RH, Lupetin AR, Dash N et al (1986) MRI in the detection of malignant infiltration of bone marrow. AJR 146:353-358

# Metastatic Bone Disease

D. Vanel

Service de Radiodiagnostique, Institut Gustave-Roussy, Rue Camille Desmoulins, 94805 Villejuif, France

## Introduction

Bone metastases occur frequently and jeopardize the length and quality of survival in cancer patients. Early detection is necessary so that treatment can be modified appropriately.

## General Information

*Frequency.* Metastases occur mainly in adults and the elderly. The most common metastases in men (60%) are from the prostate and in women from breast cancers (70%). Although the exact incidence of metastases from various tumours is difficult to determine, autopsy statistics give the following [1, 2]: 50%-80% of breast cancers, 30%-50% of cancers of the kidneys or the lungs, 30%-40% of melanomas, 50%-70% of cancers of the prostate and approximately 40% of thyroid cancers, and in children 80% of cases of neuroblastoma, 60% of Ewing's sarcoma and 25% of osteosarcoma.

*Location.* The main locations of metastases are the axial skeleton, the spine – mainly in the lumbar region – the pelvis, the ribs, the sternum, the skull and the proximal part of the long bones, in decreasing order of frequency. The high incidence of metastases to the spine emphasizes the importance of Batson's perivertebral venous system [3].

## Characteristics of Lesions

Standard radiographs are not particularly sensitive but are characteristic when positive. Metastases can be lytic, as in cancer of the kidneys, lungs, thyroid, breast or digestive tract. In the long bones, metastases are seen only if the cortex is affected. In the short bones, they can only be detected when there is considerable destruction. They may also be sclerotic or mixed, especially in the case of breast cancer [4]. Cortical destruction frequently occurs, and a fracture is possible. Extension to the soft tissues is usually minimal.

Bone tomography has been completely replaced by computed tomography (CT), which has a better spacial resolution and contrast.

CT demonstrates the lesions (sclerosis or lysis) and cortical destruction and can detect extension into the soft tissues and minimal changes in medullary density. Its sensitivity is nevertheless inferior to that of magnetic resonance imaging (MRI) which has completely replaced it in detecting and assessing the extent of a tumour. CT is often used for guiding biopsies.

Bone scintigraphy uses technetium-99$^m$-labelled pyrophosphate or diphosphonate and is extremely sensitive in detecting osteoid turnover. It explores the entire body and shows most abnormalities as areas of increased radioactive uptake. Several different types of bony abnormalities may produce increased radioactivity. In a series of 301 patients with cancer and no known metastases, one or two new abnormalities appeared at follow-up: only 11% of patients with one and 24% with two actually had metastases more frequently in the sternum and pelvis [5]. Metastatic disease typically affects the pedicles of the vertebrae, areas of ribs where traumatic fractures are uncommon such as the costovertebral junction, the skull and proximal shafts of long bones. The pelvis is also a common site of involvement.

The "superscan" is an unusual phenomenon related to widespread metastatic disease where skeletal activity is so intense that the whole skeleton avidly takes up tracer. This can be confused with a normal scan. However, there is usually some heterogeneity in the appearance and no renal activity is seen in such patients.

MRI is probably the most sensitive technique, as it can detect an intramedullary abnormality before osteoblastic activity is sufficient to be detected on bone scans [6]. Its main limitation is that it is perfomed on only part of the skeleton. The thoracolumbar spine and the pelvis are most frequently evaluated in routine screening. The basic sequence is a spin echo T1-weighted sequence in which the normal fatty marrow appears bright (high signal intensity), and metastases are darker (low signal intensity), making interpretation relatively simple in the

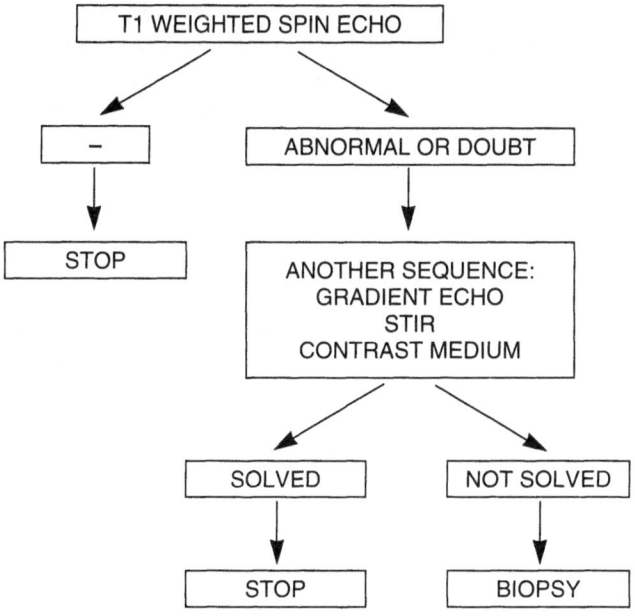

**Fig. 1.** Magnetic resonance imaging techniques

adult. When the marrow is haematopoietic, particularly in the child, it may appear heterogeneous and darker (low signal intensity) as a normal variant. Metastases may not be as apparent on T1-weighted images in the child or in the adult with this marrow pattern. On T2-weighted sequences, metastases may show high or low signal intensity or be isointense with marrow and therefore this sequence is not very useful in the adult.

Other sequences may be helpful in visualizing metastases. Gradient echo sequences profit from magnetic susceptibility, i.e. the vertebral trabeculae make the local field inhomogeneous and cause a reduction in the overall signal. This interference is compensated for in the spin echo sequence but not in the gradient echo sequence and the normal vertebrae appear black. Metastases that cause local destruction are bright.

Water-fat subtraction may be used to visualize the disappearance of fat in metastatic sites. STIR sequences show metastases as high signal intensity areas whereas normal fat is black. These sequences are, however, time-consuming and give only a limited number of levels. The injection of a contrast medium can be of help: the signal from normal marrow only changes slightly or not at all after an injection, whereas metastases absorb the contrast medium.

In summary, the basic sequence for MRI is a T1-weighted sequence with the addition or other sequences in equivocal cases (Fig. 1).

## Unusual Metastases

Distal metastases [7, 8] are rare. For metastases to the fingers and toes, lung and gastrointestinal cancers

should be considered. Cortical metastases [9] cause well-defined lysis and are most frequently due to lung cancer. Expanding "bubbly" metastases are often highly vascularized lesions and usually result from primary cancers of the kidneys and the thyroid. Metastases with extensive soft tissue components, calcification, and considerable periosteal bone formation [10, 11] may resemble a primitive bone tumour and occur most frequently with cancers of the prostate, or less frequently with cancer of the bladder or the digestive tract.

Metastases can appear synchronously with the primary tumour. They are often observed quite late on and are rarely the first sign of disease. In this case, neuroblastomas should be investigated in children, especially in those under the age of 5 years, and in young adults cancer of the kidney or thyroid, whereas in older adults, it is more likely cancer of the prostate or breast or melanomas.

## Follow-up

The follow-up of bone metastases can be conducted using skeletal scintigraphy. An interesting phenomenon which can lead to serious confusion is the so-called "flare" reaction, in which the bone scan apparently worsens and then improves or becomes stable. The flare occurs because of increased isotope uptake secondary to healing and is seen usually within the first 3 months of therapy and is gone within 6 months. On plain films of lytic lesions, the reossification of all foci without the appearance of new lesions suggests healing but osteolysis on a previously sclerotic lesion suggests progression. MRI should be perfomed in cases of spinal compression and when there is recurring pain with normal or equivocal plain films and bone scan. When the marrow becomes completely fatty, for example after radiation therapy, the result is easy to evaluate. But if a lesion persists after treatment the difference between fibrous sequels and active metastasis cannot be determined.

## Choice of Examination Technique [12] (Fig. 2)

In localized pain, conventional radiograph should be performed on the painful areas and for confirming scintigraphic abnormalities. A skeletal survey is only used as a screening examination in rare cases when scintigraphy may not be available or when patients are suspected of having purely osteolytic metastases.

Scintigraphy is the key examination, as it facilitates the study of the whole skeleton and is very sensitive for detecting lesions.

MRI is used if scintigraphy is positive and conventional X-rays are normal and may show other seats of involvement not shown on scintigraphs. A negative, local result rules out metastases [13].

In case of further doubt, a biopsy should be carried

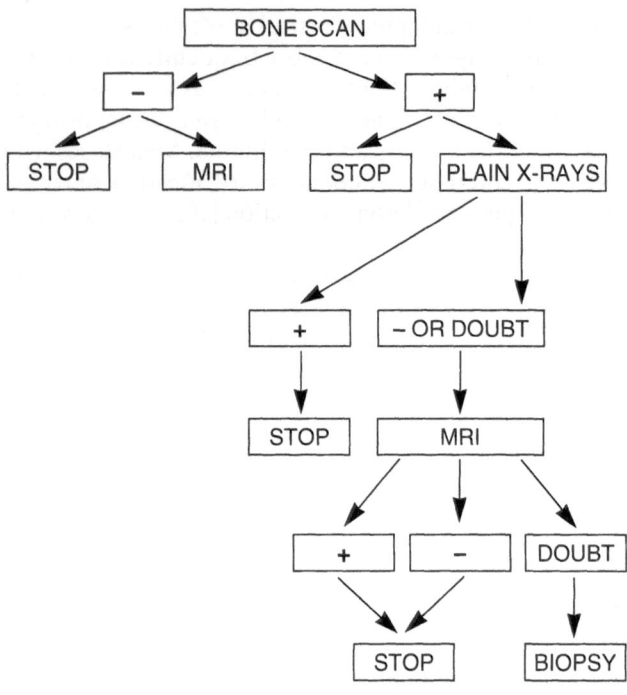

**Fig. 2.** Detection of bone metastases. *MRI*, magnetic resonance imaging

out. This is safe, simple, rapid and reliable. Metastases are usually easy to diagnose, even with cytology. A fine-needle biopsy is therefore often sufficient, guided by the most simple imaging procedure, either fluoroscopy or CT for more complicated areas such as the vertebrae [14,15].

## Strategy

The problem is different for each type of cancer, because of their varying known incidence or the agressiveness of treatment. During the initial examination of the primary tumour, the patient should be evaluated for metastases if distal spread would change the treatment, for example extensive surgery or radiation therapy, or if complementary chemotherapy would be added to treatment plan. In a series of 429 patients with bone metastases, the average survival was 5 months [16] (33% after 1 year, 17% after 2 years, and 5% after 5 years). Gastrointestinal, ears, nose, and throat and chest tumours are unresponsive to chemo- and hormonotherapy: the average survival was 2 months. In those cases, treatment regimens should be as mild as possible. In other tumours the survival may be better: hormonosensitive cancers (breast, prostate), or slowly growing tumors (adenoid cystic carcinoma, thyroid cancer).

In revealing metastases, the average survival is usually between 6 and 12 months, so the strategy must prevent the patient from costly, aggressive and useless examination. Biopsy of the metastasis should be per-

formed when the metastasis is isolated and when chemotherapy is going to be given. Searching for the primary tumour is also only useful if chemotherapy has been chosen or the metastasis seems isolated. Ultrasonography and/or CT of the abdomen are the best choices.

## Conclusion

The basic examination used in the detection of metastatic bone disease is bone scintigraphy, which is sensitive and nonspecific. Standard radiographs are used for painful areas or for checking abnormalities seen with scintigraphy, as they improve its specificity. The exact role and the best sequences for MRI are not yet clear. MRI, however, should be used in cases of doubtful diagnosis or when bone scintigraphy is normal and extensive surgery is being considered.

## References

1. Abrams HL, Spiro R, Goldstein N (1950) Metastases in carcinomas. Analysis of 1000 autopsied cases. Cancer 3:74
2. Willis RA (1941) A review of 500 consecutive cancer autopsies. Med J Aust 2:258
3. Batson OV (1940) The function of the vertebral veins and their role in the spread of metastases. Ann Surg 112:138
4. Galasko CSB (1982) Mechanisms of lytic and blastic metastatic disease of bone. Clin Orthop Rel Res 169:20
5. Jacobson AF, Cronin EB, Stomper PC, Kaplan WD (1990) Bone scans with one or two new abnormalities in cancer patients with no known metastases: frequency and serial scintigraphic behavior of benign and malignant lesions. Radiology 175:229-232
6. Avra Hami E, Tadmor R, Dally O, Hadar H (1989) Early MR demonstration of spinal metastases in patients with normal radiographs and CT and radio nuclide bone scans. J Comput Assist Tomogr 13:598-602
7. Fragiadakis EG, Panayotopoulous G (1972) Metastatic carcinoma of the hand. Hand 4:268
8. Kerin R (1958) Metastatic tumors of the hand. J Bone Joint Surg [Am], 40:263
9. Deutsch A, Resnick D (1980) Eccentric cortical metastases to the skeleton from bronchogenic carcinoma. Radiology 137:49
10. Vilar J, Lezana AH, Pedrosa CS (1979) Spiculated periosteal reaction in metastatic lesion of bone. Skeletal Radiol 3:230
11. Wyche LD, De Santos LA (1978) Spiculated periosteal reaction in metastatic disease resembling osteosarcoma. Orthopedics 1:215
12. Gold RI, Seeger LL, Bassett LW, Steckel RJ (1990) An integrated approach to the evaluation of metastatic bone disease. Radiol Clin North Am 28:471-483
13. Ramsey RG, Zacharias CE (1985) MR Imaging of the spine after radiation therapy: easily recognizable effects. AJR 144:1131
14. Hardy DC, Murphy WA, Gilula LA (1980) Computed tomography in planning percutaneous bone biopsy. Radiology 134:447
15. Mink J (1986) Percutaneous bone biopsy in the patient with known or suspected osseous metastases. Radiology 161:191
16. Stines J, Conroy T, Bey P, Schmitt C (1992) L'imagerie dans les metastases osseuses. Feuillets Radiol 32:95-116

# G.I. AND ABDOMINAL RADIOLOGY

# Radiological Workup in Oral-pharyngeal Dysphagia: Costs and Clinical Results

A. Montesi[1], M. Matei[1], A. Pisani[1], L. Provinciali[2], M. G. Ceravolo[2] and F. Mari[2]

Radiologia e Diagnostica per Immagini USL 7[1] e Clinica di Neuroriabilitazione, Università di Ancona[2], Ospedale Regionale, 60100 Ancona, Italy

## Introduction

The oral-pharyngeal swallow transports a bolus from the oral cavity through the pharynx and the upper oesophageal sphincter (UES) to the oesophagus. The structures of the oral cavity, pharynx and larynx, thirty-three head and neck muscles, and five cranial nerves are involved in swallowing. This occurs when the reflex of deglutition is triggered [1, 2].

The mechanical event of swallowing consists in the formation, containment and transport of a bolus from the oral cavity into the cervical oesophagus. This process can be functionally subdivided into four fundamental phases [3]:

1. Formation of the bolus by the tongue movements and its active, voluntary oral containment in a central groove of the tongue.
2. Horizontal transport of the bolus from the oral cavity to the pharynx and triggering of the reflex; acceptance and containment of the bolus in the orohypopharynx.
3. Vertical transport of the bolus through the pharynx and UES to the oesophagus.

The neural performance consists in the afferent transmission of the sensory impulses from the orohypopharynx with the involvement of the sensitive fibres of the V, VII and X cranial nerves, in the coordination, organization and synchronization in the swallowing centre located in the brainstem and in the efferent transmission which involves the V, VII, IX, X and XII cranial nerves [4].

Symptoms of abnormal swallow are drooling, difficulty initiating swallowing, nasal regurgitation, coughing, choking after swallow and pneumonia due to aspiration.

On the whole, the most frequent causes of this oral-pharyngeal dysphagia are:

- Motility disorders due to neurological impariment (such as stroke, cerebral vascular disease, amiotrophic lateral sclerosis, dementia, Parkinson disease, head trauma, postpolio syndrome, brain tumours etc.).
- Muscular diseases (such as dermatomiositis, miasthenya, muscular dystrophy, etc.).
- Structural lesions of the oral cavity, pharynx and larynx due to tumours and to surgery and/or radiotherapy.

In the last years the frequency of oral-pharyngeal dysphagia has apparently increased. Factors influencing a renewed clinical interest of this pathological condition are improved survival in neuromuscular diseases, increased incidence of surgery and radiation therapy in head and neck tumours, awareness of the existence of silent dysphagia, a condition in which patients with oral-pharyngeal disorders are unconscious of their disturbance, and finally the progress in the rehabilitation therapy of oral-pharyngeal dysphagia.

Therefore, the need for appropriate and objective diagnosis of oral-pharyngeal deglutition disorders is increased.

The clinical approach to oral-pharyngeal dysphagia should consist in a clinical history and physical examination of the oral-pharyngeal region.

Videofluoroscopy of deglutition of barium boluses is considered the most complete and available imaging technique for the study of the act of swallowing [5]. The entire process of deglutition can be analysed at normal speed, slow motion, frame by frame and in a back view mode.

Therefore, deficit of oral containment, horizontal transport, pharyngeal containment and vertical transport of the bolus from the pharynx to the cervical oesophagus can be evaluated [6, 7].

Aspiration, defined as the passage of food or liquid beyond the vocal cords, is the most risky swallowing disorder. Radiologically, it can be objectively assessed and the different aspiration mechanisms can be defined [8].

Occasionally, ultrasonography, videoendoscopy and scintigraphy are complementary examinations and not indicated routinely. Videofluoroscopy and contemporary manometry are recommended for the best evaluation of functional disorders.

The aim of this presentation is to evaluate the clinical results and costs of videofluoroscopic study of the act of swallowing in patients with oral-pharyngeal dysphagia. Therefore, we have investigated the predictive value of a very accurate clinical history and physical examination of the oral and pharyngeal phases of deglutition with respect to aspiration radiologically diagnosed, in order to indicate to what extent videofluoroscopy maintains a role in the first diagnostic workup of dysphagic patients.

Furthermore, we have evaluated the relationship between the radiological findings and the disability level of the patients in order to assess the physical, psychological and social consequences of radiologically demonstrated swallowing disorders.

Financial and biological costs of videofluoroscopic study of deglutition have been also considered.

## Material and Method

Ninety-two consecutive patients, 47 males and 45 females, aged from 22 to 94 years (average 62) were selected for videofluoroscopic studies of the oral-pharyngeal phases of swallowing at request of the family doctor or of a specialist, indicating disturbances related to deglutition or asking for preventive control of diseases highly linked to oral-pharyngeal dysphagia.

Ninety-two examinations were performed: four examinations were not done.

The clinical examination of the oral and pharyngeal region were performed in all cases according to the protocol outlined in Table 1. Each structure was systematically examined and any deviation from normal was noted. The clinical results were considered pathological for predictive value evaluation when at least three parameters were altered for each phase.

Clinical examination was also evaluated in terms of disability and defined, according to the International Classification of Impairments, Disabilities and Handicaps, as "any restriction or lack resulting from an impairment of ability to perform an activity in the manner or within the range considered normal for human beings" [9].

Disability is a disturbance of the whole person, while impairment is a disturbance at the organic level [9]. Disability resulting from the oral-pharyngeal impairment consists in unsatisfactory nutrition, anxiety and insecurity related to swallowing and in loss of the social and symbolic function of eating. The physical, psychological and social disabilities are the expression of the concrete involvement and suffering of the patients as a direct consequence of the swallowing disorders. Therefore, disability is an important clinical factor which influences the choice of rehabilitation therapy [10].

In order to quantify disability, a questionnaire was applied (Table 2).

The videofluoroscopic examination was performed with a tilt-table fluoroscope, tilted upright so that the patient could be examined in the erect position, in L-L and in A-P projections [11].

The radiological examination was routinely performed as follows:
- Preliminary focus on the oral-pharyngeal regions in L-L view, barium free, for a general examination of the morphological conditions and functional behav-

**Table 1.** Clinical examination

| Clinical history |
| --- |

| Nasal regurgitation |
| Coughing during swallow |
| Dysphonia |
| Dysarthria |
| Dyskinesia |

| Physical examination |
| --- |

| **Oral Phase** | Mandible |
| --- | --- |
| Lips | Lateral movements |
| Corner | Ant/sup movements |
| Closure | Masseter muscle |
| Protrusion | |
| Muscle tone | Oral sensitivity |
| Anterior leakage | |
| Tongue | *Pharyngeal phase* |
| Motility | Swallow reflex |
| Force | Soft palate motility |
| Bolus formation | Pharyngeal reflex |
| Oral clearance | Hyoid-laryngeal motility |
| Posterior leakage | |

**Table 2.** Questions related to disabilities resulting from dysphagia

| | Score |
| --- | --- |
| **Physical disability** | |
| *Inability to attain satiety* | |
| Hungry or thirsty after meals | 1 |
| *Inability to obtain nutritional requirement* | |
| Frequency of dysphagia | 1-3 |
| Frequency of complete obstruction | 1-2 |
| Meal duration > 40 min | 1 |
| Vomiting at meals | 1 |
| **Psychological disability** | |
| *Inability to feel secure when eating* | |
| Anxiety for dysphagia | 1 |
| Panic feeling during meals | 1 |
| Hopelessness with meals | 1 |
| Insecure feeling when eating | 1 |
| *Inability to control eating situation* | |
| Unpredictable obstruction | 1 |
| Lack of control of eating | 1-3 |
| **Social disability** | |
| *Inability to take part in the symbolic function of eating* | |
| Avoids dinner invitations | 2 |
| Increased dysphagia when together with others | 1 |
| Difficulty in taking part in conversation at meal time | 1 |
| Alienation when eating | 1 |
| *Inability to enjoy various kinds of food* | |
| Avoidance of certain kinds of food | 1 |
| Special diet | 2 |
| Maximum sum | 24 |

Patients scoring 0 to 8 were considered to have no or mild disability, those scoring 9 to 16 to have moderate, and those scoring 17 to 24 to have severe disability.

**Table 3.** Protocol of the radiological study of deglutition

| Routine | IF retention/penetration aspiration with 5 ml L-L | IF retention/penetration aspiration with 15 ml L-L |
|---|---|---|
| Fonation, barium-free | | |
| 5 ml L-L | Then | Then |
| 10 ml L-L | 10 ml L-L in flexion | 10 ml L-L flexion |
| 15 ml L-L | 5 ml A-P | 10 ml L-L |
| 15 ml L-L | 5 ml A-P for oesophagus | 10 ml A-P for oesophagus |
| 10 ml L-L | 5 ml A-P for oesophagus | 10 ml A-P for oesophagus |
| 10 ml L-L for oesophagus | Solid bolus A-P | Solid bolus in A-P |
| 10 ml L-L for oesophagus | Solid bolus L-L | Solid bolus in L-L |
| If necessary Valsalva | Solid bolus L-L in flexion | Solid bolus in flexion |
| Solid bolus L-L | | |
| Solid bolus extension | | |
| 15 ml L-L: 3 quickly | | |
| repeated swallows | **If necessary:** | **If necessary** |
| | 10 ml supraglottic degl. | 10 ml supraglottic degl. |
| | 10 ml Mendelsohn manoeuvre | 10 ml Mendelsohn manoeuvre |
| | 5 ml head rotation to right | 5 ml rotation to right |
| | 5 ml head rotation to left | 5 ml rotation to left |
| | 5 ml head inclination to right | 5 ml inclination to right |
| | 5 ml head inclination to left | 5 ml inclination to left |

L-L, latero-lateral view; A-P, anterior-posterior view; degl., deglutition.

iour of anatomical structures during fonation and saliva deglutition.

– Examination of oral containment of boluses of different volume.

– Examination of the oral-pharyngeal regions during the passage boluses varying in volume and consistency and analysis of the oral and pharyngeal structure motility.

A summary of the radiological examination is seen in Table 3.

Two examiners evaluated the results of dynamic imaging, individually and in cooperation. Patients were excluded from this study if severe aspiration during radiological examination occurred, if tracheostomy enabled radiological evaluation, or if patient compliance was lacking. Patients were informed beforehand about the risks of the examination and their written consent was requested.

Clinical pathological findings in the oral and pharyngeal phases were compared with the occurrence of radiologically diagnosed aspiration. Using the Contingency Table Analysis, the positive predictive value (PPV) and the negative predictive value (NPV) of the clinical findings were computed. The analysis was repeated, dividing the total number of patients into three groups characterized by different levels of disability.

The costs of clinical and radiological examination were based on the following financial factors: equipment, personnel, materials and examination time.

Biological costs consists in radiation exposure of the patients and operators; the actual dose of radiation delivered to the patient in a videofluoroscopic study of deglutition is highly dependent on the operator, the machine and the individual patient. The most relevant factors that influence the dose a patient receives are patient size, density of the body part examined, location of tissue (within the field or near the beam entrance, near the beam exit), tube kilovoltage, dose-rate level settings, electronic magnification, X-ray field size, and fluoroscopy duration. The considerable variation in local variables makes it extremely difficult to estimate the dose from a videofluoroscopic study of deglutition; nevertheless, it is recommended that a reliable method is used to calculate organ doses for thyroid, active bone marrow, and lungs per minute of fluoroscopy in each projection [12].

## Results

The clinical and radiological examinations were evaluated separately for the oral and pharyngeal phases of swallowing. The predictability of the clinical history and physical examination for aspiration detected by radiology is illustrated in Table 4.

These data show that there is no significant difference in terms of PPVs between the oral and pharyngeal clinical examination (respectively, 70% and 67%) and show that in 30%-33% of the cases (false negatives), aspiration is not correctly predicted by the clinical history and

**Table 4.** Predictive values of clinical examination

| | Phase of swallowing | |
|---|---|---|
| | Oral (%) | Pharyngeal (%) |
| PPV | 70 | 67 |
| FN | 30 | 33 |
| NPV | 77 | 72 |
| FP | 23 | 28 |

PPV, positive predictive value; NPV, negative predictive value; FN, false negative; FP, false positive.

**Table 5.** Predictive values of clinical examination for each disability level

| Disability | Oral phase of swallowing | | | | Pharyngeal phase of swallowing | | | |
|---|---|---|---|---|---|---|---|---|
| | PPV | FN | NPV | FP | PPV | FN | NPV | FP |
| None/mild | 66% | 34% | 79% | 21% | 40% | 60% | 73% | 27% |
| Moderate | 70% | 30% | 87% | 13% | 75% | 25% | 87% | 13% |
| Severe | 77% | 23% | 43% | 57% | 75% | 25% | 37% | 63% |

PPV, positive predictive value; NPV, negative predictive value; FN, false negative; FP, false positive.

physical examination. Therefore, the radiological results can adjust the underestimation of a very accurate clinical evaluation of dysphagia, approximately in one third of the cases.

In contrast, in 23% and 28% of the cases of oral and pharyngeal examinations (false positives), respectively, the radiological results can correct the overestimation of the clinical evaluation. In addition, the PVs of clinical history and physical examination for an unsafe swallow (aspiration) related to disability level are shown in Table 5.

In the clinical examination of the oral phase of swallowing an increase of PPVs in the three groups of disability occurs (66%, 70% and 77%, respectively). Specifically, increased severity of the disability is associated with increased percentage of PPV of the clinical examination. In the three groups of patients the clinical history and physical examination of the oral phase failed to predict aspiration in 34%, 30% and 23% of the cases (false negatives), respectively. When disability was severe, the NPV of the clinical history and physical examination of the oral phase was fairly low (43%), caused by 57% clinically overestimated cases (false positives).

In the clinical examination of the pharyngeal phase of swallowing the PPV was low in patients with none or mild disability (40%), while patients with moderate and severe disability were most likely to aspirate (75%). In the three groups of patients the clinical history and physical examination of the pharyngeal phase failed to predict aspiration in 60%, 25% and 25% of the cases (false negatives), respectively. When disability was severe the NPV of the clinical history and physical examination of the pharyngeal phase was low (37%), caused

by 63% clinically overestimated cases (false positives). These data demonstrate that disability due to dysphagia strongly influences the predictiveness of the clinical examination. Therefore, the role of videofluoroscopy in the objective diagnosis of aspiration at different levels of disability is underlined. In fact, in the group of patients with no or mild disability, 34% of false negatives for aspiration in the oral phase and 60% of false negatives in the pharyngeal phase can be correctly diagnosed by the radiological examination, and, in the group of patients with severe disability, 57% of false positives for aspiration in the oral phase and 63% in the pharyngeal phase can be correctly ruled out by videofluoroscopy.

The rehabilitation therapy of patients with swallowing disorders is based on the evaluation of the functional impairment of deglutition and on the consequent level of patient disability; therefore, both clinical and radiological examinations are part of an integrated diagnostic approach in oral-pharyngeal dysphagia.

Videofluoroscopy is capable to demonstrate not only aspiration, but also other swallowing disorders such as oral leakage, swallowing reflex abnormalities, abnormal motility of the tongue, abnormal motility of the pharyngeal constrictor wall, penetration, retention, etc. [7].

The results showed that, among the 50 patients who did not aspirate during videofluoroscopy, 18 showed no pathological patterns, 22 showed an impairment either during the oral or pharyngeal phase, whereas 10 had alterations during both phases.

The diagnosis of an oral phase impairment was based more often on the detection of either anterior or posterior leakage, whereas the pharyngeal phase impairment was more frequently related to the presence of swallowing reflex alteration or retention or penetration, either alone or in combination. The distribution of disability in the three groups with different radiological patterns is described in Table 6.

In summary, these data suggest that abnormal radiological findings, when aspiration is not included, do not have a direct relationship with the disability of the patients. In fact, moderate or severe disability is present in seven of 18 patients without radiological abnormalities; in contrast three of ten patients showing alterations during both the oral and pharyngeal phases had only none or mild disability.

**Table 6.** Relationship between radiological finding and disability level

| Disability level | Radiological pattern | | | Total patients (n) |
|---|---|---|---|---|
| | No alterations | Impairment of at least one phase | Impairment of both phases | |
| None or mild | 11 | 12 | 3 | 26 |
| Moderate | 6 | 7 | 5 | 18 |
| Severe | 1 | 3 | 2 | 6 |
| Total patients | 18 | 22 | 10 | 50 |

**Table 7.** Financial cost of a videofluoroscopic examination of oral-pharyngeal swallowing

|  | Cost (Dollars) |
| --- | --- |
| Clinical examination | 14 |
| Equipment | 2.7 |
| Materials | 32 |
| Personnel | 43 |
| **Total cost** | **92** |

Finally, Table 7 shows the average financial cost of a videofluoroscopic examination of oropharyngeal swallowing in our department.

## Discussion

The videofluoroscopic examination of the oral-pharyngeal phases of deglutition is widespreading because of a renewed interest in oral and pharyngeal dysphagia. Therefore, an evaluation of the clinical results and considerations of costs are essential in order to define the cost-effectiveness of radiology in the diagnostic workup of dysphagia.

Aspiration is the most risky swallowing disorder and radiology is a very reliable technique to ascertain and to rule it out [13]. Hence videofluoroscopically detected aspiration has been the gold standard for the clinical evaluation of dysphagic patients in our investigation.

The results of our study reveal that an accurate clinical examination has a high positive predictivity for aspiration: 70% in the oral phase and 67% in the pharyngeal one.

Nevertheless, videofluoroscopy can be considered essential in the first diagnostic workup of dysphagia because in 30%-33% of the cases the clinical history and physical examination fail to predict aspiration and in 23%-28% of the cases the clinical suspicion of unsafe swallowing is unfounded.

Disability resulting from oral-pharyngeal dysphagia consists in disturbance of the whole person which is affected as a direct consequence of the swallowing disorders [9]. Our data demonstrate that the disability level due to dysphagia strongly influences the predictiveness of the clinical history and physical examination. Therefore, the role of videofluoroscopy in the objective diagnosis of aspiration at different levels of disability is pointed out. For example, in the groups of patients with severe disability videofluoroscopy can rule out aspiration in more than half of the subjects in whom clinical parameters suggest aspiration in the oral phase and in two thirds in the pharyngeal phase.

In our study swallowing abnormalities detected by radiological examination are not completely related to the patient disability; in fact, radiology may demonstrate abnormal findings with mild disability, and, in contrast, may show irrelevant findings in the oral and pharyngeal phases in patients suffering from severe disability.

Financial cost of videofluoroscopy is relatively low. Radiation dose measurement are recommended in the thyroid, lungs, and active bone marrow.

In conclusion, even the most accurate clinical investigation based on a check list history, physical examination and disability evaluation requires an additional videofluoroscopic study performed by radiologists experienced in the clinical workup of dysphagia and in the risk of radiation exposure. Futhermore, when there is a discrepancy between radiological investigation and disability score, one has to keep in mind that videofluoroscopy estimates the functional impairment of swallowing, whereas disability involves the patients personally, both influence the rehabilitation approach.

## References

1. Bosma JF, Donner MW, Tanaka E, Robertson D (1958) Anatomy of the pharynx, pertinent to swallowing. Dysphagia 1: 23-33 (1985)
2. Donner MW, Bosma JF, Robertson DL (1985) Anatomy and physiology of the pharynx. Gastrointest Radiol 10: 196-212
3. Montesi A, Pisani AM, Matei M (1994) La meccanica della degiutizione. Perona (in press)
4. Kennedy JG, Kent RD (1985) Physiological substrates of normal deglutition. Dysphagia 3:24-37
5. Curtis DJ, Ekberg O, Montesi A (1991) Swallowing: a radiological perspective. Gastroenterol Int 4: 47-54
6. Dodds WJ, Stewart ET, Logemann JA (1990) Physiology and radiology of the normal oral and pharyngeal phases of swallowing. AJR 154: 953-963
7. Dodds WJ, Logemann JA, Stewart ET (1990) Radiologic assessment of abnormal oral and pharyngeal phases of swallowing. AJR 154: 965-974
8. Terry PB, Fuller SD (1989) Pulmonary consequences of aspiration. Dysphagia 3: 179-183
9. Gustafsson B, Tibbling L (1991) Dysphagia, an unrecognized handicap. Dysphagia 6: 193-199
10. Langmore SE, Miller RM (1994) Behavioral treatment for adults with oropharyngeal dysphagia. Arch Phys Med Rehabil 75: 1154-1160
11. Montesi A, Pesaresi A, Antico E, Piloni V (1988) Lo studio radiologico dinamico con videoregistrazione delle fasi orale e faringea della deglutizione normale. Radiol Med 75: 166-172
12. Beck TJ, Gayler BW (1990) Image quality and radiation levels in videofluoroscopy for swallowing studies: a review. Dysphagia 5: 118-128
13. Logemann JA (1983) Evaluation and treatment of swallowing disorders. College-Hill, San Diego, CA

# Ischaemic Bowel Disease: Radiographic and Imaging Features

J. Pringot

Department of Medical Imaging, Cliniques Universitaires St Luc, Avenue Hippocrate 10, 1200 Brussels, Belgium

Bowel ischaemia is a clinical and pathophysiological concept relating functional and structural bowel disorders to inadequate blood supply to the small intestine and/or colon. Depending on many variables, including the onset and duration of the injury, the area and length of bowel affected, the vessel involved and the mechanism of ischaemia, different clinical, pathological and radiological forms or entities are encountered. Colonic ischaemia is the most common form of bowel ischaemia but acute mesenteric ischaemia has the worse prognosis mainly because the diagnosis is often delayed. Acute mesenteric venous thrombosis is considered apart from the other acute mesenteric ischaemic syndromes on the basis of differences in clinical manifestations and in prognosis.

Today cross-sectional imaging plays an important role in the work-up of patients suspected of having bowel ischaemia prior to angiography, colonoscopy or serial contrast enemas, which remain an integral part of an appropriate evaluation.

## Acute Mesenteric Ischaemia and Infarction [1-6]

Acute mesenteric arterial ischaemia only accounts for approximately one third of all intestinal ischaemias but is responsible for the majority of deaths. Prompt recognition and aggressive therapy are required if the fatality rate is to be lowered. Occlusive arterial mesenteric ischaemia commonly associated with atherosclerotic cardiovascular disease is due either to superior mesenteric artery (SMA) emboli from atrial or mural thrombus or to thrombosis of SMA. Nonocclusive mesenteric ischaemia represents ischaemia from splanchnic vasoconstriction in response to decreased cardiac output, hypovolaemia, dehydration, hypotension or use of vasopressor agents.

The pathophysiological changes caused by acute mesenteric arterial ischaemia are consistent and independent of the aetiology of the ischaemia. Low SMA flow initially produces openings of the collateral vascular pathways that tend to maintain adequate intestinal flow. If diminished flow is prolonged, however, active vasoconstriction develops and can persist even after the initial cause of the ischaemia has been corrected, leading to irreversible intestinal damage. Histological changes are seen in experimental intestinal ischaemia after 12 h consisting in partial loss of the intestinal villi, followed after 24 h by submucosal and intramural haemorrhage and later by intense inflammatory reaction.

Abdominal pain is present in a majority of patients but suggests this condition only when sudden and severe in onset and associated with forceful evacuation of intestinal contents. Early identification of acute mesenteric ischaemia requires attention to patients at risk for the disorders and relies on the aggressive use of mesenteric arteriography.

### Radiographic and Imaging Findings

At an early stage of bowel ischaemia, plain films of the abdomen may reveal normal findings and an abdomen free of gas due to spasm of the muscularis propria of the damaged intestine. Later in the ischaemic period, the muscle, while still viable, will lose its contractile function, and much of the spasm will cease. An "ileus" of the ischaemic segment will cause the bowel gas pattern in this segment to remain virtually identical from hour to hour or day to day (Fig. 1). Thickening of the mucosal folds and thumbprints due to extravasation of blood in the submucosa may be seen on a plain film. The viable and functioning bowel above the ischaemic segment may not be able to force its peristaltic bolus of gas through a long, atonic, ischaemic segment, and a clinical and radiographic picture of progressive diffuse small bowel ileus may develop (Fig. 1). If the intestinal ischaemia persists the mucosa infarcts, allowing intestinal gas to dissect the mucosa from the serosa and to penetrate in the mesenteric and portal veins with resulting intestinal pneumatosis and gas in the mesenteric and portal veins. Finally, with persisting ischaemia, full-thickness or transmural infarction of the wall occurs with consecutive peritoneal irritation and more pronounced diffuse ileus, and the bowel may perforate with resulting free intraperitoneal air.

Computed tomographic findings in the abdomen sug-

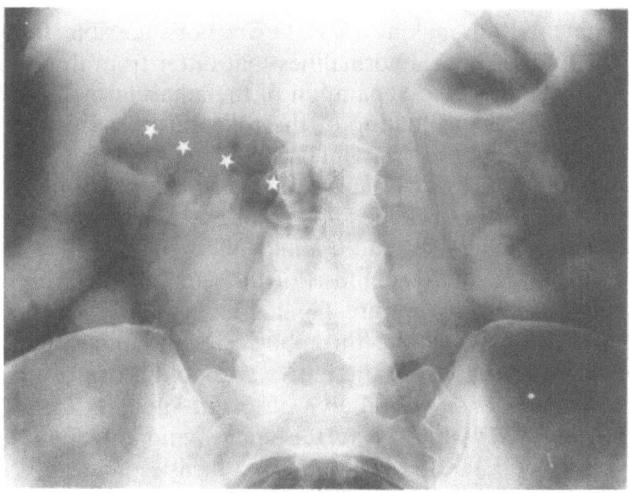

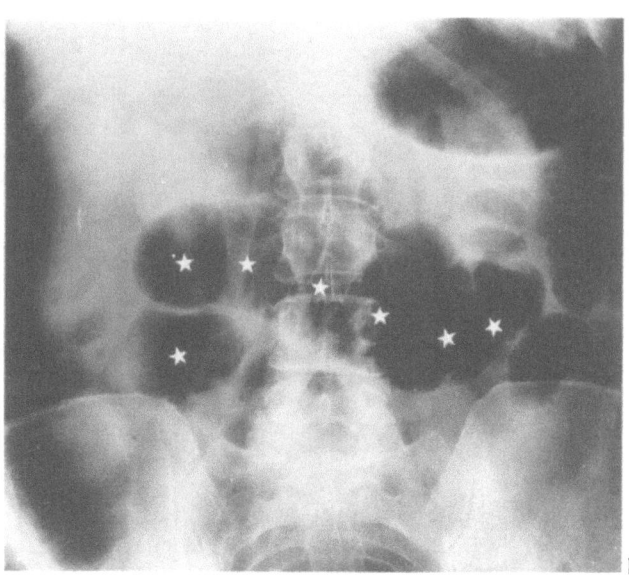

**Fig. 1 a, b.** Acute mesenteric infarction. **a** Initial abdominal plain film shows localized ileus of small bowel (*stars*) with blurred and thickened folds. Two days later, the ileus is more pronounced (*stars*) and more widespread.

**b** Laparotomy showed nonresectable infarcted small bowel

gestive of acute ischaemia include dilated, fluid-filled loops of thick-walled bowel that demonstrate persisting postcontrast enhancement. Patchy low density may be seen within the wall. However, in obstructive ischaemia, contrast-enhanced CT may show thin-walled, nonenhancing intestine as well as the site of the SMA occlusion (Fig. 2). A variable quantity of fluid may be present in the peritoneal cavity. With bowel infarction, portal or mesenteric venous gas, intramural air, and free intraperitoneal air may be seen.

In the absence of intestinal ileus, colour Doppler sonography may demonstrate thin or thick adynamic

bowel and associated reduced flow in one or two visceral arteries, findings which are suggestive of mesenteric ischaemia (Fig. 3).

In occlusive ischaemia, mesenteric arteriography is useful to define the type, degree and site of the arterial occlusion (Fig. 2) and permits treatment decisions regarding infusion thrombolytic therapy, embolectomy, or other surgical options. In patients with suspected low-flow state ischaemia whose condition does not respond to restoration of normal cardiac output, angiography may demonstrate reflex mesenteric vasoconstriction which may be reversed by intraarterial infusion of papaverine.

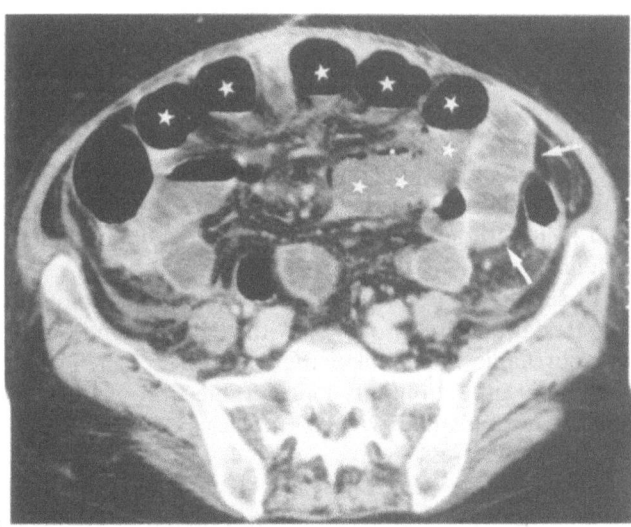

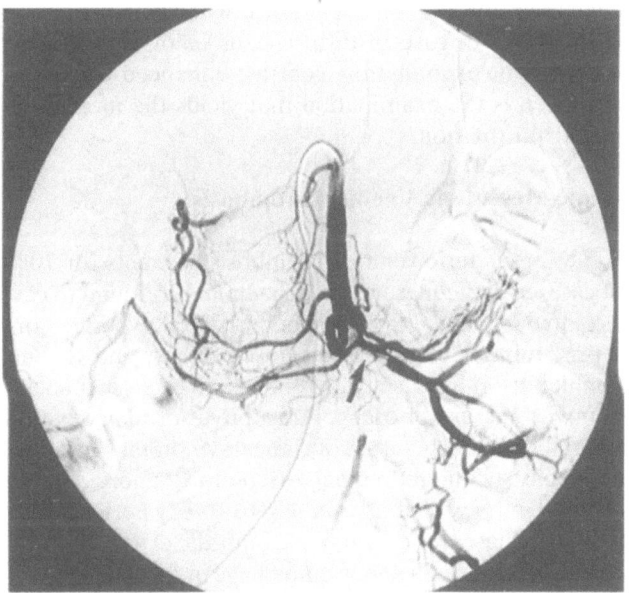

**Fig. 2 a, b.** Resectable acute mesenteric infarction. **a** Contrast-enhanced computed tomography shows diffuse small bowel ileus with enhancing proximal loops in the left flank (*arrows*) and thin-walled nonenhancing loops more distally (*stars*).

**b** Arteriography of the superior mesenteric artery shows partial occlusion of an arterial branch (*arrow*)

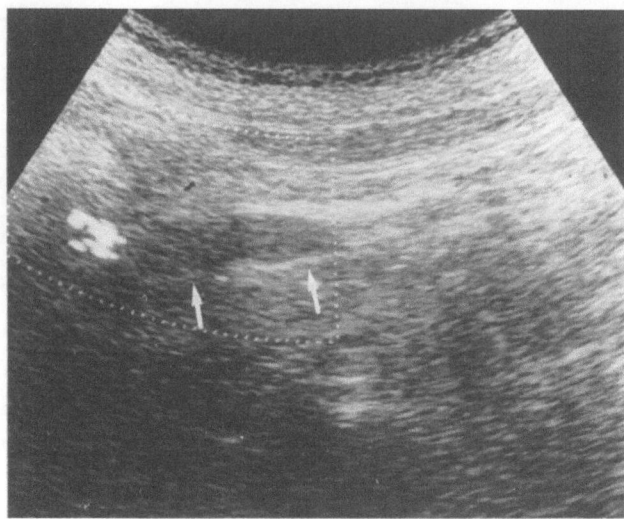

**Fig. 3.** Resectable acute mesenteric infarction, Colour Doppler sonography shows absence of flow in superior mensenteric artery (*arrows*). Arteriography confirmed the proximal superior mesenteric occlusion of the SMA and subsequent surgery was performed

## Diagnostic Strategy

When acute ischaemia is suspected, plain abdominal filming is the usual first examination. Thereafter, the radiologist may suggest an ultrasound examination of the upper abdomen with colour Doppler, intravenous, contrast-enhanced, dynamic CT or angiography of visceral vessels, depending on the findings from the initial plain film of the abdomen.

If a sonographic examination is performed and the results suggest mesenteric ischaemia, mesenteric arteriography is strongly indicated, particularly if history and clinical findings are in accordance with ischaemia at an early stage. In case of diffuse ileus or of inconclusive sonographic examination, contrast-enhanced CT of the abdomen is the examination that yields the most diagnostic information.

### Acute Mesenteric Venous Thrombosis

Acute mesenteric venous thrombosis accounts for 10% of cases of acute mesenteric ischaemia. It is found in cases of hypercoagulability, carcinoma, portal hypertension, sepsis, tumour compression, direct injury, and thrombophlebitis. It has also been reported to occur in association with the use of oral contraceptives or may develop spontaneously. The onset of clinical symptoms is gradual and consists in abdominal discomfort, anorexia and changes in bowel habits over a 7- to 10-day period.

Acute mesenteric venous thrombosis causes marked congestion, oedema and haemorrhage in the damaged intestine and, ultimately, mucosal necrosis and the mesentery is greatly thickened. Plain films may be normal or, in typical cases, may show rigid, fixed, thick-walled bowel

segments, thus making a specific diagnosis possible. Barium studies show abnormalities that differ from those of arterial ischaemia. Separation of the adjacent loops and thickening and blunting of the mucosal folds are both more pronounced. Marginal scalloping and thumbprinting are more constant and a pattern consisting of transitional zones of thickened folds is often seen.

Ultrasound (US) and CT may allow preoperative diagnosis of acute thrombosis of the superior mesenteric vein by showing features analogous to those found in other forms of venous thrombosis, for instance, a high-density thrombus on the native scan and a rim of wall enhancement, a central area of low attenuation (representing clot within the vessel lumen), and an extensive venous collateral circulation on contrast-enhanced CT scanning (Fig. 4). If thrombosis of the superior mesenteric vein is limited and does not involve the distal venous branches, the venous collateral circulation may prevent small bowel infarction. The CT pattern of small bowel infarction is characterized by symmetric thickening and persistent enhancement of the bowel wall. Streakiness of the mesentery adjacent to the infarcted small bowel may be seen. In case of thrombosis of peripheral mesenteric veins, a haemorrhagic infarction of the bowel wall may occur that is characterized by a sharply defined circular wall thickening of homogeneous density and that is indistinguishable (in the absence of pertinent clinical history) from intramural intestinal haemorrhage. Symmetric small bowel wall thickening is easily detected by real-time US, which may be used as a screening procedure in patients with nonspecific acute abdominal symptoms. However, the venous thrombus (appearing as an echogenic filling of the lumen of the vein) may be more difficult to detect with US in the absence of associated thrombosis of the portal vein.

## Segmental Ischaemia of the Small Bowel [6]

Segmental or focal ischaemia of the small intestine is an uncommon but distinct entity that, like ischaemic colitis, has been defined on the basis of clinical, radiological and histopathological findings as well as experimental evidence.

In segmental ischaemia the clinical and radiological manifestations are associated with acute oedematous or haemorrhagic intestinal damage in cases of so-called segmental infarction and considerable fibrous thickening of the intestinal wall in the cases of so-called ischaemic strictures.

### Acute Segmental Ischaemia or Infarction

The extent of the intestinal lesions, and in particular the depth to which the necrosis penetrates, depend on the territorial extension and the duration of the ischaemia. Most patients have pain. Mild bleeding or reversible ob-

**Fig. 4 a, d.** Computed tomographic scan demonstrates acute mesenteric venous thrombosis (*arrowheads*; **a, b**), small bowel infarction characterized by thickened, dense bowel wall (*arrows*) and streaky oedematous mesentery (*broad arrows*; **b-d**) as well as minor ascites and focal hypodensity of probable liver infarction (*star*; **a**). Reproduced from [6] with permission

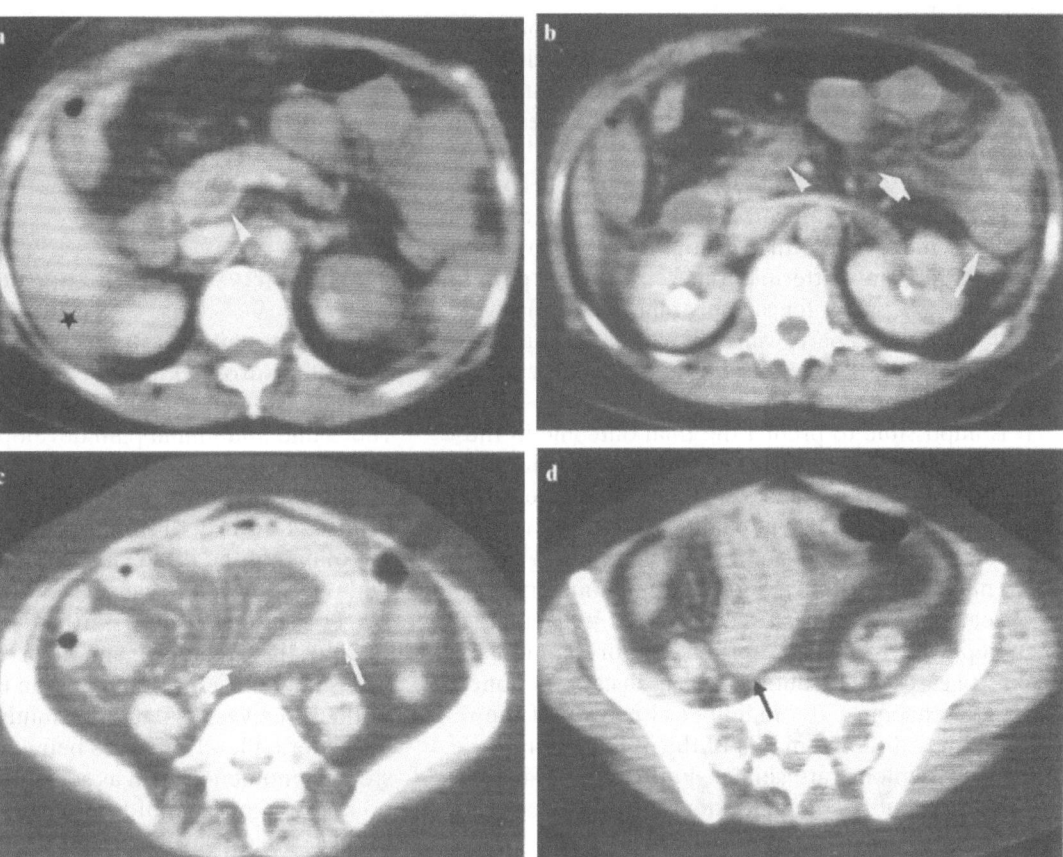

struction may be observed. Peritoneal signs, when present, suggest transmural necrosis or perforation.

Plain films of the abdomen commonly show nonspecific air patterns in the intestine. Not infrequently, however, they show more suggestive features such as oedematous mucosa in an air-filled bowel segment, an airless bowel segment, or a narrowed, rigid, air-filled loop separated from the others and from which the mucosal folds are noticeably absent (Fig. 5).

Barium studies of the small intestine performed in the absence of or after regression of the dynamic ileus reveal the intestinal damage in virtually all cases (Fig. 5). The entire bowel may be involved, but more commonly the damage is located in the mid-or distal portions or both. The length of the usually one damaged segment has been diversely reported as 7-10 cm or more. Spasm associated with the separation and uncoiling of the damaged loop, which remains mobile when the abdomen is palpated, is

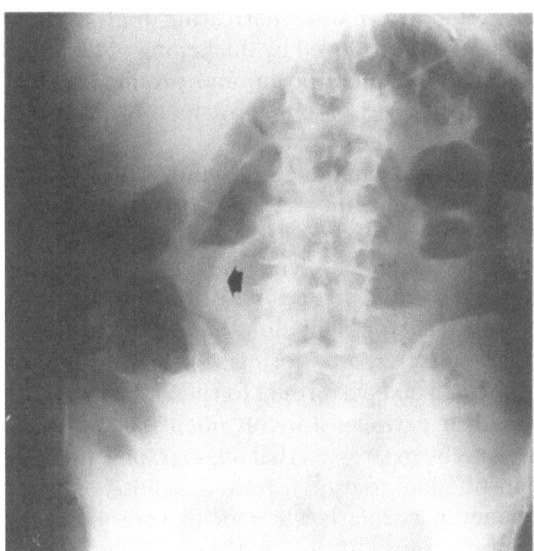

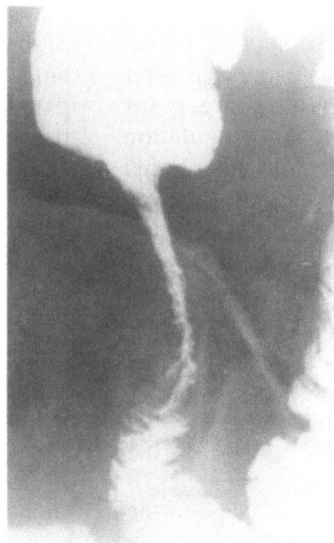

**Fig. 5 a, b.** Acute segmental mesenteric ischaemia. **a** Plain film of the abdomen shows distended loops and, on the right side, short, narrowed, rigid, air-filled loop (*broad arrow*). **b** Two days later after regression of ileus, barium examination demonstrates distension of the small bowel proximal to a short stenosis which appears concentric and tapered with complete blurring of mucosa fold. Reproduced from [6] with permission

a common finding. Dilatation and delayed emptying of the damaged segment are also observed, especially when there is extensive ulceration of the intestinal mucosa. A variety of morphological patterns have been described: (1) slight to moderate dilatation associated with either a blunted or spiky bowel contour or with a smooth contour and a homogeneous appearance of the barium column; (2) relative narrowing with a scalloping of the bowel contour, a thumbprint pattern, a transverse ridging pattern, or symmetrical picket-fence appearance; and (3) severe, concentric, tapered narrowing with complete blurring of the mucosal folds. Sometimes different patterns are associated in the same patient.

It is impossible to predict the final outcome in these cases, because a barium examination is unreliable in evaluating the depth of necrosis or potential viability of the ischaemic segment. On healing, the bowel may return to normal or nearly normal, even in cases of tapered narrowing, within a period of time ranging from 1 to 6 weeks or even more. Recurrence of ischaemia has been reported to occur after surgery or spontaneous healing in cases of vasculitis as well as in cases of nonobstructive ischaemia. The radiological pattern of the recurrence may differ from that of the initial lesion.

CT may demonstrate similar, but less extensive features as in the more common extensive acute mesenteric infarction.

Mesenteric angiography in cases of nonocclusive ischaemia often shows aspecific arteriosclerotic changes in major mesenteric arteries but may occasionally reveal a thrombotic or embolic occlusion of a medium-calibre arterial branch or even localized arterial changes in cases of vasculitis, such as the very characteristic nodularity and beaded appearance of the arteries occurring in periarteritis nodosa.

### Fibrous Ischaemic Strictures

Strictures caused by ischaemia are rare clinical entities. They may occur as a result of acute segmental ischaemia or after occlusion by extrinsic compression of the vascular supply to a region of the bowel, as may occur after herniography for an inguinal hernia or after surgery for a strangulated hernia or for internal strangulation caused by adhesions, invagination, blunt abdominal trauma with intestinal contusion, or a mesenteric tear.

Symptoms of obstruction usually occur after a latent period of 2-16 weeks. The radiographic appearance is that of a single, rigid, tubular narrowing 5-30 cm in length with regular flat borders gradually tapering off at either end toward the relatively dilated adjacent bowel loop. Because of the asymmetric fibrosis occurring in the transitional zone between the tubular structure and the normal segment, the antimesenteric border may become sacculated or pseudodiverticular.

The diagnosis of segmental ischaemic damage in the intestine depends on clinical findings as well as on small

bowel barium study. The radiological differential diagnosis includes a variety of conditions that cause segmental oedema, haemorrhage in the bowel wall, or a concentric stricture, in particular, intramural haematoma, radiation enteritis, Crohn's disease, intestinal tuberculosis and malignant lymphoma.

## Chronic Mesenteric Ischaemia [7, 8]

Chronic mesenteric arterial insufficiency may produce a clinical syndrome known as abdominal, mesenteric, or intestinal angina. Patients present with weight loss, diarrhoea and abdominal pain developing within 2 h of eating.

Although many entities may cause intestinal angina, arteriosclerotic occlusion or severe narrowing of the origin of two of the three visceral vessels is overwhelmingly the most common cause. It may occur after aneurysm surgery and has been described secondary to compression by the arcuate ligament or coeliac ganglion. Patients may have intestinal angina even with the orifices of the three vessels patent or minimally narrowed if the mesenteric blood supply is being diverted by a vascular steal phenomenon such as seen in mesenteric arteriovenous fistula or arterial-to-arterial steals in compression of the coeliac axis, in occlusion of the lower aorta and in occlusion of the portal vein causing compensatory increased hepatic artery flow.

### Radiographic Findings and Diagnosis

The radiographic findings on small bowel examination are nonspecific and include malabsorption pattern, thickened fold pattern, focal ulcer, focal stricture and recurrent small bowel obstruction. The small bowel study may appear normal in patients with intestinal angina, particularly those without malabsorption.

The diagnosis of coeliac axis compression syndrome may be suggested by CT when narrowing or effacement of the coeliac axis is produced by thickening of the crura anterior to the abdominal aorta, and prominent peripancreatic collateral vessels, and poststenotic dilation of the celiac trunk are seen.

Radiographic confirmation of the clinical diagnosis of chronic intestinal ischaemia depends on arteriography demonstrating absence or severe flow impairment of two of the three vessels supplying the bowel. Lateral arteriography is essential to see the orifice of the three vessels. If lateral aortography does not show narrowing of the orifice, selective superior mesenteric and coeliac arteriography must be performed to rule out mesenteric vascular steal or peripheral involvement of the SMA. However, it has been stressed that angiographic findings alone are insufficient to establish the diagnosis of arterial insufficiency, particularly when the diagnosis of coeliac axis compression syndrome is uncertain and has to rely on physiological information. Colour Doppler US may show abnormal mesenteric blood flow but there is no clinical data showing its value as an accurate predictor of chronic mesenteric insufficiency.

Recently, it has been suggested that magnetic resonance imaging (MRI) measurements of superior mesenteric venous blood oxygen saturation could be used for determining the degree of SMA occlusion. Arteriography may also play an alternative therapeutic role to vascular surgery by allowing balloon dilatation of a stenosis.

## Colonic Ischaemia [9-12]

The term colonic ischaemia is used today to describe a pathophysiological process that can lead to a variety of clinical conditions. Regardless of cause, all ischaemic injuries to the colon produce the same spectrum of damage, with reversible and irreversible abnormalities further categorized as (1) reversible ischaemic colopathy (submucosal or intramural haemorrhage), (2) transient ulcerating ischaemic colitis, (chronic ulcerating ischaemic colitis (4) ischaemic colonic stricture, (5) colonic gangrene, and (6) fulminant colitis. Colonic ischaemia is the most common form of intestinal ischaemia and is seen approximately twice as often as acute mesenteric ischaemia, in contrast to which it has typically a less severe presentation and decreased mortality.

Approximately 9% of patients with this disease are older than 60 years of age and have evidence of systemic atherosclerotic disease, which suggests a relation to degenerative changes in the vascular tree, but abnormalities on angiography have only rarely correlated with clinical disease. Oral contraceptives and cocaine use are responsible for a substantial number of cases in the younger population. The great majority of ischaemic events are "spontaneous", occurring without occlusion of a major vessel or any periods of low iatrogenic cardiac output and are attributed to low flow states, small vessel disease or both. An iatrogenic cause (surgery, use of vasopressin, birth control pills) or a site of vascular occlusion are recognized in only 5% of total cases. However, up to 20% of patients with colonic ischaemia have an associated and potentially obstructing colonic lesion such as a stricture, carcinoma, foecal impaction or segment of diverticulitis.

Colonic ischaemia usually presents with the sudden onset of crampy, mild, left-lower abdominal pain and followed within 24 h by the passage of blood mixed with the stool.

## Pathology

The morphological changes of the colon vary with the duration and severity of the ischaemic insult. The mildest changes are submucosal and mucosal haemorrhage and oedema which may be either resorbed (in reversible colopathy) or followed by the formation of multiple ulcers producing the pattern of transient or reversible segmental ulcerating colitis. More severe injury results in extensive mucosal necrosis and oedematous thickening of the submucosa, which is progressively replaced by granulation and fibrous tissue. In more severe and prolonged ischaemia, there is damage to the muscularis propria, replacement of the muscularis propria with fibrous tissue and formation of a fibrous scar. In the most severe ischaemic damage, there is transmural infarction of all layers of the bowel with gangrene and perforation.

### Radiography and Imaging Findings

In a patient with suspected colonic ischaemia abdominal plain films may be normal or nonspecific or may show a colon cut-off sign due to spastic contraction of the diseased colonic segment and presence of air in the rest of the colon, a thumbprinting pattern or a tubular narrowing of the colon against a column of air or even free peritoneal air in case of perforation.

The characteristic finding on contrast enema is "thumbprinting" or pseudotumours. A segmental distribution of these findings, with or without ulceration, is very suggestive of colonic ischaemia (Fig. 6). Any part of the bowel may be affected, but the splenic flexure, descending colon and sigmoid are the most common sites. Segmental colitis associated with a distal tumour or other potentially or partially obstructing lesions is also characteristic of ischaemic disease.

It is imperative to obtain the initial diagnostic study early in the course of the disease because thumbprinting will disappear within days as the submucosal haemorrhages are either resorbed or evacuated into the colon when the overlying mucosa ulcerates and sloughs. Barium enema performed 1 week after the initial study should reflect the evolution of the disease, either by a return to normal or by the replacement of the thumbprints with a segmental ulcerative colitis pattern.

In approximately one half of patients, symptoms subside within 24-48 h, and clinical and roentgenographic evidence of healing is seen within 4 weeks. One third of all cases of colonic ischaemia exhibit only reversible colonic haemorrhage and oedema while 16% of all cases of colonic ischaemia manifest a transient colitis. Sometimes, with severe tissue damage the entire mucosa may slough as a tube, yet several months later the colon may revert to normal (Fig. 6). More severe, but still reversible ischaemic damage may take from 1 to 6 months to resolve. In about one half of patients with colonic ischaemia, the ischaemic damage is too severe to heal and the patient will develop irreversible disease. In approximately two thirds of such patients colonic ischaemia follows a protracted course, developing into either chronic segmental ischaemia colitis or ischaemic stricture. Strictures may develop over weeks to months, may be tran-

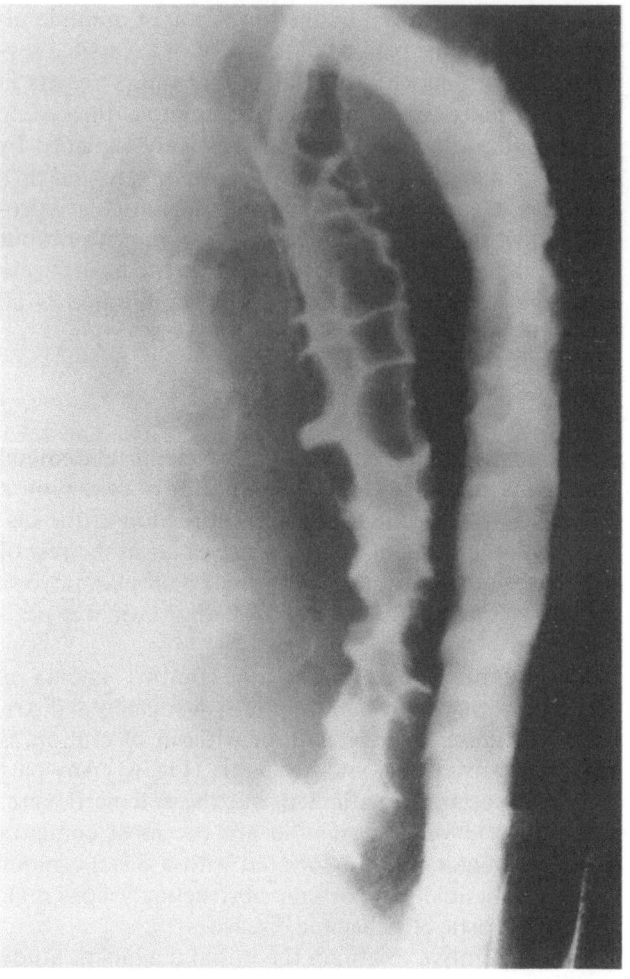
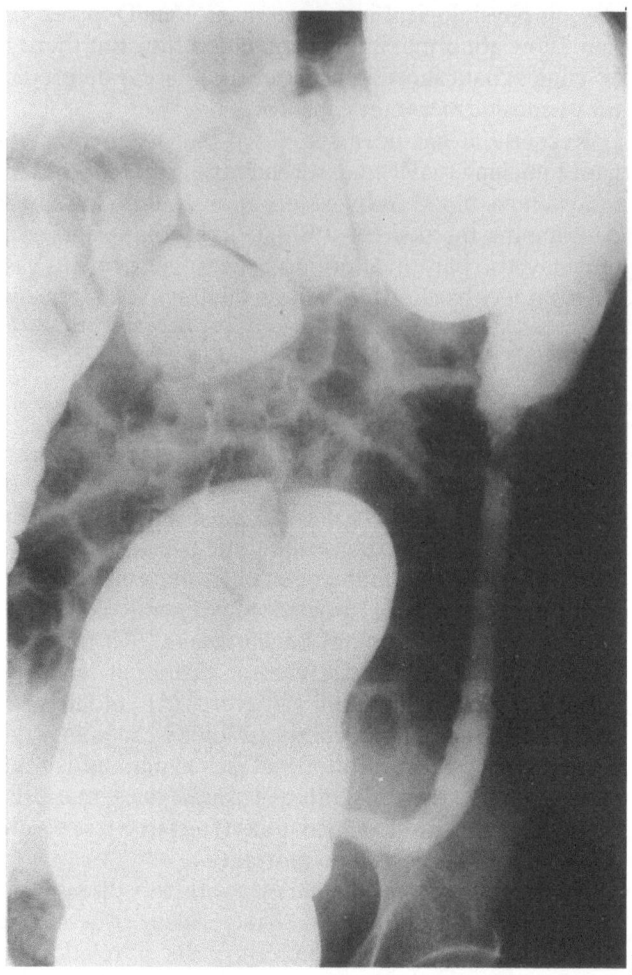

**Fig. 6 a, b.** Patterns of ischaemic colitis in two different patients. **a** Typical thumbprinting of the splenic flexure. **b** Segmental tubular narrowing of the descending colon

sient or persistent, and may be clinically silent or produce progressive bowel obstruction. In the remaining one third, signs and symptoms of an intra-abdominal catastrophe such as gangrene (with or without perforation) occur.

Sonography or CT may demonstrate aspecific thickening of the colonic wall as well as the segmental distribution of the involvement and, consequently, may be useful prior to colonoscopy or barium enema when colonic ischaemia is not suspected clinically (Figs. 7, 8). Doppler studies are usually normal because at the time of the examination the period of ischaemia has passed and blood flow to the affected segment has returned to normal. Angiography seldom shows significant occlusions or other abnormalities and is rarely (after aortic surgery) indicated in patients with colonic ischaemia.

**Diagnosis and Differential Diagnosis**

In patients who are acutely ill with abdominal pain and distention, colonic ischaemia must be differentiated from acute mesenteric ischaemia. Rectal bleeding due to

colonic ischaemia must be distinguished from bleeding due to diverticulosis, vascular ectasias and neoplasm. The new onset of colitic symptoms in an elderly patient is likely to be due to colonic ischaemia, but infectious colitis and inflammatory bowel disease must also be excluded.

A combination of roentgenographic (if necessary serial contrast enemas), colonoscopic and clinical findings may be necessary to establish the diagnosis of colonic ischaemia. In fact, persistence of thumbprints on serial barium studies suggests a diagnosis other than colonic ischaemia, such as carcinoma, lymphoma or amyloidosis. Thus, sequential barium enemas or colonoscopy together with observation of the clinical course are necessary to confirm the diagnosis of colonic ischaemia and to determine the outcome of the ischaemic injury.

Roentgenographic findings of universal colonic involvement, loss of haustrations, or pseudopolyposis occur with colonic ischaemia but are more typical of chronic idiopathic ulcerative colitis. The presence of multiple skip lesions, linear ulcerations or fistulas suggests Crohn's disease.

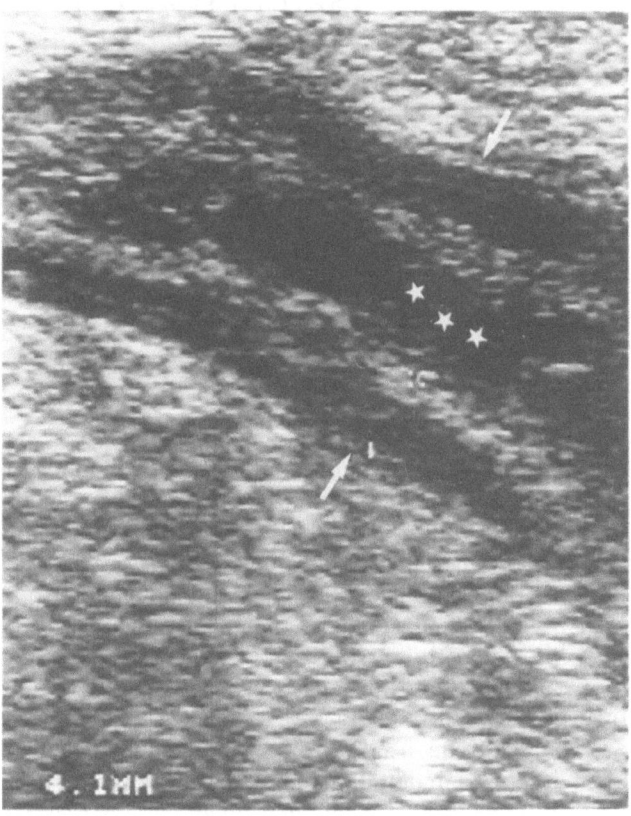

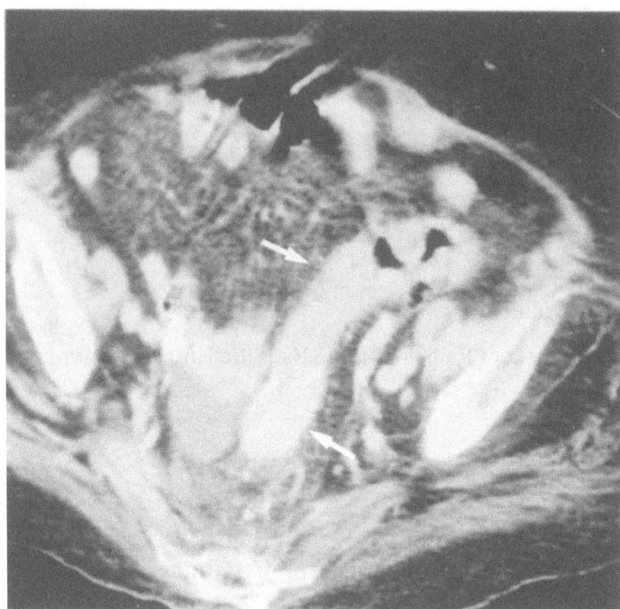

**Fig. 8.** Contrast-enhanced computed tomography shows concentric wall thickening of the sigmoid colon with hypodense enhancement of the submucosa (*arrows*)

**Fig. 7.** Abdominal sonography shows concentric wall thickening of the descending colon (between *arrows* and *stars*)

## Selected References

*Acute mesenteric ischaemia and infarction*

1. Lund EC, Han SY, Holley HC, Berland LI (1985) Intestinal ischemia,. comparison of plain radiographic and computed tomographic finding. Radiographics 8: 1083-1108
2. Kalga RN, Sammartano RJ, Boley SJ (1992) Aggressive approach to acute mesenteric ischaemia. Surg Clin North Am 72: 157-182
3. Klein HM, Lensing R, Klosterhalgen B, Töns C, Gunther RW (1995) Diagnostic imaging of mesenteric infarction. Radiology 197: 79-82
4. Danse EM, Van Beers BE, Goffette P, Dardenne AN, Laterre PF, Pringot J (1996) Acute intestinal ischaemia due to occlusion of the superior mesenteric artery: detection with Doppler sonography. Ultrasound (in press)
5. Rahmouni A., Mathieu D, Golli M, Douek P, Anglade MC, Caillet H, Vasile N (1992) Value of CT and sonography in the conservative management of acute splenoportal and superior mesenteric venous thrombosis. Gastrointest Radiol 17: 135-140

6. Pringot J, Bodart P (1989) Segmental ischaemia of the small bowel. In: Margulis AR, Burhenne HJ (eds) Alimentary tract radiology, vol 1, 4th edn. Mosby St, Louis, pp 800-806

*Chronic mesenteric ischaemia*

7. Scholz FJ (1993) Ischemic bowel disease. Radiol Clin North Am 31: 1208-1211
8. Li KCP, Whitney WS, McDonnell CH, Fredrickson JO, Pelc NJ, Dalman RL, Brooke Jeffrey R (1994) Chronic mesenteric ischaemia: evaluation with phase-contrast cine MR imaging. Radiology 190: 175-179

*Colonic ischaemia*

9. Pringot J, Goncette L, Gilbeau JP, Bodart P (1978) Plain film and contrast enema in ischemia of the colon. J Belg Radiol 61: 253-259
10. Brandt L, Boley S, Kauvar DJ (1992) Colonic ischaemia. In: Winaver SJ (ed) Management of gastrointestinal disease. Gower, New York, pp 2302-2315
11. Iida M, Matsui T, Fuchigami T, Iwashita A., Yao T, Fujishima M (1986) Ischemic colitis serial changes in double-contrast barium enema examination. Radiology 159: 337-341
12. Philpotts LE, Heiken JP, Westcott MA, Gore RM (1994) Colitis: use of CT findings in differential diagnosis. Radiology 190: 445-449

# Disorders of the Small Intestine

D.J. Nolan

Department of Radiology, John Radcliffe Hospital, Oxford OX3 9DU, UK

## Introduction

An increasing number of radiologists use enteroclysis as the technique of choice for examining the small intestine. During enteroclysis the barium suspension is introduced directly into the small intestine through a duodenal tube. This permits a large volume of the barium contrast medium to fill the intestine. The intestinal distension obtained with enteroclysis makes it easier to identify any abnormality that is present. Enteroclysis is accurate at identifying morphological abnormalities with a sensitivity of 93.1% and a specificity of 96.9% [1].

The 10- or 12-Fr gauge radiopaque tube is passed via the nose to the stomach and manipulated through the pylorus and duodenum so that the tip lies in the distal duodenum or proximal jejunum. The barium suspension, diluted to 18%-20% weight/volume is infused at about 75 ml per minute. Radiographs (Fig. 1) are taken at high kilovoltage (110-120 kV). Compression is applied to separate the intestinal loops and spot views are taken of the terminal ileum, pelvic loops of ileum and any other segments that require further evaluation.

The technique used by the author has previously been described in detail [2] and is similar to the method devised by Sellink. The radiologist can quickly become skilled at performing and interpreting enteroclysis. When a 10-Fr tube is used most patients experience only minor discomfort [3]. The radiation dose to the patient during enteroclysis is similar to that of other barium examinations.

## The Abnormal Intestine

Crohn's disease is the most common disorder of the small intestine. A combination of different radiological signs is seen in most patients [4]. The radiological signs of Crohn's disease include fissure ulcers, discrete ulcers, longitudinal ulcers, sinuses and fistulae. Long longitudinal ulcers are seen on the mesenteric borders of the distal ileum and, although an uncommon finding, are characteristic of Crohn's disease. The distal ileum and ileum at ileocolic anastomosis sites are the usual location of fissure ulcers, sinuses and fistulae. Fistulae pass from the diseased intestine to adjacent loops of small intestine, colon, urinary bladder and occasionally to the skin or vagina.

Dilute barium is ideal for outlining fissure ulcers, sinuses and fistulae. Cobblestoning is a frequent and characteristic appearance seen in Crohn's disease and mostly results from a combination of longitudinal and transverse ulceration (Fig. 2). Narrowing of the lumen is common, frequently resulting in stricture formation. Strictures may be single or multiple and often cause some degree of obstruction, indicated by proximal di-

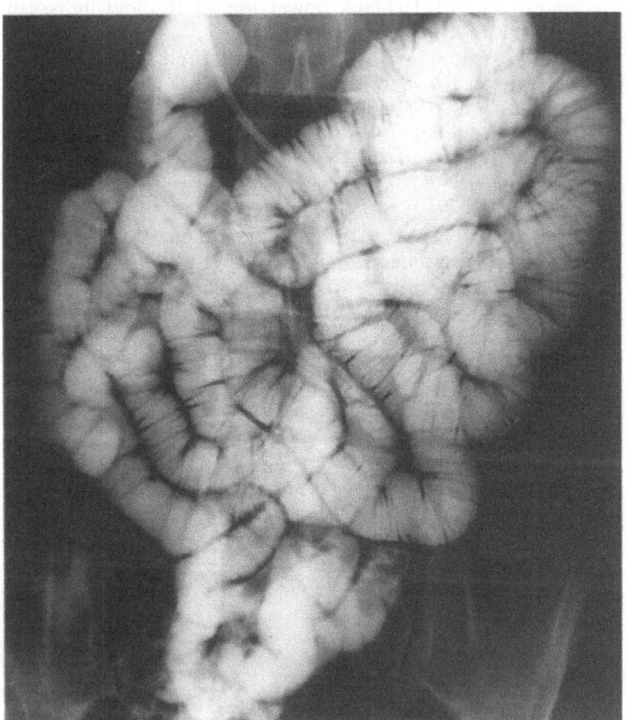

**Fig. 1.** Enteroclysis examination showing normal small intestine outlined with barium suspension

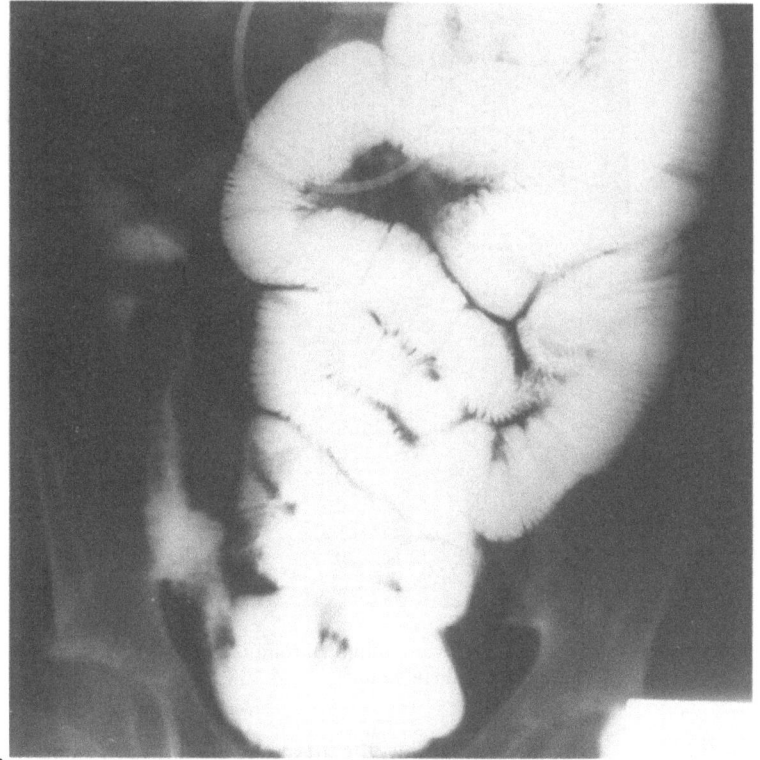

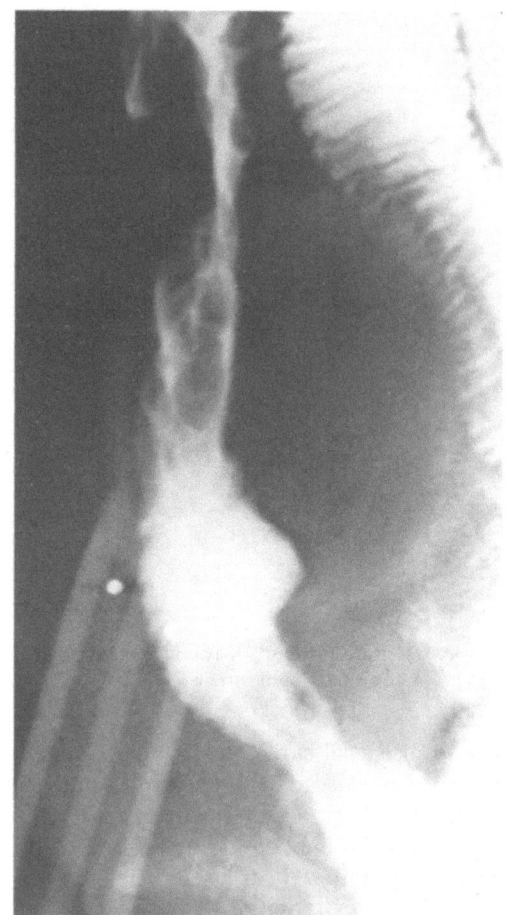

a

b

**Fig. 2 a, b.** Ileal Crohn's disease. **a** All the small intestine is outlined with barium. There is an irregular stricture of the terminal ileum causing some degree of obstruction. **b** A spot view of the terminal ileum showing the tight stricture at the distal end and cobblestoning in the more proximal part

latation of the intestine. Other signs include thickening and distortion of the valvulae conniventes and evidence of discontinuity of the disease process, as shown by asymmetrical involvement and skip lesions. Pseudodiverticula are characteristically seen in segments of asymmetrical involvement.

Neoplasms are uncommon in the small intestine and as a result malignant neoplasms are often detected at a late stage. Enteroclysis is proving to be a reliable method for detecting primary neoplasms. Neoplasms present with nonspecific symptoms such as abdominal pain, gastrointestinal bleeding, intestinal obstruction and intussusception.

Leiomyomas are the most frequently encountered benign neoplasm. They mostly present with acute bleeding. Leiomyomas may grow into the intestinal lumen or they may grow outwards. Intraluminal leiomyomas are mostly seen radiologically as a round intraluminal filling defect, whereas a serosal neoplasm is seen as a mass on the serosal surface displacing adjacent loops of intestine. Lipomas rarely cause symptoms and are shown as intramural or submucosal lesions. Hamartomas are a developmental anomaly and are present in large numbers in the Peutz-Jeghers syndrome. Adenomatous polyps are uncommon and rarely cause symptoms. They are seen at enteroclysis as small sessile or pedunculated filling defects.

The most frequently encountered malignant neoplasms are carcinoma, carcinoid tumours, lymphoma and leiomyosarcoma. Primary carcinomas are mostly seen in the jejunum and the radiological features are similar to those of carcinoma of the colon, characteristically shown as stricture formation with mucosal destruction and shouldered margin, a polypoid mass or an ulcerating lesion [5]. Carcinoid tumours are usually located in the ileum, particularly the distal ileum, and are mostly seen as single or multiple small intramural or intraluminal filling defects (Fig. 3) [6]. They occasionally present as strictures. There may be extensive mesenteric fibrosis at the time of presentation compressing adjacent loops of intestine and making it impossible to identify the primary tumours. Lymphomas are mostly seen in the ileum, are frequently multiple and have a variety of radiological appearance, including strictures with characteristic signs of malignancy, mass lesions with broad-based ulceration or cavitation, and sometimes polypoid lesions [7]. The highly characteristic aneurysmal dilatation is a very occasional finding. Leiomyosarcoma is less frequently seen and is usually shown as a large mass with a central cavity outlined by barium.

Secondary neoplasms may involve the intestine by directly invading from adjacent organs, lymphatic extension, peritoneal seeding and embolic metastases [8].

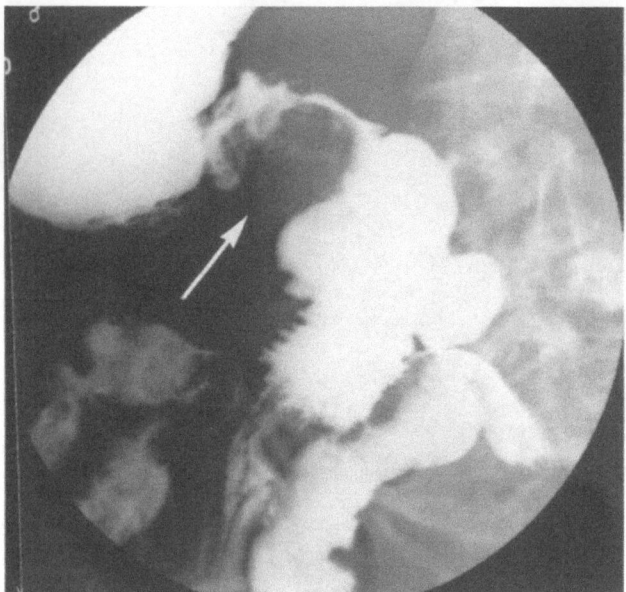

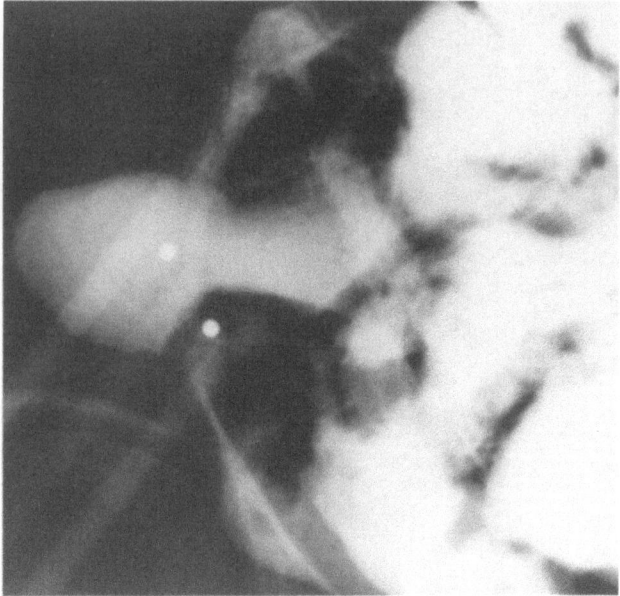

**Fig. 3.** Carcinoid tumour. A round intramural filling defect is seen in the terminal ileum (*arrow*)

**Fig. 4.** Meckel's diverticulum. Barium is seen outlining a blind-ending sac in the distal ileum

Spread of caecal carcinoma to the terminal ileum, frequently shown as an ileal stricture, is an example of lymphatic spread. Blood-bourne metastases are uncommon, with metastatic melanoma being one of the most frequently encountered. Metastatic melanoma may present as a solitary cavitating mass or single or multiple small nodules.

Chronic radiation enteritis is an uncommon complication of abdominal radiotherapy and mostly involves the pelvic loops of ileum. The patient can develop symptoms of chronic radiation damage to the small intestine any time from the end of treatment up to 25 years later. The characteristic radiological appearances include thickening of the valvulae conniventes, strictures, mural

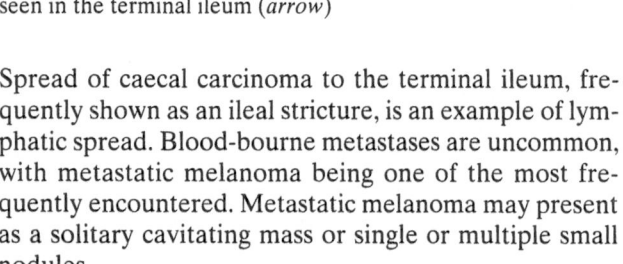

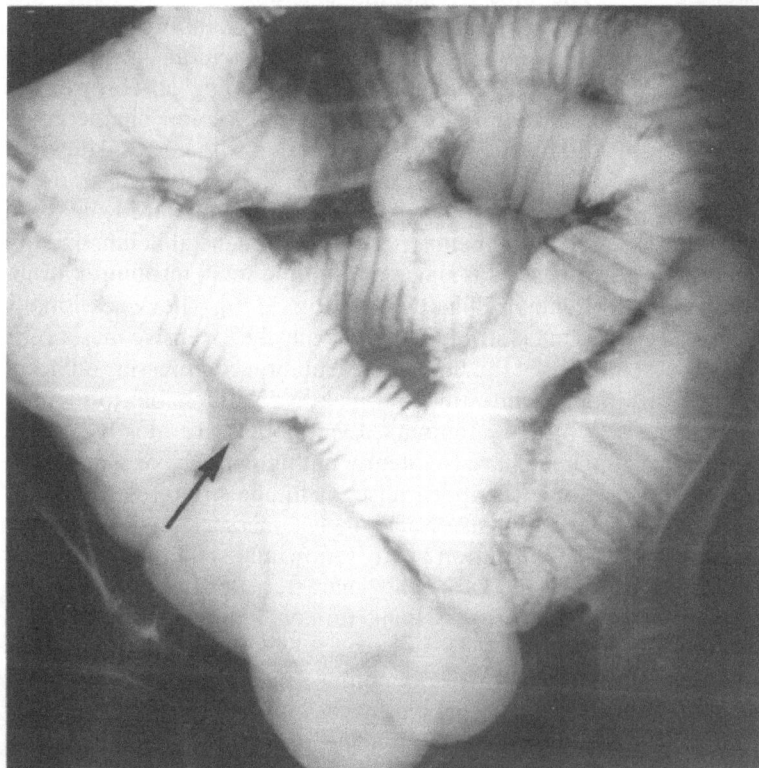

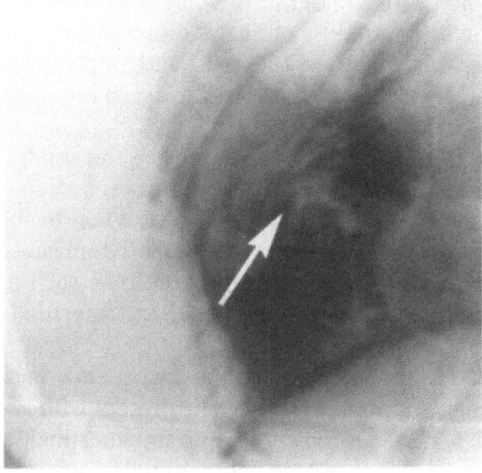

**Fig. 5.** Intestinal obstruction due to adhesions.
**a** Small intestine is dilated throughout most of its length. An apparent area of narrowing is noted in a segment overlying the right sacroiliac joint (*arrow*). **b** A spot compression view shows the acute transition from dilated intestine to collapsed loops (*arrow*). Only a small amount of barium is passing through this narrowing

thickening, mucosal tacking, adhesions and effacement of the mucosal pattern [9].

Intestinal tuberculosis is rare in Europe. The distal ileum is the most frequent site of involvement and in many cases is seen on barium studies as a tight stricture of the terminal ileum causing obstruction. There is often distortion of the ileocaecal junction and contraction of the caecum. In some cases multiple ileal strictures are seen. The appearances of intestinal tuberculosis may be indistinguishable from Crohn's disease.

Diverticula are an uncommon finding in the small intestine. Jejunal diverticulosis is an acquired disorder and may present with malabsorption and megaloblastic anaemia. Jejunal diverticula are shown on barium studies as large outpouchings from the jejunum. Meckel's diverticulum is a developmental anomaly and is present in about 1%-2% of the population. Complications include bleeding and intestinal obstruction. Radiologically, Meckel's diverticulum is seen as a blind-ending sac, varying considerably in size and shape, arising from the antimesenteric border of the ileum (Fig. 4). Acquired ileal diverticula are few in number and are seen as small outpouchings arising from the terminal ileum.

Progressive systemic sclerosis (scleroderma) may involve the small intestine. Dilatation, diminished peristalsis, wide-necked sacculations and the characteristic 'hidebound' appearances are well shown on enteroclysis [10].

Other disorders that may be shown well on enteroclysis include intestinal ischaemia, intramural haemorrhage, nonsteroidal antiinflammatory drug (NSAID) enteropathy, intestinal lymphangistasia and Whipple's disease.

Enteroclysis can play a valuable role in suspected intestinal obstruction when plain radiographs are inconclusive or further information is required about the site or cause of obstruction. Barium is safe to use in patients with small intestinal obstruction. The obstruction site is identified by the sharp transition in calibre between distended proximal intestine and the distal collapsed loops (Fig. 5). The cause of the obstruction may be obvious from the appearances of the obstructing lesion. In closed-loop obstruction, the closed-loop may be outlined with barium, prompting urgent surgical treatment [11]. Enteroclysis is useful in the postoperative period for differentiating obstruction from ileus.

## Conclusion

It is important for the radiologist to know how to perform enteroclysis as it is an excellent technique for showing the characteristic appearances of morphological disorders of the small intestine. By adopting the enteroclysis technique the radiologist can play a more constructive and interesting role in evaluating the small intestine.

## References

1. Dixon PM, Roulston ME, Nolan DJ (1993) The small bowel enema: a ten year review. Clin Radiol 47: 46-48
2. Nolan DJ, Cadman PJ (1987) The small bowel enema made easy. Clin Radiol 38: 295-301
3. Traill ZC, Nolan DJ (1995) Technical note: intubation fluoroscopy times using a new enteroclysis tube. Clin Radiol 50: 339-349
4. Nolan DJ, Gourtsoyiannis NC (1980) Crohn's disease of the small intestine: a review of the radiological appearances in 100 consecutive patients examined by a barium infusion technique. Clin Radiol 31: 597-603
5. Papadopoulos VD, Nolan DJ (1985) Carcinoma of the small intestine. Clin Radiol 36: 409-413
6. Jeffree MA, Barter SJ, Hemingway AP, Nolan DJ (1984) Primary carcinoid tumours of the ileum: the radiological appearances. Clin Radiol 35: 451-455
7. Gourtsoyiannis NC, Nolan DJ (1988) Lymphoma of the small intestine: radiological features. Clin Radiol 39: 639-645
8. Meyers MA (1981) Intraperitoneal spread of malignancies and its effect on the bowel. Clin Radiol 32: 129-146
9. Mendelson RM, Nolan DJ (1985) The radiological features of radiation enteritis. Clin Radiol 36: 141-148
10. Nolan DJ (1992) The small intestine. In: Grainger RG, Allison DJ (eds) Diagnostic radiology: an Anglo-American textbook of organ imaging, 2nd edn. Churchill Livingstone, Edinburgh, pp 883-908
11. Maglinte DDT, Herlinger H, Nolan DJ (1991) Radiological features of closed loop obstruction: analysis of 25 confirmed cases. Radiology 179: 383-387

# Defecography in Anorectal Functional Disorders

P. Mahieu

Service de Radiologie et d'Imagerie Médicale, Institut Chirurgical, Marie-Louise Square 59, 1040 Brussels, Belgium

## Introduction

The proper treatment of functional disorders of rectal evacuation requires that the diagnosis is as accurate as possible. To supplement anamnesis and clinical examination, techniques such as anorectal manometry and electromyography have been developed. Radiology makes its contribution through defecography.

As early as 1964, Burhenne emphasized the fact that after the barium enema the evacuation of the contrast material occurs without the radiologist making use of this moment in the examination, which in fact can provide much very useful diagnostic information [1]. Even though some of the first radiologists did study the evacuation of liquid barium [1, 2], there were others who preferred to render the faeces opaque by having their patients eat meals with barium sulphate added for 3 consecutive days [3]. This rather impractical technique was modified by administering a more dense barium mixture to the patients rectally [4]. Radiocinematography was then used as a means of recording [4, 5]. This technique involves the inconvenience of relatively high irradiation and the need for a sophisticated apparatus which is no longer widely available. More recently, two methods of opacification have been developed: balloon proctography [6] and defecography [7-10].

## Method

### Technique

The anorectal system is made opaque before both the static and the dynamic examination.

Defecography [7-10] begins with opacification of the rectum with a paste composed of a mixture of liquid barium and potato starch. After heating, this mixture forms a paste with the usual semisolid consistency of the faeces. A volume of about 250 ml of this paste is introduced into the rectum by means of an injector. To make the anal canal opaque the paste is continuously injected while the extremity of the injector is progressively drawn out through the anus. For improved coating and for a sharper outline of the rectal mucosa, a concentrated suspension of barium is injected into the rectum before the paste. In order to improve the quality of the radiographs, a special seat, conceived and utilized since 1978 [7], permits the collection of the contrast material evacuated during the examination. This seat is composed of a set of superposed air chambers, filled with water and connected with one another by a plexiglass cylinder. The central orifice is equipped with a disposable plastic bag, which is thrown away immediately after the examination. Thus the procedure can take place in hygienic conditions, completely acceptable both for the patient and the medical staff.

### Static Examination

Thanks to the technique described, it is possible to carry out a static examination in profile with the patient in a sitting position. The static examination aims essentially at determining the position of the anorectal junction in relation to the pubococcygeal line, the anorectal angle (ARA) at rest and the behaviour of the anal sphincter, also at rest.

The pubococcygeal line has most often been described as the line connecting the anterior and superior edges of the pubic symphysis to the distal end of the coccyx [11]. The length of a perpendicular line beginning at the pubococcygeal line and descending to the anorectal junction provides a measure of the pelvic floor descent at rest. Measurement of the same line during straining and the difference between the length of the lines during straining and at rest yields the pelvic floor descent during straining.

Evaluation of the ARA provides a good measure of the tonic activity of the puborectal muscle. This muscle forms a sling, attaching at the level of the pubic symphysis and supporting the anorectal junction posteriorly. This muscle is tonically contracted at rest and induces an angulation, the ARA, between the axis of the anal canal and the axis of the rectum, which is taken to be the line

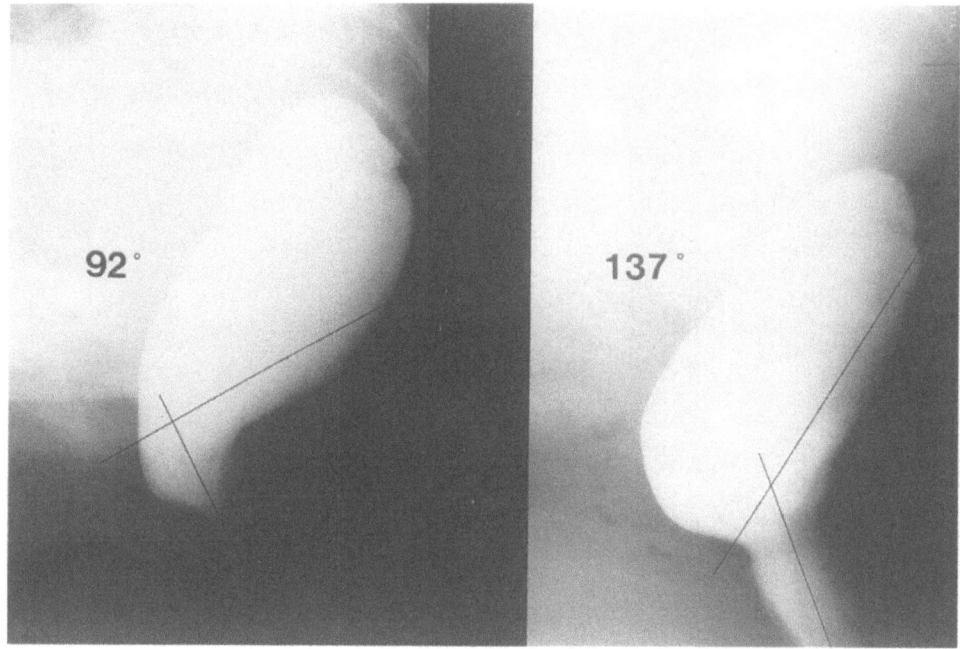

**Fig. 1.** Normal anorectal angle. The mean value is 92° at rest (*left*) and 137° (*right*) if the axis of the rectum is drawn as a line tangential to the posterior aspect of the distal part of the rectal ampulla. The width of the anal canal can be measured during evacuation (*right*)

tangential to the posterior edge of the distal part of the rectal ampulla (Fig. 1).

The important role of the puborectal muscle in anal continence, described by Parks et al. [11], is based on the flap valve mechanism: at rest, the muscle is contracted and allows the anterior distal rectal aspect to take up a position opposite to the internal end of the anal canal, rather like a lid. Any increase in abdominal pressure reinforces the efficiency of the lid. When the puborectal muscle relaxes, which normally occurs during voluntary straining, the ARA opens, the valve phenomenon can no longer take place and the rectum can be emptied due to increased abdominal pressure. The valve phenomenon must be considered together with the complementary role of the anal sphincter itself in order to fully explain faecal continence.

The behaviour of the anal sphincter at rest and during strain can be evaluated by measuring the width of the anal opening, which is an indirect indication of its muscular tonicity or relaxation (Fig. 1).

### Dynamic Examination

The dynamic study is an essential part of the overall examination because it can reveal the functional anomalies of the anorectal system during and at the end of evacuation. It appraises not only the movements of the rectum and of the anal canal, but also the speed of rectal evacuation, the significance of any possible residue, the value of the ARA during the process of emptying, the degree of resistance offered by the muscular pelvic floor to the pressure produced to obtain rectal evacuation and the width of opening of the anal canal.

## Results

### Static Examination

*Pubococcygeal Line and Pelvic Floor Descent*

When Parks described the syndrome of the descending perineum [11], he made the measurements on patients reclining in a left lateral position. This seems less physiological than the sitting position, as in lateral position the pelvic floor is not under pressure. Furthermore, the left lateral reclining position does not facilitate rectal evacuation.

On average, the normal pelvic floor does not descend more than 3.5 cm during straining compared with its position at rest [12]. This value is thus taken as the maximum normal limit for pelvic floor descent during straining. In our experience, the normal value of the pelvic floor descent at rest is 8.5 cm [13].

*Anorectal Angle*

The value of the ARA at rest has been described as varying from 60° to 105° [14]. Our personal series [8, 9] indicated a mean ARA of 92° in a group of 56 patients at rest. In the same normal group, the mean ARA during straining was 137° (Fig. 1). An increase of the ARA at rest is observed in incontinence. In a group of 19 incontinent patients, the mean ARA was 130° at rest, 38° more than in the normal patients [9]. However, the existence of an external rectal prolapse or of an intra-anal rectal intussusception is also associated with a significant increase of the ARA at rest [10].

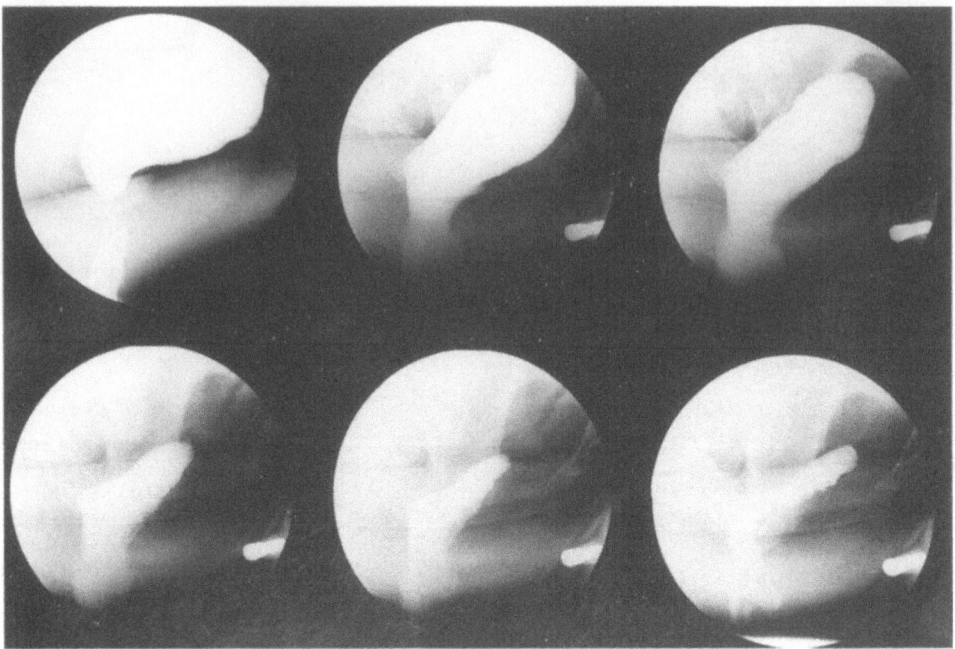

**Fig. 2.** Normal defecogram shows increase of the anorectal angle, attenuation of the imprint due to the puborectal muscle, broad opening of the anal canal, emptying of the rectal lumen and short descent of the pelvic floor

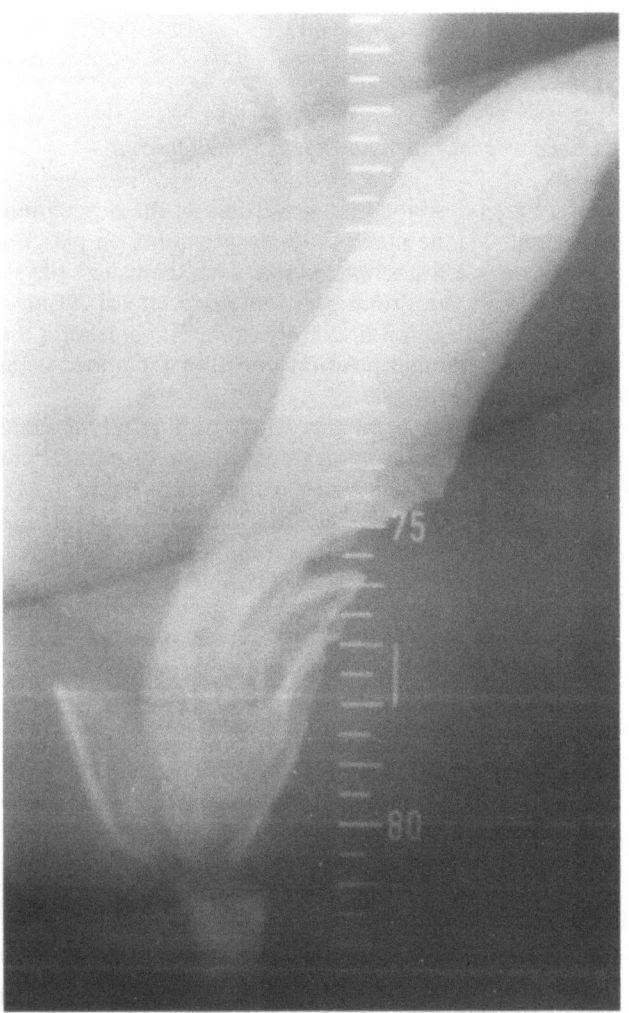

**Fig. 3.** Circumferential rectal intussusception

### Anal Sphincter

The behaviour of the anal sphincter can be roughly appraised on the basis of its width. In incontinence, the anal canal can be visualized at rest, wider than normal.

## Dynamic Examination

### Normal Defecogram

During rectal evacuation, the following signs are consistently observed in normal patients and can be taken as the criteria for a normal defecogram: an increase in the ARA, on average from 92° to 137°; diminution of the imprint left by the puborectal muscle at the level of the posterior aspect of the anorectal junction; broad opening of the anal canal; complete or practically complete emptying of the rectum; and appropriate resistance by the pelvic floor to the forces exerted to achieve the evacuation of the rectal contents [9] (Fig. 2).

### Main Radiologically Detectable Disorders of Rectal Evacuation

*Intussusception and Prolapse of Rectum.* According to some authors [5], complete rectal prolapse only constitutes the end point, the last degree of severity, of the phenomenon of invagination of the rectal wall. In our opinion, different stages can be distinguished. Simple rectal intussusception corresponds to simple invagination of the rectal wall. This invagination is identified radiologically by the development of a fold which is either lateral, most often anterolateral [10], or circumferential right from the outset. The fold becomes progressively

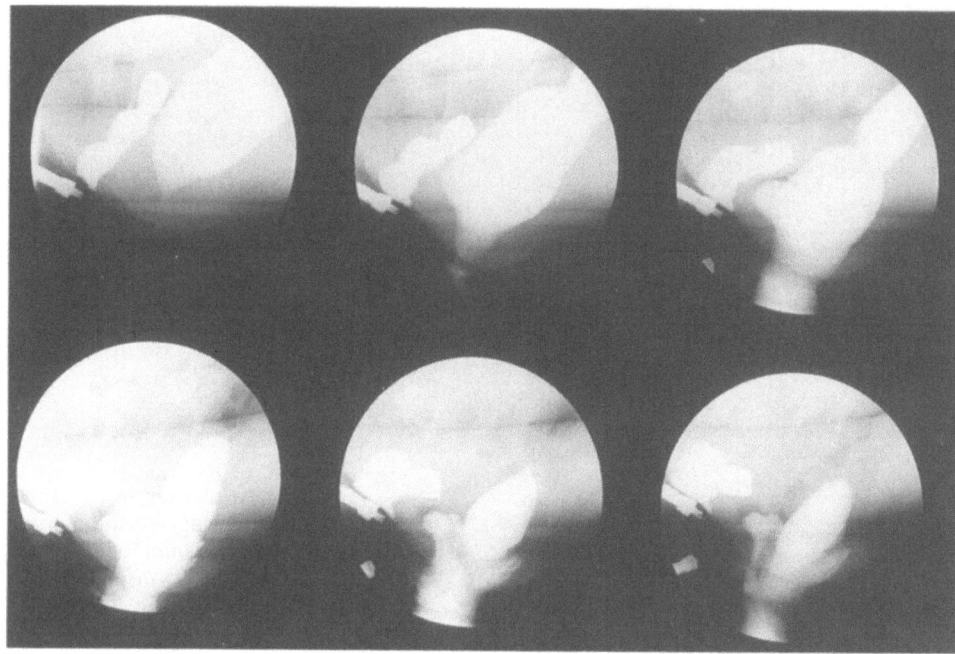

**Fig. 4.** Association of rectal intussusception and rectocoele

accentuated and constitutes the starting point for an invagination which remains localized in the rectal lumen
(Figs. 3; see also Fig. 6). In rectal intra-anal intussusception the invagination goes beyond the internal anal margin and extrudes into the anal canal without exterioriz-
ing (Fig. 4). Finally, external rectal prolapse consists of
the exteriorization of the invagination through the anal
canal (Fig. 5). This exteriorization may be spontaneously reversible, the prolapse shrinking as soon as the
straining stops, or manual intervention in the patient
may be necessary after the emptying of the rectum.

*Rectocoele.* Radiologically, a rectocoele is seen as a
bulging of the anterior rectal wall and of the rectovaginal
septum under the abdominal pressure which pushes the
fecal bolus forward (Fig. 5, top right view). This bulging
creates an anterior rectal sacculation in which contrast
medium is sequestred while the rest of the rectal lumen is
evacuated. As soon as the straining ceases, the elasticity of
the rectal walls leads the opaque sequestrum back to the
rectal lumen. The persistence of a rectal residue then
causes a new urge to evacuate a short time after the first
evacuation.

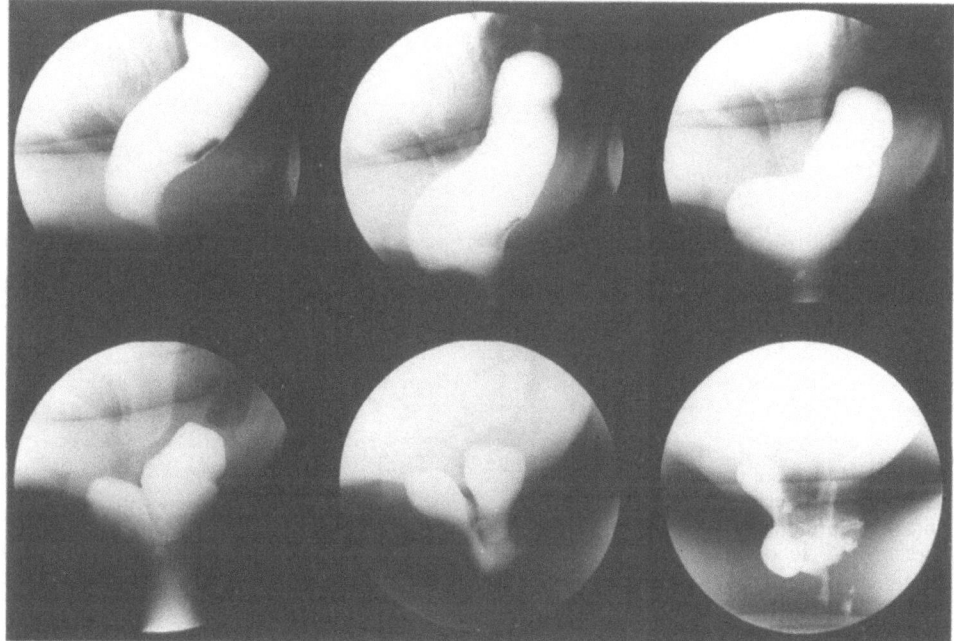

**Fig. 5.** Circumferential intra-
rectal intussusception. The an-
nular fold created by the rectal
invagination penetrates into
the anal lumen at the end of
evacuation

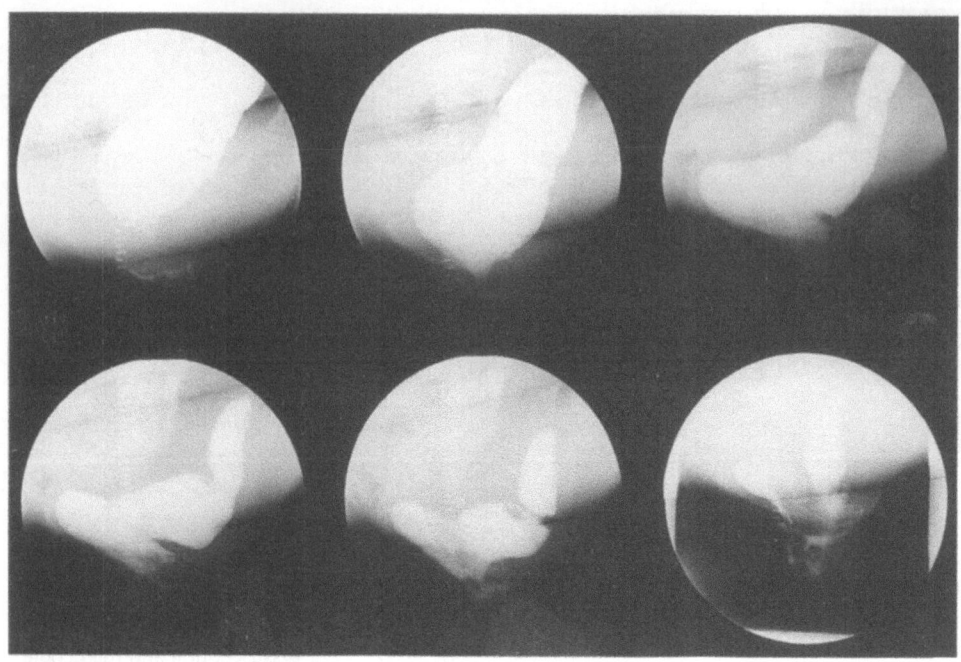

**Fig. 6.** External rectal prolapse. An anterior rectal intussusception passes through the anal canal and produces a rectal external evagination hanging under the anus. Note the associated rectocoele appearing on the third image

*Association of Intussusception and Rectocoele.* A rectocoele is often associated with a discrete anterior rectal intussusception. More rarely, it may be associated with a circumferential intussusception (Fig. 4). It is, moreover, conceivable that this image simply corresponds to a mucous prolapse rather than to a true intussusception affecting the entire thickness of the rectal wall.

*Dyskinesia of the Puborectal Muscle.* Dystinesia of the puborectal muscle most often consists in a hypertonia which can be intermittent or constant during the entire period of straining. It appears radiologically as an accentuation of the posterior impression at the level of the anorectal junction and as an absence of increasing, or even a diminution, of the value of the ARA during straining (Fig. 7). This hypertonia constitutes an obstacle to normal rectal evacuation, which leads to a more intense and prolonged straining despite the resistance linked to the abnormal contraction of the puborectal muscle. Some authors [15] regard this as the probable origin of the solitary rectal ulcer syndrome. In a personal series of 43 patients presenting with a solitary rectal ulcer, we found only four cases of functional disorders of the puborectal muscle in the form of hypertonia, but 19

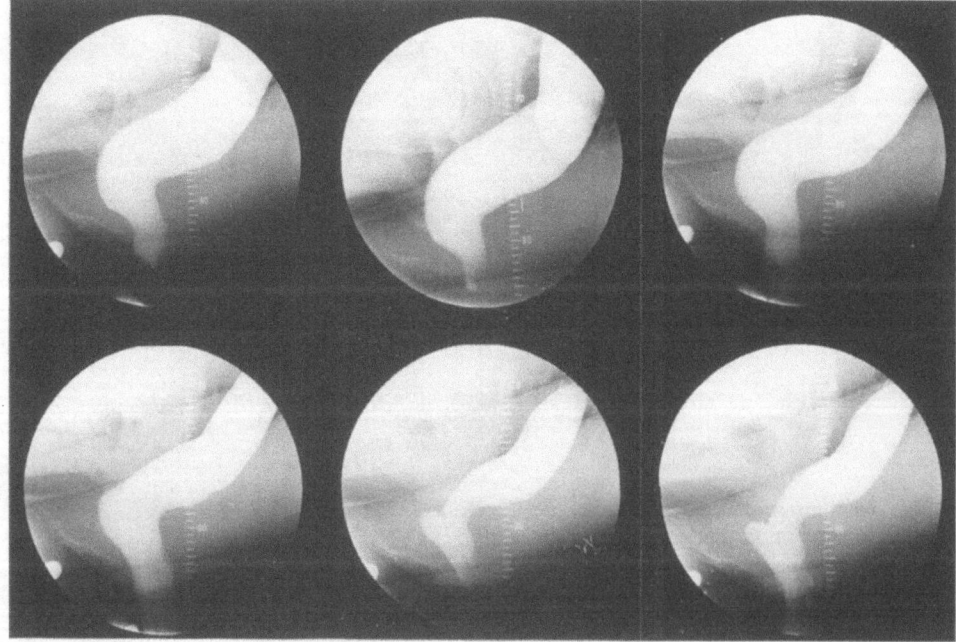

**Fig. 7.** Dyskinesia of the puborectal muscle. During evacuation, the imprint due to the puborectal muscle decreases at the first stage (*second image*) and then increases suddenly, altering the rectal evacuation

external rectal prolapses, five rectal intussusceptions and 5 intra-anal rectal intussusceptions [16].

*Descending Perineum.* Pelvic floor descent of a value above 3.5 cm during straining seems to be pathological [12]. This abnormal descent of the pelvic floor during straining is usually observed in patients presenting with the syndrome of the descending perineum [11].

## Conclusion

Defecography is a practical routine investigative procedure – probably even more so in specialized units – for the detection of intussusception and rectal prolapse, rectocoele, dysfunction of the puborectal muscle and syndromes of the descending perineum and solitary rectal ulcer. It allows the clinician to make a choice between medical and surgical treatment and can also play a role in the monitoring of the surgical treatment and in the long-term evaluation of its efficacy.

## References

1. Burhenne HJ (1964) Intestinal evacuation study: a new roentgenologic technique. Radiol Clin (Basel) 33: 79-84
2. Brown B (1965) Defecography or anorectal studies in children including cinefluorographic observation. J Can Assoc Radiol 16: 66-76
3. Phillips SF, Edwards DAW (1965) Some aspects of anal continence and defecation. Gut 6: 396-405
4. Kerremans R (1969) Morphological and physiological aspects of anal continence and defecation. Arscia, Brussels
5. Broden B, Snellman B (1968) Procidentia of the rectum studied with cineradiography: a contribution to the discussion of causative mechanism. Dis Colon Rectum 11: 330-347
6. Preston DM, Lennard-Jones JE, Thomas BM (1982) The balloon proctogram. Br J Surg 71: 29-32
7. Mahieu P, Pringot J, Vanheuverzwyn R, Goncette L (1981) Les prolapsus du rectum: apport du lavement baryté et de la défécographie. Acta Gastroenterol Belg 44: 501-512
8. Mahieu P (1983) La Défécographie. Description d'une technique simplifiée et apport diagnostique. Ann Gastroentérol Hepatol (Paris) 19: 345-350
9. Mahieu P, Pringot J, Bodart P (1984) Defecography: I. Description of a new procedure and results in normal patients. Gastrointest Radiol 9: 247-251
10. Mahieu P, Pringot J, Bodart P (1984) Defecography: II. Contribution to the diagnosis of defecation disorders. Gastrointest Radiol 9: 253-261
11. Parks AG, Porter NH, Hardcastle JD (1966) The syndrome of the descending perineum. Proc R Soc Med 9: 477-482
12. Mahieu PHG (1987) Defecography in ano-rectal defecation disorders. In: Cola B, Morganti I (eds) Advances in coloproctology. Monduzzi, Bologna, pp 743-747
13. Bartram Cl, Mahieu P. Radiology of the pelvic floor. In: Henry M, Swash M (eds) Proctology and the pelvic floor. Butterworths, London, pp 151-186
14. Hardcastle JD, Parks AG (1970) A study of anal incontinence and some principles of surgical treatment. Proc R Soc Med 63: 116-118
15. Rutter KPR, Riddell RH (1975) The solitary ulcer syndrome of the rectum. Clin Gastroenterol 4: 505-530
16. Mahieu PHG (1986) Barium enema and defaecography in the diagnosis and evaluation of the solitary ulcer syndrome. Int J Colorect Dis 1: 85-90

# Imaging of Focal Lesions of the Liver: Ultrasonography, Computed Tomography and Magnetic Resonance Imaging

M. Lüning

Am Oskar-Ziethen-Krankenhaus, Fanningerstrasse 32, 10365 Berlin, Germany

## Introduction

There are the three main goals in the diagnosis of focal liver lesions: detection, evaluation of localization and extension and characterization. The rapid development of the three cross-sectional imaging procedures in recent years has significantly influenced the reliability of diagnostic accuracy concerning all these aspects. Unfortunately, a defintive diagnostic decision frequently cannot be made by only one of the methods; a combined application is needed in most cases.

This chapter will concentrate on the different techniques and on the characterization of the most common benign tumours as well of hepatocellular carcinoma (HCC) as the most common malignant lesion of the liver. The description of the pathological findings is based to a great degree on publications by C. Powers and P. R. Ros [1].

## Modalities

### Sonography

Sonography is widely available, inexpensive and a sensitive method for the detection of liver lesions. Depending on the patients' condition and the localization of the region of interest, the highest frequency transducer (usually 3 MHz) has to be used. Because of small acoustic windows (subcostal, intercostal) a sector scanner is preferred to a linear scanner.

Colour Doppler imaging does not only provide information on the direction of blood flow and flow rates, it may also give insight into the vascularization of the different hepatic tumours [2]. Sonography with intraarterial infusion of microbubbles, the combination of sonography and angiography, is an invasive procedure for the differentiation of liver masses but seems to be promising [3].

### Computed Tomography

There are different techniques used for detection and characterization of focal liver lesions. Unenhanced computed tomography (CT) should always be the first step in examination. However, its sensitivity is only about 50%. By intravenous injection of water-soluble contrast material, the contrast between hepatic lesion and parenchyma is increased; local blood supply and especially the vascularization of the liver tumours is reflected [4].

### Contrast CT

Regarding dosage of contrast medium (CM), timing and image acquisition, different techniques are used for contrast enhancement on the liver, depending on the diagnostic goal.

### Screening of Liver Masses

- Incremental dynamic CT.
  Variant 1: Administration of CM in a biphasic mode. Short bolus of 50 ml at 5 ml/s and subsequently infusion of 120 ml at 1 ml/s.
  Variant 2: Administration of CM in 2 uniphasic mode. Bolus of 120 - 150 ml at 2 - 3 ml/s.
  Start of image acquisition 45 s after beginning of injection with 8- to 10-mm scans continuously through the entire liver [4].
- Dynamic CT arterial portography. Tip of catheter at the proximal superior mesenteric or splenic artery. Administration of 100-200 ml CM at 2-3 ml/s. Start of image acquisition 5-10 Hz after injection (portal phase). Incremental techniques.
- Dynamic CT hepatic arteriography. Tip of catheter at the proper hepatic artery distal to the gastroduodenal artery. Multiple boluses of 7-10 ml at 2 ml/s. Incremental technique.
- Delayed iodine scanning. Image acquisition 4-6 h after injection of CM (minimum 60 g).
  With all these incremental techniques, the entire liver can be viewed by uni- and biphasic spiral scanning in about 10-20 s.

## Characterization of Liver Masses

– Single level dynamlc CT. Selection of a region of interest (focal lesion). Administration of 60-100 ml CM at 5-8 ml/s. Start of image acquisition 13-15 s after injection (4-6 scans/min during the first 2 min, one image after 3, 4 and 5 min).

## Magnetic Resonance Imaging

The nature and quality of magnetic resonance imaging (MRI) depend very strongly on a multiplicity of different parameters. Spin echo pulse sequences are most widely used and are accepted as the standard technique. T1-weighted images (short TR and short TE) provide a good depiction of anatomical details, while the T2-weighted images (long TR and long TE) provide better contrast and therefore are more reliable in lesion detection. Both are essential for the characterization of liver lesions.

The so-called gradient echo technique, with a very short TR and a smaller flip angle, help in reducing acquisition time and motion artefacts (combined with breath-hold technique). Routine transverse MR: 8- to 10-mm slice thickness; 1- to 2-mm interslice spacing.

Paramagnetic contrast agents (e.g. gadolinium-DT-PA) are increasingly being used to characterize liver tumours. The incremental or single level technique is similar to the corresponding CT techniques.

# Hepatic Lesions

## Hepatocellular Adenoma

### Pathological Findings

Hepatocellular adenoma (HCA) is rare benign hepatic tumour. Most are seen in women of child-bearing age, which is linked to oral contraceptives; HCA is rare in men and is related to the use of anabolic steroids. They are 5-8 cm in diameter. In 15%-20% of cases a thin fibrous (peudo-) capsule. Large pericapsular and intratumoral vessels. Tumor composition of fat- and glycogen-rich hepatocytes formed in cords is similar to normal liver. Kupffer cells exist. Paucity of bile dusts and portal tracts. Often haemorrhage (most common histopathologic finding) or infarction [5].

### Imaging Findings

There are only few reports on the diagnostic critera for HCA. Sonographically these tumours, in most cases, are of mixed echogenicity and heterogeneous in texture; sometimes they are hypoechoic, less frequently isoechoic. Areas of hypoechogenicity can be due to haemorrhage. A hypoechoic halo may be detected in very rare cases [6].

On unenhanced CT, adenomas are hypodense or iso-dense because of fat and glycogen contained within the liver. If there is bleeding into the tumour, there are hypodense or hyperdense areas (depending on the age of haemorrhage). After bolus CM administration, there is a distinct and rapid enhancement of the solid tumour compartments, similar to focal nodular hyperplasia (FNH; see below) but with a more prolonged decline. The (pseudo-)capsule sometimes may demonstrate a hyperdense rim on delayed scans.

The appearance of adenomas on MRI is variable. Because of the tumour composition, with cells resembling normal hepatocytes, adenomas and FNH may be isointense or hypointense on T2-weighted images (Fig. 1) and isointense or hyperintense on T1-weighted images. Some of the adenomas are nearly isointense on T1-weighted and T2-weighted images. Hyperintensity on T1-weighted images can be due to fatty infiltration and increased glycogen content. The capsule appears as a hypointense rim. Most adenomas enhance in the arterial phase.

It may be difficult to distinguish HCAs from HCC because there may be (pseudo-)capsule necrosis and haemorrhage in both [7]. Heterogeneity of signal helps to differentiate HCA from FNH [5].

## Focal Nodular Hyperplasia

### Pathological Findings

FNH is a tumour-like formation, perhaps a response to arteriovenous malformation It is the second-most common benign tumour found predominantly in the third to fifth decades of life, more frequently in women. It is usually smaller than 5 cm and solitary. Sometimes giant tumours replace an entire lobe of the liver, and pedunculation is not a rare occurrence.

FNH consists of nodules from hyperplastic hepatocytes, small bile ducts, fibrous bands, vessels and Kupffer

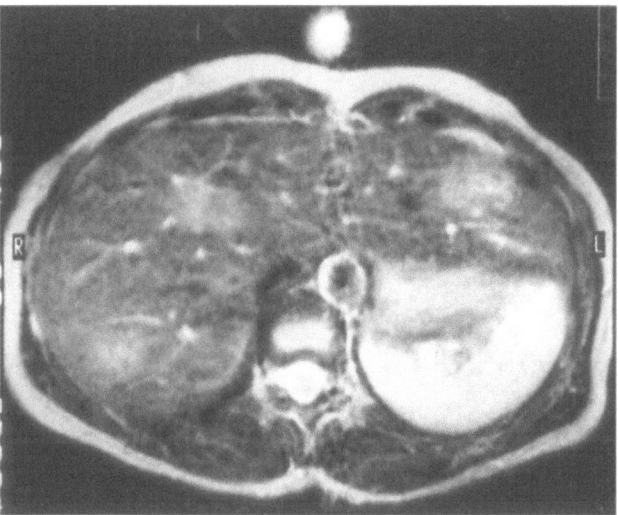

**Fig. 1.** Uncharacteristic features of three hepatocellular adenomas on T2-weighted image

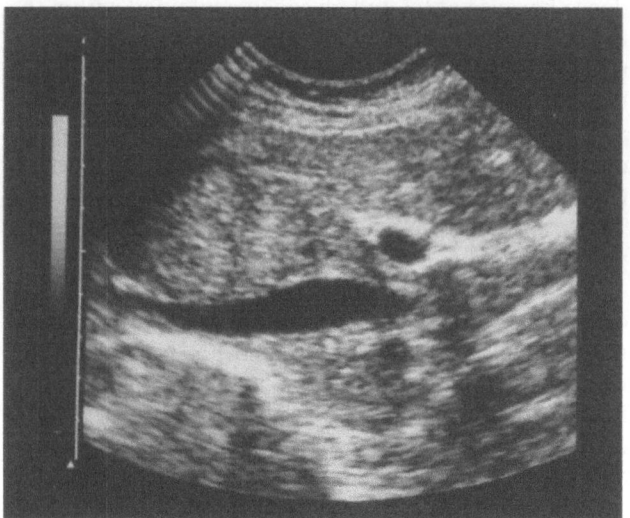

**Fig. 2.** Sonographic characteristics of focal nodular hyperplasia of the caudate lobe of the liver

cells. There is no capsule. In 70% of the cases there is a central scar, but only exceptionally are areas of a haemorrhage seen. Tumours are solitary in about 90% of cases.

The characteristic central scar, caused by fibrotic tissue and obliteration of central tumour vessels, is detectable by all the three cross-sectional procedures but most sensitively by MRI and CT.

*Imaging Findings*

Although the appearance of FNH on sonograms is highly variable, the hypo- and isoechogenicity and the central scar as a strongly hyperechoic area are the dominant features (Fig. 2). A faint hypoechoic halo can very rarely be seen. Colour Doppler sonography can be very useful, as it is noninvasive and provides a reliable diagnosis by depicting the large central artery at the scar.

On unenhanced CT images FNH are usually slightly hypodense or isodense. Central scars can be depicted in about 50% of the cases as hypodense structures. In dynamic CT of the liver the combination of rapid contrast enhancement with a peak during the first 20 s and rapid decrease to isodensity to the liver is considered to be a relatively reliable finding. The central scar may remain hypodense (Fig. 3), but on delayed scans the scar almost always enhances. Fibrous septa detected on precontrast scans as hypodense bands show hyperdensity on postcontrast images. Differentiation from adenomas and HCC (the latter with the same contrast behaviour, scars and septa) may be difficult.

Varying MRI signal intensities for FNH have been described in the literature. Most commonly there is isointensity of the homogenous lesions on T1-weighted and only slight hyperintensity (or isointensity) on T2-weighted images. The central scar shows hypointensity on T1-weighted and hyperintensity on T2-weighted and in about 60% of cases on postcontrast images [8]. After bolus administration of gadolinium-DTPA, the gradient echo images show contrast behaviour which is very similar to that of dynamic CT. A characteristic appearance can be demonstrated on plain gradient echo images (flow sensitive). There are dilated vessels surrounding the lesion in a very typical manner ("octopus sign") in about 70% of the cases of FNH, which have only exceptionally been found in other focal lesions [9]. On dynamic MRI scans after i.v. bolus injection of Gd-DTPA, there is a strong enhancement of the lesion in the arterial phase.

**Cavernosus Haemangioma**

*Pathological Findings*

The most common benign hepatic tumour is cavernosus haemangioma, with an incidence of approximately 15%.

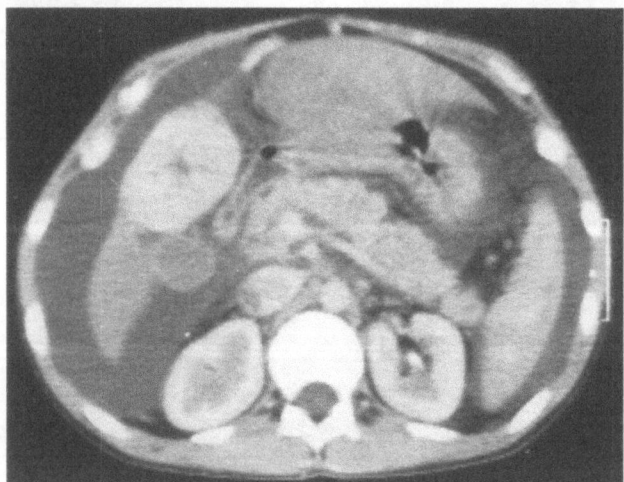

a

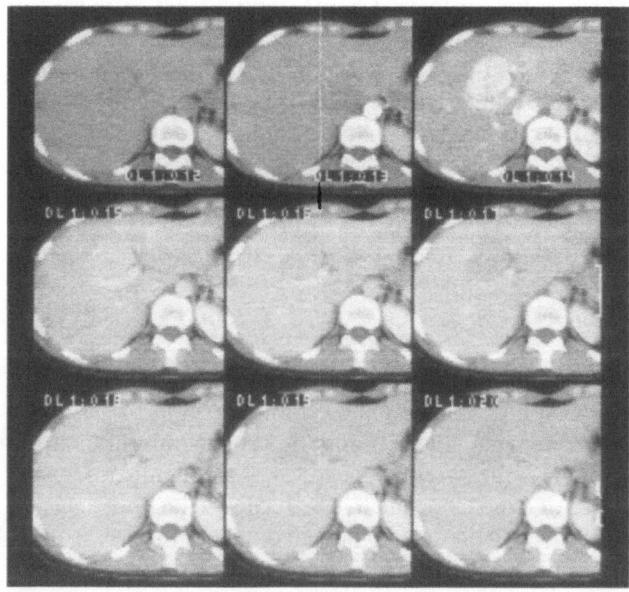

b

**Fig. 3 a, b.** Evidence of focal nodular hyperplasia on dynamic computed tomography (**a**) and with a central scar remaining hypodense on the delayed scan (**b**)

It can occur at any age and is eight to nine times more common in women than in men.

The tumour is composed of multiple vascular lakes and channels of various sizes lined by a single layer of endothelial cells and separated by connective tissue. The

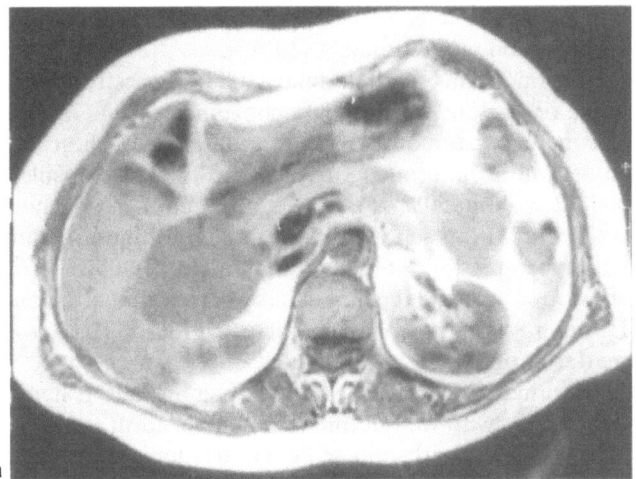

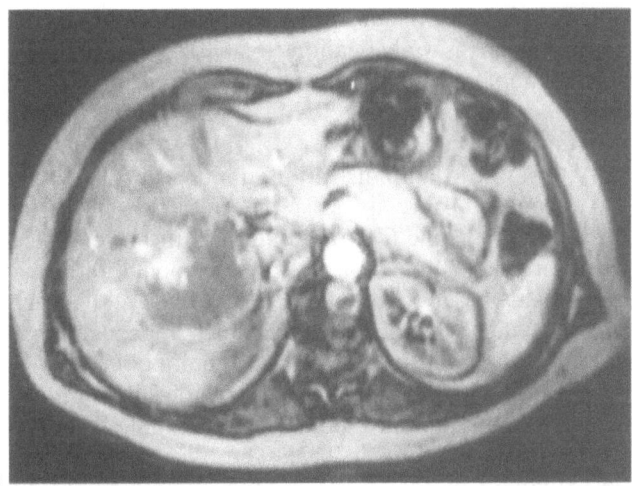

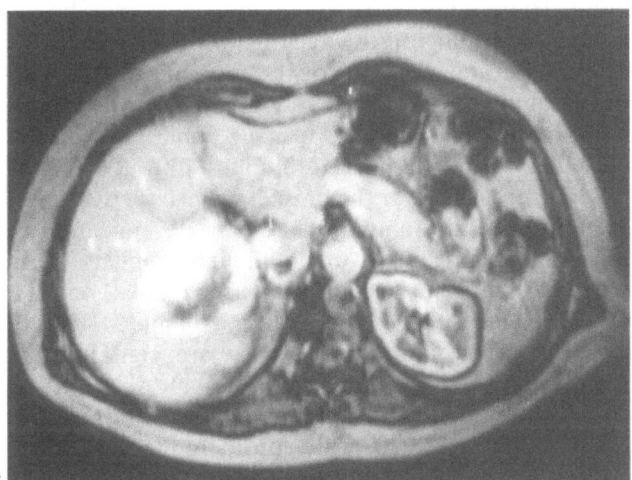

**Fig. 4 a-c.** Selected images from a dynamic hypointense precontrast (**a**) magnetic resonance imaging in haemangioma; with the typical fill-in phenomenon postcontrast (**b, c**)

slow blood flow supports thrombosis, hyalination and fibrosis. Most tumours are solitary, ranging in size from a few millimetres to over 20 cm.

*Imaging Findings*

Haemangiomas are usually well-defined hyperechoic masses with acoustic shadowing, most frequently depicted in the proximity of blood vessels or in subcapsular regions of the liver. They may be hypoechoic. Large haemangiomas (especially "giant haemangiomas") can show an inhomogeneous texture.

On unenhanced CT scans they are seen as hypodense, lobulated lesions, sometimes with small, more hypodense areas most probably caused by degenerative alterations. Following bolus CM administration, characteristic patterns of an early patchy uptake of CM at the periphery and the centropetal fill-in phenomenon up to isodensity to the liver can be registered in about 65% of the cases. Small lesions (less than 2 cm) may show complete enhancement. In large tumours, degenerative areas do not enhance and show cleft-like configurations. Globular enhancement (76%) with enhancement isodense with the aorta (72%) are characteristic findings [10].

On two-phase dynamic incremental CT there are different types of cavernous haemangioma enhancement. Lesions with homogeneous high attenuation in the first phase are difficult to distinguish from other hypervascular lesions (e.g. HCC, FNH [11]).

On T1-weighted MRI, haemangiomas show hypointensity with relatively smooth margins. Because of their long T2 values, they are more hyperintense on T2-weighted images than most malignancies. This "light-bulb sign" guarantees reliable diagnoses in more than 90% of all cases. Problems may arise with very small and very large haemangiomas, but also in differentiating these tumours from hypervascularized metastases of endocrine tumours. Sometimes haemangiomas appear heterogeneous because of thrombosis, fibrosis or haemorrhage. A dynamic contrast MRI study, therefore, is recommended in all these cases. Here, again, the contrast behaviour is very similar to that of dynamic CT, characterized by the fill-in phenomenon (Fig. 4). The unique homogeneous hyperintensity of haemangiomas on delayed postcontrast images helps to differentiate them from hypervascularized metastases.

**Hepatocellular Carcinoma**

*Pathological Findings*

HCC is the most common primary liver malignancy. The age of presentation is 70-80 years. Most of the cases are associated with underlying cirrhosis of the liver. There are three major patterns of growth: single and massive, nodular or multifocal, and diffuse. Lesions frequently show necroses and haemorrhage, if large. Microscopically, most HCCs are well differentiated, with malignant hepatocytes arranged in cords or trabeculae. The cytoplasma of hepatocytes often contains fat and glycogen. Well-differentiated HCCs frequently have a fibrous (pseudo-) capsule. The arterial blood supply is from the periphery to the centre. Vascular invasion (hepatic and portal veins) is common.

## Imaging Findings

All the pathomorphological patterns of HCC, such as fatty degeneration, increased copper content, haemorrhage, fibrosis, calcifications, capsule and signs of liver

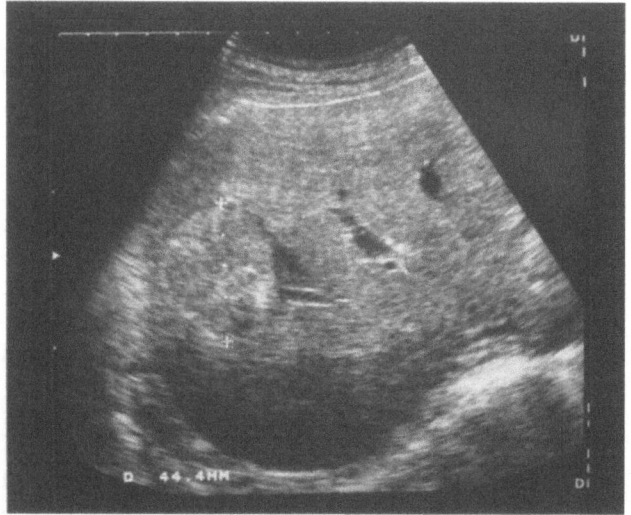
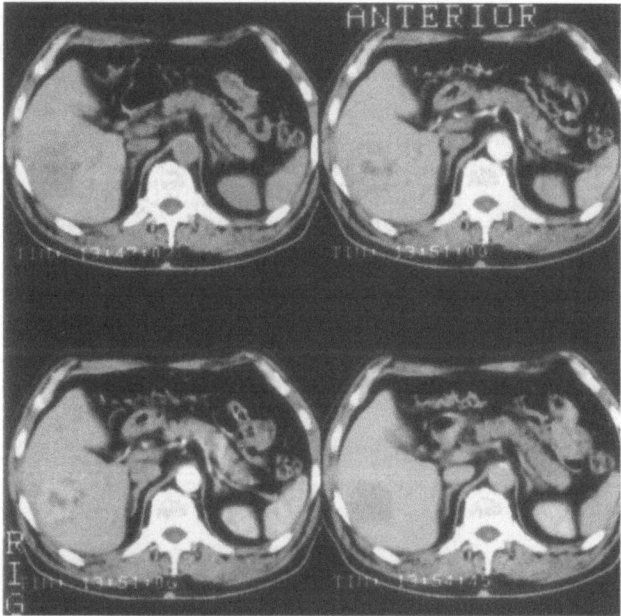

**Fig. 5 a, b.** Encapsulated hepatocellular carcinoma sonographically (**a**) and in same patient on dynamic computed tomographic scans (**b**)

cirrhosis, have to be taken into account in diagnosing these tumours. Therefore, a halo, septations and signal inhomogeneities of a liver mass seen on sonograms, CT and MRI indicate the presence of HCC. Moreover, a characteristic finding caused by the expansively growing form of HCC beside the fibrous capsule is the multinodular appearance with daughter nodules and nodular composition of the tumours [12, 13].

On sonograms small nodular HCC are mostly hypoechoic or present with mixed echogenicity (Fig. 5a). As size increases, tumours tend to become hyperechoic and to assume a heterogeneous texture. Fibrous capsules, visible in about 50% of all cases, are seen as hypoechoic rings and fibrous septa as hypoechoic intratumoural linear structures [5]. Nonencapsulated (infiltrative) HCC show areas of mixed echogenicitiy. The value of colour Doppler sonography for characterization of HCC is a matter of debate.

On unenhanced CT scans, HCC is usually a hypodense mass with well-defined (expansive form) or more often with unsharp and irregular borders (infiltrative form). Hyperdense structures in the hypodense tumour may be caused by haemorrhage; hypodensity represents areas of necrosis. Calcifications (5%-10%) are most sensitively depicted on CT. A hypodense peripheral rim may by occasionally detected by the expansive form of the tumour.

After i.v. CM administration, nonnecrotic structures are enhanced. There are three types of time-density behaviour in dynamic CT: rapid and significant enhancement (arterial; 30%), retarded enhancement (40%), and no enhancement (avascular; 30%) [14]. In the early phase of the dynamic study, capsules appear as high-density or low-density rings around the tumour.

About 70% of the HCC are depicted as hypointense on T1-weighted images, the remainder being hyper- or isointense in equal parts [12]. The hyperintensity can be explained by fat and/or copper content of the tumour. Hyperintense or hypointense areas may be detected, depending on the age of the haemorrhage. On T2-weighted images most of the tumours are hyperintense (about 90%). In actively growing HCC, the tumours show small nodules fusing to one tumour complex. Together with the intratumoural fibrous septa the latter is reponsible for the mosaic pattern seen in about 20%-50% of the tumours. The capsule appears as a low-intensity ring on T1-weighted images and as a double ring (inner low signal and outer high signal) on most of T2-weighted images (Fig 5b). In dynamic MRI studies, the capsule and vibrous septa are high-intensity structures.

Daughter nodules, the multinodular appearance, capsules and fibrous textures are considered to be very important prognostic factors and can be most sensitively depicted by MRI and sonography. Both these methods, including colour Doppler sonography, are also more sensitive in diagnosing a vascular invasion.

## Small HCC

*Pathological Findings*

Nodular tumours less than 3 cm in diameter are considered small HCCs. They have a fibrous capsule and mosaic macroscopic pattern caused by small nodules separated by septa. The tumour is moderately to poorly differentiated and has necrotic areas and fatty degeneration.

*Imaging Findings*

Sonographically most small HCC are hypoechoic with a hypoechoic halo (capsule) and posterior acoustic enhancement. On Doppler sonography a high-velocity signal is registered which is caused by arteriovenous shunting.

On CT images, small HCCs appear as well-defined, hypodense lesions with ring enhancement on postcontrast scans when a capsule is present. The most common type of enhancement after CM administration is the rapidly enhanced tumour with a quick decline of density.

"In hepatocarcinogenesis of the cirrhotic liver, a regenerating nodule might be the first step in the development of hepatocellular carcinoma, going through phases of adenomatous hyperplasia and early HCC in a multistep fashion" [15].

## Adenomatous Hyperplastic Nodule

*Pathological Findings*

Adenomatous hyperplastic nodule (AHN) is also referred to as hyperplastic nodule, adenomatoid hyperplasia and macroregenerative nodule. It is larger (> 1 cm in diameter) than other regenerative nodules of cirrhotic liver that accumulate iron or fat. The lesion is benign but has a greater malignant potential than other nodules. The blood supply is via the portal vein. There is no capsule, and histologically they are portal areas blood vessels and bile ducts. This entity is divided into three histological types [15]:
- Adenomatous hyperplasia without atypia
- Atypical adenomatous hyperplasia
- Adenomatous hyperplasia with malignant foci

The third type is considered to be an early stage of HCC ("nodule within a nodule"). Early HCC is nonencapsulated and has a rapid growth, with an average doubling time of 29 weeks for diameter and 9.5 weeks for volume [16]. It is composed of well-differentiated hepatocytes.

*Imaging Findings*

Sonographically AHN appear as hypoechoic lesions, often surrounded by a thin hyperechoic ring. On CT scans

AHN ist usually isodense and without enhancement after i.v. CM administration; therefore in most cases they are not detectable. On T1-weighted images these lesions are hyperintense, on T2-weighted image hypo- and sometime isointense to the liver. The presence of a low-signal intensity nodule with a small focus of increased signal intensity of T2-weighted images suggests a focus of malignancy ("nodule within a nodule" = regenerative nodule with a small focus of HCC [13]).

# References

1. Powers C, Ros PR (1994) Hepatic mass lesions. In: Haaga JR et al (eds) Computed tomography and magnetic resonance imaging of the whole body. Mosby, St. Louis
2. Tomita S (1991) Color doppler imaging in hepatic disease, Med Rev 37: 32-38
3. Kudo M, Tomita S, Tochio H et al (1992) Sonography with intraarterial infusion of carbon dioxide microbubbles (sonographic angiography): value in differential diagnosis of hepatic tumour. AJR 158: 65-74
4. Foley WD (1989) Dynamic hepatic CT. Radiology 170: 617-622
5. Chung KY, Mayo-Smith WW, Saini S et al (1995) Hepatocellular adenoma: MR imaging features with pathologic correlation. AJR 165: 303-308
6. Wernecke K, Vasallo P, Bick U, Diederich S, Peters PE (1992) The distinction between benign and malignant liver tumors on sonography: value of a hypoechoic halo. AJR 159: 1005-1009
7. Paulson EK, Mc Clellan JS, Washington K et al (1994) Hepatic adenoma: MR characteristics and correlation with pathologic findings. AJR 163: 113-116
8. Vilgrain V, Flejou JF, Arrive L et al (1992) Focal nodular hyperplasia of the liver: MR imaging and pathologic correlation in 37 patients. Radiology 184: 699-703
9. Marchal GJ, Pylyser K, Tshibwabwa-Tumba EA et al (1985) Anechoic halo in solid liver tumours: sonographic, microangiographic, and histologic correlation. Radiology 156: 479-483
10. Leslie DF, Johnson CD, Johnson CM et al (1995) Distinction between cavernous hemangiomas of the liver and hepatic metastases on CT: value of contrast enhancement patterns. AJR 164: 625-629
11. Hanafusa K, Ohashi I, Himeno Y, Suzuki S, Shibuya H (1995) Hepatic hemangioma: findings with two-phase CT. Radiology 196: 465-469
12. Honda H, Onitsuka H, Murakami J et al (1992) Characteristic findings of hepatocellular carcinoma: an evaluation with comparative study of US, CT and MRI. Gastrointest Radiol 17: 245-249
13. Taylor AJ, Carmody TJ, Quiroz FA et al (1994) Focal masses in cirrhotic liver: CT and MR imaging features AJR 163: 857-862
14. Lüning M, Paris S, Mutze S, Wenig B (1993) Tissue characterization by imaging procedures: comparison between benign and malignant liver tumours. In: Reiser M, Stendel A, Hirner A, Kania U (eds) Lebertumoren und portale Hypertension. Radiologische und chirurgische Aspekte. Springer, Berlin Heidelberg New York
15. Choi BI, Takayasu K, Han MC (1993) Small hepatocellular carcinomas and associated nodular lesions of the liver: pathology, pathogenesis, and imaging findings. AJR 160: 1177-1187
16. Sadek AG, Mitchell DG, Siegelman ES, Outwater EK, Matteucci T, Hann HWL (1995) Early hepatocellular carcinoma that develops within macroregenerative nodules: growth rate depicted at serial MR imaging. Radiology 195: 753-756

# Pancreatic Tumours

A.L. Baert, S. Gryspeerdt and L. Van Hoe

Department of Radiology, University Hospitals K.U.L., Herestraat 49, 3000 Leuven, Belgium

## Introduction

The current armamentarium of noninvasive radiographic imaging of the pancreas includes ultrasonography (US), computed tomography (CT), magnetic resonance, imaging (MRI), and endoscopic retrograde cholangiopancreaticography (ERCP). The development of these new imaging techniques has improved the ability to diagnose pancreatic carcinoma preoperatively and is discussed in this chapter.

## Anatomoclinical Aspects of Pancreatic Tumours [1]

*Ductal adenocarcinoma* of the exocrine pancreas comprises about 90% of all cases of pancreatic malignancies. The majority of ductal adenocarcinomas (60%-70%) are located in the head of the pancreas, thus producing early clinical symptoms because of the proximity of the common bile duct. Tumours of the body and tail of the pancreas produce clinical symptoms at the more advanced stage.

*Anaplastic carcinomas* are in the most cases variants of duct-derived carcinomas; however, their appearance is so distinctive and their behaviour so aggressive that they should be differentiated from ordinary ductal adenocarcinomas. There is a distinct male predeliction.

Histologically *intraductal pancreatic tumours* may be considered as papillary growths of ductal epithelium with varying amounts of mucin production.

*Cystic neoplasms* of the pancreas are uncommon tumours. Most of the cystic tumours are epithelial neoplasms and can be divided into two distinct morphological types: microcystic (serous type) and macrocystic (mucinous type). Microcystic cystadenomas are invariably benign. Although macrocystic neoplasms are divided into the categories benign and malignant, it is well known that macrocystic cystadenomas may coexist with and/or develop into cystadenocarcinomas. Microcystic cystadenoma is observed primarily in middle-aged and elderly patients, while macrocystic cystadenoma is found in a younger group, predominately in women.

Papillary cystic neoplasms are found in young women. It is important to differentiate this entity since the malignant potential is low and the prognosis excellent.

*Endocrine tumours* make up a small fraction of all pancreatic neoplasms. They can be classified into two groups: clinically inactive and active tumours. Clinically inactive tumours are frequently large and often have already metastasized to the liver at the time of diagnosis. Clinically active tumours are typically small at time of diagnosis. The most common endocrine tumour of the pancreas is the insulinoma, followed by glucagonoma, gastrinoma, vipoma and somatostatinoma.

*Benign mesenchymal tumours* of the pancreas are extremely rare and include lymphangioma, haemangioma and neurilemoma. Primary sarcomas of the pancreas are also extremely rare.

Most malignant *lymphomas* involving the pancreas originate in the peripancreatic or retroperitoneal liver nodes. Cases of pancreatic plasmacytoma and plasma cell granuloma have been reported.

## Modalities and Technique

### Ultrasound

Initially, patients are scanned in the supine position using a 3.5-5 MHz probe. Visualization of the pancreas is improved if patients are scanned after a prolonged fast, if the patient drinks water, or by evaluating patients in the upright position. Both the fluid-filled duodenum and the gastric antrum can be used as an acoustic window for evaluating the pancreatic body; the spleen serves as an acoustic window for the pancreatic tail.

### Computed Tomography

Helical or spiral CT is currently considered the state-of-the-art CT technique [2]. Optimal opacification of the pancreas is obtained at 32 s after administration of 150 ml bolus infused at 5 ml/s. Depending on the acquisition volume, a collimation of 4 or 8 mm and pitch 1 is used. Dual-phase helical CT scanning allows the pancreas to be visualized during the arterial phase and the liver during the portal venous phase. Oral administration of diluted iodinated or barium sulphate contrast medium delineates the duodenum and small bowel.

## Magnetic Resonance Imaging

The T1-weighted, fat-suppressed spin echo imaging and fast, low angle shot (FLASH) gradient echo (GRE) sequence provides the best delineation of the panceatic parenchyma and tumoural lesions [3]. Dynamic gadolinium-enhanced spin echo sequence with the breath-hold technique offers excellent contrast between normal pancreas and pancreatic tumours [4]. Recently, MR cholangiopancreaticography has emerged as a very promising tool for the noninvasive evaluation of the pancreaticobiliary tree. Various techniques employing heavily T2-weighted fast spin echo sequences as well as three-dimensional, fast spin echo MR have been described and are under investigation [5].

## Endoscopic Retrograde Cholangiopancreaticography

Besides the behaviour and morphology of the tumour itself, the radiographic quality is a major factor limiting the sensitivity of ERCP in the diagnosis of pancreatic carcinoma. To diagnose carcinoma of the pancreas, one must be able (a) to see the small details of the obstructed or encased duct; (b) to distinguish, by assessing the distention of surrounding ducts, between poor filling and true obstruction; and (c) to visualize adequately the pancreatic ducts, and preferably the biliary ducts as well.

## Differential Diagnosis of Pancreatic Carcinoma

Although ductal adenocarcinoma represents more than 90% of all pancreatic tumours, one must make certain that the tumour being visualized is not one which has a potentially better prognosis. Cystic neoplasms and islet cell tumours, although accounting for only a small fraction of pancreatic neoplasms, are particularly important to recognize. These two entities will therefore also be discussed, besides the more common ductal adenocarcinoma.

### Ductal Adenocarcinoma [6]

*Ultrasound.* Local mass and/or change in echo texture is the most sensitive sonographic feature in the detection of pancreatic carcinoma (Fig. 1a). Dilatation of the pancreatic duct, bile duct dilatation and gallbladder enlargement are associated findings. Tumour encasement and obstruction of the peripancreatic arteries and veins can be identified in some cases.

*Computed Tomography.* CT demonstrates the tumoural mass most frequently as a (segmental) hypovascular enlargement of the pancreas (Fig. 1b, c). Associated findings are dilatations of the bile duct and/or pancreatic

**Fig. 1 a-d.** Ductal adenocarcinoma of the pancreatic head. **a** Ultrasound. A hypoechoic lesion in the head of the pancreas (*arrow*). **b-c** Spiral computed tomography (CT) scan of the pancreas. **b** CT before IV iodinated contrast administration, showing enlargement of the pancreatic head. Linear soft tissue structures are visible ventral to the pancreatic tail, representing retro-obstructive pancreatitis. **c** CT after IV iodinated contrast administration. The pancreatic head has a lower degree of enhancement due to the presence of tumour (*arrow*). The dilated pancreatic duct is clearly visible after contrast enhancement. **d** T1-weighted, fat-saturated magnetic resonance imaging, spin echo sequence. The tumour exhibits a low signal intensity on T1-weighted, fat-suppressed spin echo images (*arrow*)

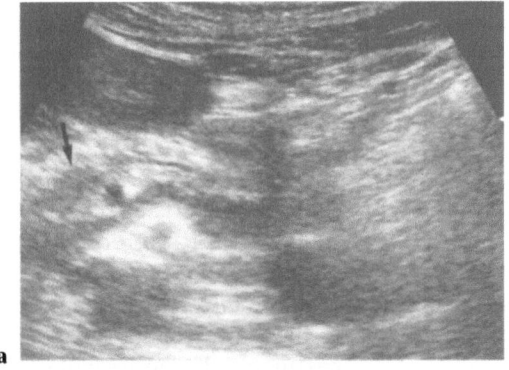
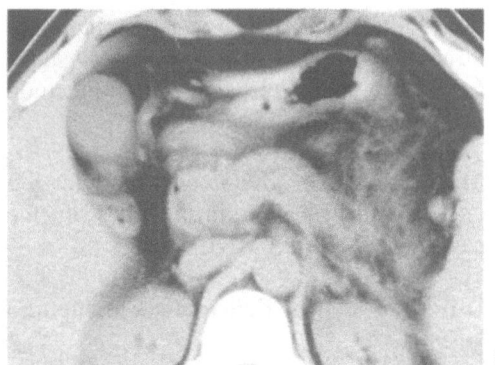
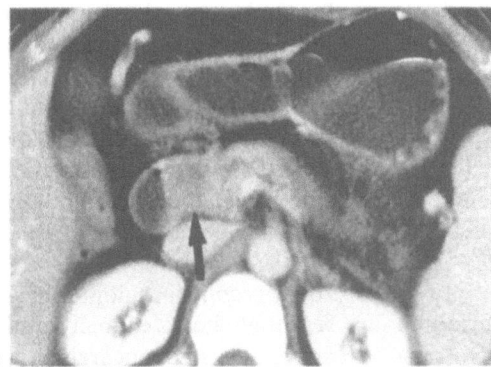
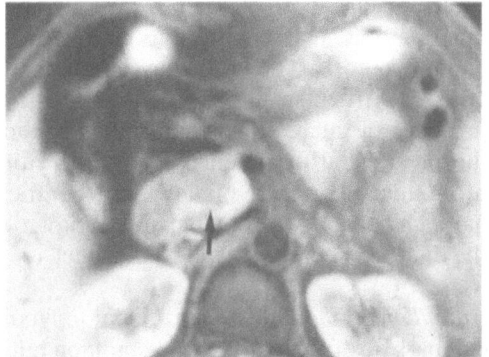

duct (double duct sign), obstructive pancreatitis, atrophy of the gland, and postobstructive pseudocysts. Spiral CT ideally demonstrates the hypovascular nature of the lesion.

*Magnetic Resonance Imaging*. MRI findings of pancreatic ductal adenocarcinoma are a low signal intensity of the tumour on T1-weighted, fat-suppressed, spin echo images (Fig. 1d). In patients in whom pancreatic carcinomas are associated with chronic pancreatitis, tumour margins are less distinct on fat-suppressed, T1-weighted images because nontumoural portions are also hypointense.

*Angiography*. Angiography is used prior to surgery to demonstrate whether the tumour can be removed or not. Irregular narrowing of the arterial lumen is characteristic of pancreatic adenocarcinoma in most cases; however, when the tumour is more extensive, changes may be difficult to differentiate from those produced by chronic pancreatitis. Veins are invaded and occluded early.

*Endoscopic Retrograde Cholangiopancreaticography*. There are three diagnostic features of carcinoma of the pancreas: (1) the encased duct; (2) the obstructed duct with side-branch filling; and (3) the double duct sign with a rat tail obstruction of the pancreatic duct and partial obstruction as well as impression of the common bile duct.

## Other Epithelial Tumours of Ductal Origin

On US or CT the presence of a large pancreatic tumour with multiple areas of decreased reflection or attenuation due to tissue necrosis associated with multiple enlarged abdominal adenopathies may suggest anaplastic carcinoma. Differential diagnosis includes pancreatic sarcoma and lymphoma.

*Mucinous adenocarcinoma* is characterized by the presence of cystic intratumoural spaces which can be visualized by US, CT and MRI.

## Differentiation of Pancreatic Carcinoma from Benign Disease

Acute or chronic pancreatitis with a focal mass is the main pathological condition to be considered in differential diagnosis. The following findings suggest pancreatitis: (a) irregular dilatation of pancreatic duct; (b) the presence of dilated ducts and small pseudocysts within the intraductal or parenchymal calcifications; (d) less pronounced degree of atrophy of the pancreatic parenchyma; and (e) gradual, not abrupt, obstruction of the dilated pancreatic hand or bile duct.

*Ampullary carcinoma* is an irregular polypoid intraluminal mass obstructing the distal common bile duct. Imaging modalities show an abrupt obstruction of the common bile duct and the pancreatic duct without an associated mass lesion.

## Cystic Neoplasms of the Pancreas

*Microcystic and Macrocystic Adenoma or Adenocarcinoma*

*Ultrasound*. On ultrasound cystic elements can be clearly identified (Fig. 2a). If the cysts are small, the lesion is predominantly reflective; if they are larger, a multiloculated cystic mass is seen. Calcifications may be identified. The differential diagnosis is from the following pancreatic cystic lesions: pseudo-cyst, papillary cystic tumour, mucinous adenocarcinoma, congenital cyst, cystic islet cell tumour, vascular tumours, cystic metastasis, pancreatic sarcoma.

*Computed Tompgraphy* [7]. The *microcystic cystadenoma* is a well-encapsulated, ovoid or multinodular mass (Fig. 2b-d). Its cystic portion is often multilocular, with (innumerable) cysts varying between 0.1 and 2 cm. It often has a solid portion with central septae. The solid portion may enhance after contrast administration. A stellar burst calcification is almost specific, though very rare. Demonstration on double phase spiral CT of a small cystic portion containing innumerable small cysts and a hypervascular solid portion suggests serous cystadenoma.

The *macrocystic cystadenoma or cystadenocarcinoma* is a well-encapsulated, round or lobulated mass. Its cystic portion is more often unilocular. If multilocular, it frequently shows one large cyst with smaller daughter cysts. Its solid portion has a dominant fibrous wall which frequently shows papillary projections and/or convolutions. Calcification is occasionally seen.

*Magnetic Resonance Imaging* [8]. MRI demonstrates the same characteristics, except for the calcification as mentioned for CT. Moreover, the shape of the external lobulation is more apparent on T2-weighted images. *Macrocystic cystadenomas* or cystadenocarcinomas tend to have an irregular, oval shape due to daughter compartments. Large irregular cystic spaces are separated by thick septa. Differences in intensity between compartments are suggestive though not specific findings of mucinous cystic neoplasms.

*Microcystic cystadenoma* frequently possesses a central scar. Delayed enhancement of the scar may be observed on contrast-enhanced FLASH images. The lesion has a smooth or nodular contour and does not invade adjacent organs.

*Angiography*. Angiographically it is not possible to differentiate between microcystic and macrocystic cystadenoma or cystadenocarcinoma (Fig. 2e). Characteristical-

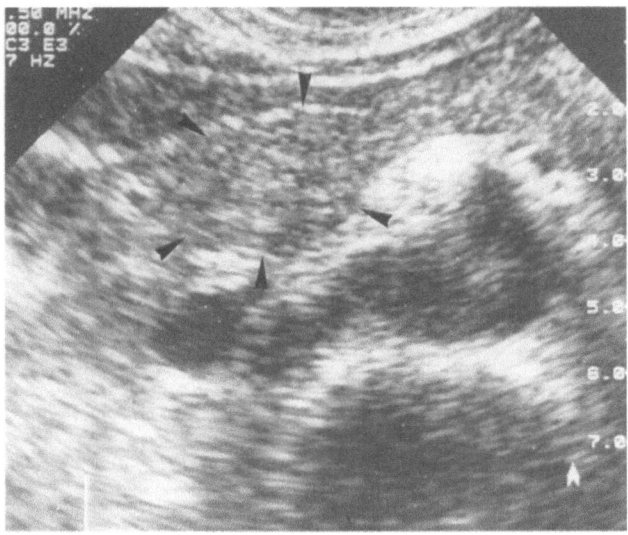

a

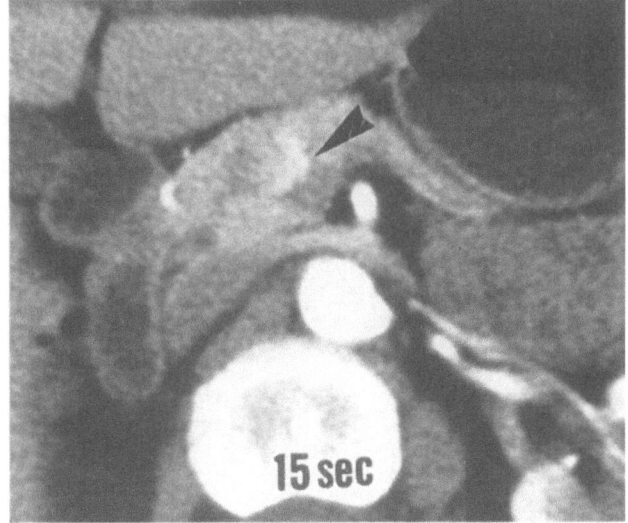

c

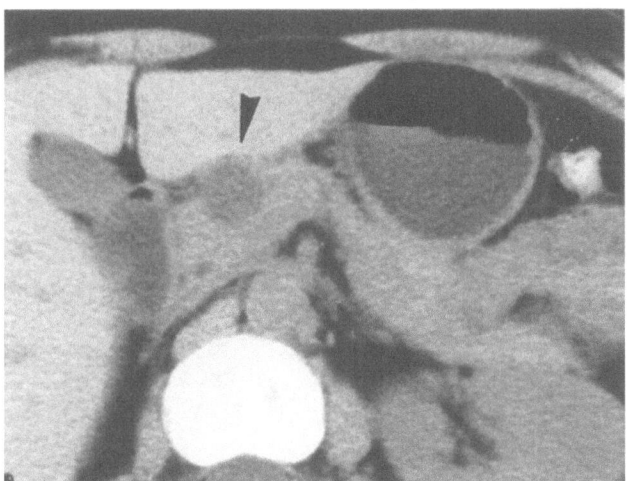

b

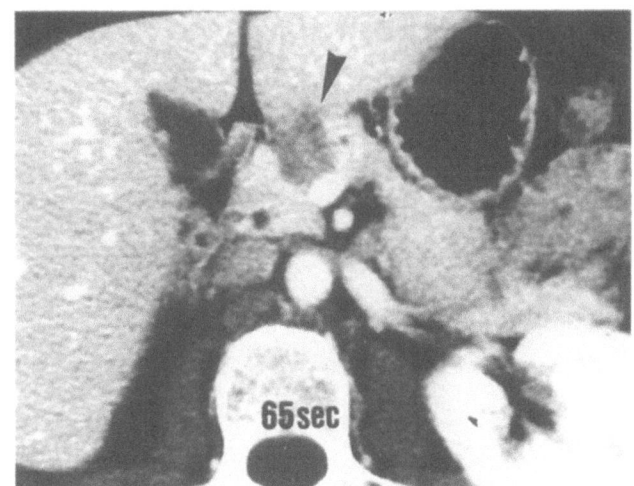

d

**Fig. 2 a-e.** Serous cystadenoma. **a** Ultrasonography. There is an enlargement of the pancreatic head (*arrowheads*) due to the presence of a hyperechoic lesion. **b-d** Double phase spiral computed tomography (CT). **b** Plain CT shows a hypodense lesion in the pancreatic body (*arrowhead*). **c** Arterial phase images (15 s after contrast administration) show peripheral enhancement, which excludes the diagnosis of pancreatic (pseudo)cyst (*arrowhead*). **d** Parenchymal phase images: the tumour appears as a hypodense mass. Angiography confirms peripheral ring enhancement (*arrow*)

e

ly the pancreatic vessels are displaced around the tumour and not encased as in pancreatic adenocarcinoma. Cystic components within the tumour stand out as defects during the parenchymal phase. Angiography may show the small hypervascular component in microcystic cystadenoma.

## Other Cystic Neoplasms

Papillary cystic neoplasms are large tumours showing extrapancreatic growth. The lesions are sharply defined with a mixture of solid and cystic portions that can be identified on CT, US and MRI.

Intraductal pancreatic tumours show cystic dilatation and mucin production, with or without a visible tumoural lesion. Intraductal mucus has been reported on ERCP studies in cases of ductectatic, mucinous cystadenoma and cystadenocarcinoma.

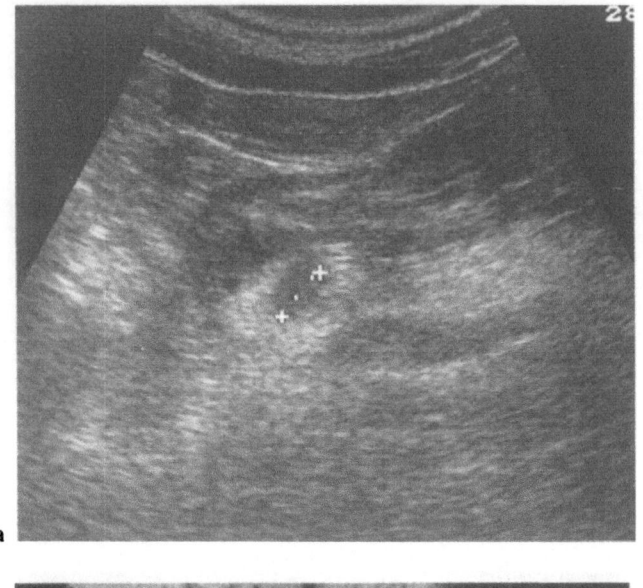

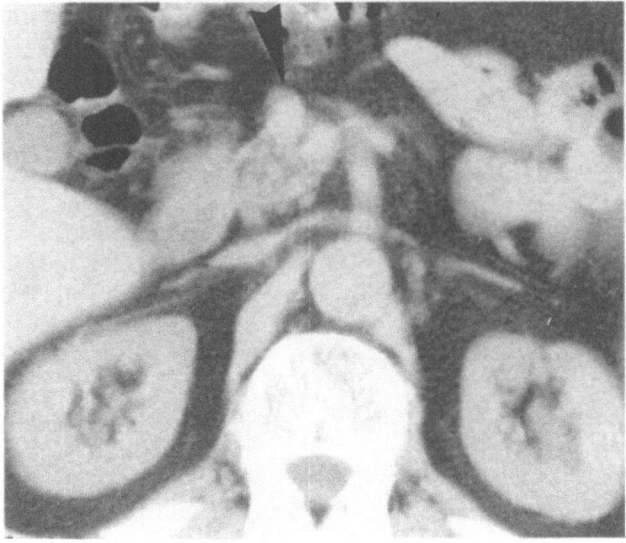

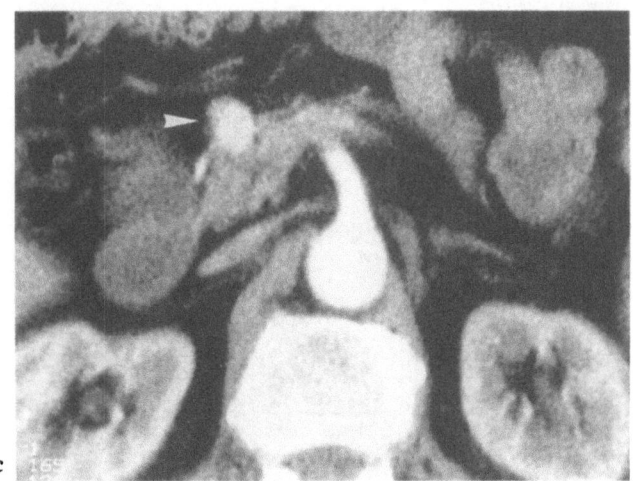

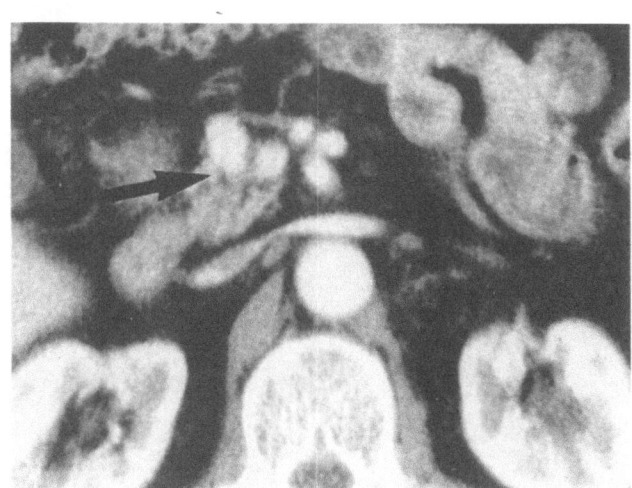

**Fig. 3 a-e.** Insulinoma of the pancreatic head. **a** Ultrasonography. A small hypoechoic area is present in the ventral portion of the pancreatic head. **b-d** Double phase spiral computed tomography (CT). **b** CT before administration of iodinated contrast medium. There is diffuse fatty replacement of the pancreatic head, and a small round area with increased attenuation and bulging of the ventral border (*arrowhead*). **c** First spiral CT 15 s after IV contrast administration clearly shows the hypervascular nature of the tumour (*arrowhead*). **d** Second spiral CT 65 s after IV administration still shows the hypervascular nature of the tumour. The tumour is, however, more difficult to differentiate from adjacent vascular structures when compared to arterial phase images. **e** Angiography confirms the presence of a small hypervascular tumour (*arrowhead*)

## Endocrine Tumours

*Ultrasound.* On US endocrine tumours are usually well defined, round and oval in shape and generally appear hypoechoic (Fig. 3a). Cystic endocrine tumours have been reported. Important features which allow inactive endocrine tumours to be differentiated from adenocarcinoma are calcifications (present in 20% of the cases) and the large volume.

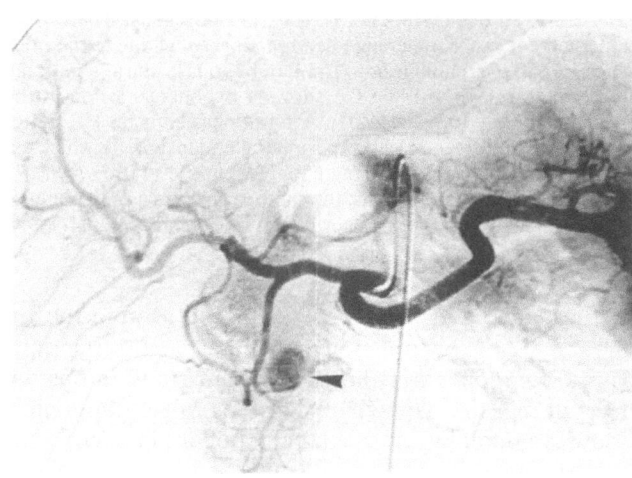

*Computed Tomography.* Islet cell tumours may be detected as small hypervascular lesions on CT (Fig. 3 b-d), Double phase spiral CT has been reported to improve the detection of active endocrine tumours, [9]. Hypervascular liver metastases are frequently present in non-active neuroendocrine tumours.

*Magnetic Resonance Imaging* [10]. Islet cell tumours are visualized on MRI as hypointense tumours on T1-weighted, fat-suppressed spin echo images. Gadolinium-enhanced images show the hypervascular nature of these tumours. Gastrinomas have been shown to exhibit high intensity on fat-suppressed, T2-weighted images.

*Arteriography*. An islet cell tumour is characterized by a hypervascular mass usually supplied by normal-sized arteries (Fig. 3e). The tumour stains in late arterial phase and the staining remains long into the venous phase.

## Conclusion

US serves as a primary screening tool for all pancreatic neoplasms. Angiography still plays a central role in the localization of islet cell tumours of the pancreas. Most other pancreatic neoplasms are preferably diagnosed by CT and/or MRI. ERCP, though an invasive imaging modality, still remains an invaluable procedure in patients suspected of having pancreatic carcinoma. Prior to surgery, angiography is used to show the resectability of tumours.

## References

1. (1989) Pancreas and periampulary region. In: Juan Rosai (ed) Ackermans' surgical pathology. Mosby, St. Louis, pp 757-788
2. Hollett MD, Jorgensen MJ, Jeffrey RB Jr (1995) Quantitative evaluation of pancreatic enhancement during double phase spiral CT. Radiology 195: 359-361
3. Semelka RC, Asher SM (1993) MR imaging of the pancreas. Radiology 188: 593-602
4. Gabat T, Marsui O, Kadoya M et al (1994) Small pancreatic adenocarcinomas: efficacy of MR imaging with fat suppression and gadolinium enhancement. Radiology 193: 683-688
5. Soto JA, Barish MA, Yucel EK et al (1995) Pancreatic duct: MR cholangiopancreatography with a three-dimensional fast spin-echo technique. Radiology 196: 459-464»
6. Baert AL, Riguats H, Marchal G (1994) Ductal adenocarinoma. In: Baert AL, Delorme G (eds) Radiology of the pancreas. Springer, Berlin Heidelberg New York, pp 129-172
7. Itai Y, Moss AA, Ohtomo K (1989) Computed tomography of cystadenoma and cystadenocarcinoma of the pancreas. Radiology 145: 419-425
8. Minami M, Itai Y, Ohtomo K et al (1989) Cystic neoplasms of the pancreas: comparison of MR imaging with CT. Radiology 171: 53-56
9. Van Hoe L, Gryspeerdt S, Marchal G, Baert AL (1995) Helical CT for the preoperative localization of islet cell tumors of the pancreas value of arterial and parenchymal phase images. AJR 165
10. Carison B, Johnson DH, Stephens DH et al (1993) MRI of pancreatic islet cell carcinoma. J Comput Assist Tomogr 17 (5): 735-740

# Imaging an Abdominal Mass in Children: Concepts and Challenges

U.V. Willi

Division of Radiology, University Children's Hospital, Steinwiesstr. 75, 8032 Zürich, Switzerland

## Introduction

The majority of abdominal masses in children are benign and a large number of them are cystic. A cystic mass is almost always benign, especially in the young child. In a vast majority, the cystic mass originates from the urinary tract and is due to some obstructive lesion, especially in a newborn or infant. Solid or heterogenic malignant abdominal masses are often characteristic of the child's age. The origin of an abdominal mass may be a malformation, a neoplasia, trauma (including an iatrogenic lesion) or an inflammatory or metabolic process.

With a modern "armamentarium" of imaging tools at our disposal, it has become paramount to make the right choice of prompt, noninvasive, safe and cost-effective diagnosis. On the other hand, if one is limited to the more easily accessible imaging modalities (i.e. X-ray and ultrasonography) it is important to know what is technically possible, i.e. the strengths and limits of these procedures, in order to reach a reliable diagnosis.

## Clinical and Anatomical Features

The child's history, age, sex and clinical presentation are imporant parameters in the evaluation of an abdominal mass. The mass may be the only sign, with no additional symptom. This is common in nephroblastoma, which usually presents as a large abdominal mass without pain, and the child is apparently in good health, while, for example, in neuroblastoma and lymphoma the child is more likely to be ill. In an inflammatory mass, the signs and symptoms are usually those of an inflammatory (i.e. infectious) disease. Abdominal pain, although highly nonspecific, is the most frequent symptom in abdominal disease, whether or not there is an anatomical correlate. Pain may be present in a mass due to trauma or malformation. Severe illness, loss of weight and/or appetite, functional abnormality of an organic system, systemic disease and fever, although signs of significant disease, are nonspecific in the presence of an abdominal mass and do not indicate malignancy per se. In urinary reten-

tion, the full bladder may present as a large midline mass in the lower abdomen. Although various pathophysiological causes are possible, a pelvic tumour (pre- or retrorectal mass) then must be excluded.

Any attempt to diagnose and characterize an abdominal mass should aim at identifying the anatomical site of origin of the mass. For a practical differentiation, it seems useful to localize a mass in the peritoneal or retroperitoneal space, in the pelvis, anterior abdomen or liver (Table 1). One should also try to decide whether the mass is in the abdomen, chest or in both areas (e.g. neuroblastoma). Pelvic masses should be differentiated as prerectal, rectal and retrorectal. With regard to the characterization of the mass, it may be solid, cystic or mixed; it may be simple or complex, benign or malignant.

## Imaging of an Abdominal Mass

In the clinical diagnosis or suspicion of an abdominal mass, a plain radiography of the abdomen with the child in recumbent position is recommended as the first imaging approach. This will often demonstrate the location, size and density of the mass, its effect upon adjacent structures, and its possible interference with the gastrointestinal and/or urinary tracts (i.e. disturbance of bowel motility, obstruction of the urinary tract, etc.). There may be skeletal or other abnormalities and calcifications associated with the mass. Some of these findings may be a diagnostic clue (e.g. calcifications in teratoma) and can easily be missed on ultrasonography. Information from the preliminary abdominal radiograph and the subsequent ultrasonographic evaluation is often

**Table 1.** Differential location of an abdominal mass

Peritoneum vs retroperitoneum
Renal vs nonrenal location
Pelvis vs anterior abdomen
Liver vs extrahepatic location
Abdomen vs chest

considerably easier, more rapid and more rewarding. It must be emphasized that the child's history, the clinical findings and occasional laboratory tests are of the same order of importance in view of a quick and satisfying diagnostic result.

Ultrasonography then follows as the most versatile and most effective method of a first look at the inside of the child's abdomen, and, in many instances, all that is needed for a preliminary diagnosis based on anatomical facts. Often, a specific diagnosis becomes quite probable by the morphological information gained by ultrasonography. The next step to prove a given hypothesis is the biopsy.

One tends to forget that the strength of ultrasonography is the anatomical definition of organ structures and not of their functional capacity. There are exceptions to this. For instance, the increased size of the kidney combined with a normal echogenicity of its thinned parenchyma and obstruction of the upper urinary tract may be indicative of preserved renal function, especially in the young child. The possibility of demonstrating blood flow and normal or preserved perfusion characteristics of a specific organ by means of Doppler techniques is another means to add functional information to the image as well as to expand anatomical understanding. Sophisticated information as to the vascular anatomy and segmental differentiation has become possible in hepatic tumours.

Ultrasonography is also the only imaging tool with which organ movement (i.e. from respiration) can provide diagnostic information. Free movement of the liver over a renal or suprarenal mass from nephro- or neuroblastoma indicates that the peritoneum is likely to be intact in this area. It is more difficult to observe free movement between an adrenal neuroblastoma and the adjacent kidney, which might be a prognostically useful sign in view of the excision of the tumour without the need to endanger or compromise the ipsilateral kidney. In this case, additional information is gained by Doppler evaluation of the main renal vasculature. In the case of a very large mass or if the respiratory movement is reduced due to pain, the criteria of free movement between organs are more difficult or impossible to obtain. In follow-up studies of an abdominal mass, further criteria become available, i.e. consistency or change of the echogenicity and size, shape and location of the mass. In a haematoma, the echo characteristics usually change within days, which is not the case in a solid tumour unless there is acute bleeding into the tumour.

## Further Imaging Considerations

Beside the information gained from Doppler sonography, functional (i.e. pathophysiological) aspects of an abdominal mass or its associated organ involvement may be obtained by conventional radiographic/fluoroscopic contrast studies, and exquisitely by scintigraphy. Biliary scintigraphy may be considered in the case of a cystic hepatic mass related directly or indirectly to the biliary tract. Skeletal scintigraphy is useful in the evaluation of metastatic disease, i.e. staging of a neuroblastoma or some other malignant abdominal tumour. Meta-iodobenzylguanidine (MIBG) scintigraphy is helpful in demonstrating the various forms of neuroectodermal tumours.

Computed tomography (CT), if available and used with proper technique, is of great help in many instances. It characterizes the abdominal mass, defines the site of its origin and shows with high precision the extent and spread of a malignant tumour. This includes the demonstration of enlarged lymph nodes possibly involved in the malignant process. By the uptake of contrast material, the degree of perfusion of the mass can be estimated and the involvement of organic systems adjacent to the tumour can be assessed. CT is the most accurate and easiest means of diagnosing nephroblastoma and its spread and further complications within the abdomen (and thorax). In nephroblastoma, CT is best complemented by two-dimensional and Doppler ultrasonography for evaluation of venous tumour spread up to the right atrium. CT is excellent for the diagnosis and staging of abdominal lymphoma and other infiltrative abdominal tumours.

Although involvement of the spinal canal by neuroblastoma is common, only in a minority of patients is there a neurological abnormality. Yet the evaluation by magnetic resonance imaging (MRI) in neuroblastoma has become the modality of choice, if available. Another area of indication for evaluation by MRI is the pelvis in the presence of a solid or cystic mass, especially if due to some malformation (e.g. hydro- or haematometrocolpos) or neoplasia. Because of the need for immobility, the pelvis and retroperitoneum are better suited for evaluation by MRI than the anterior abdomen, which is more exposed to physiological motion from the heart and from respiration. With cardiac and respiratory gated rapid sequences, the imaging technique of the anterior abdomen can be considerably improved.

## Biopsy

In a potentially malignant mass, histological proof or characterization is usually required prior to a decision for therapy (immediate or secondary excision after initial chemotherapy). In recent years, transcutaneous biopsy under direct vision has becom common in children. In many instances, ultrasonographic guidance of the procedure is possible. CT may be used as an alternative and is highly recommended in lesions more difficult to reach because of their relatively small size or more problematic location (e.g. paravertebral).

**Table 2.** Common malignant abdominal tumours in the child

Neuroblastoma
Nephroblastoma
Lymphoma
Germ cell tumours
Soft tissue sarcoma (rhabdomyosarcoma, primitive neuroecto-
   dermal tumour, Ewing sarcoma)

**Table 3.** Differential diagnosis of nephroblastoma

Nephroblastoma (favourable and unfavourable histology)
Nephroblastomatosis (precursor of nephroblastoma, often bila-
   teral)
"Clear cell sarcoma" (i.e. "bone metastasizing tumour of kidney")[a]
Rhabdoid renal tumour (sarcoma)[a]
Renal cell carcinoma
Transitional cell carcinoma
Malignant renal lymphoma
Neuroblastoma (intrarenal)
Congenital mesoblastic nephroma (benign)
Multilocular cystic nephroma (benign)

[a] High-grade malignancy.

**Table 4.** Tumours of the ovary

Germ Cell
   Seminoma (i.e. dysgerminoma)
   "Mature" teratoma (20% malignant)
   "Immature teratoma (all malignant)
   Embryonal carcinoma
   Yolk sac tumour (usually high malignancy)
   Choriocarcinoma

Specialized gonadal stroma
   Granulosa-thecal cell tumour
   Sertoli cell tumour

Others
   Rhabdomyosarcoma
   Neuroectodermal tumour
   Lymphoma, leukaemia

## Malignant Abdominal Masses in the Child

The most common malignant abdominal masses are of embryological origin, i.e. neuroblastoma and nephroblastoma (Wilms tumour), followed in frequency by lymphoma, germ cell tumours and soft tissue sarcoma (Table 2). Although it is usually possible in a retroperitoneal tumour to demonstrate renal or extrarenal origin, there are occasional difficulties in differentiating between neuroblastoma and nephroblastoma. As stated above, the child with a nephroblastoma is usually "healthy"; the child with a neuroblastoma is ill. The differential diagnoses of a nephroblastoma are listed in Table 3. In lymphoma, leukaemia has to be considered as an alternative diagnosis. Both of these may represent a differential diagnosis to rhabdomyosarcoma. Depending on the differentiation, germ cell tumours are benign in many instances. With regard to the ovary, the differential diagnoses of malignant germ cell tumours are listed in Table 4. The soft tissue sarcomas comprise the rhabdomyosarcomas, the primitive neuroectodermal tumour (PNET) and the Ewing sarcoma.

## Summary

The prompt diagnosis and characterization of an abdominal mass in the child is the aim of the paediatric radiologist. Awareness of the specific paediatric conditions (pathophysiology, changing anatomy of the growing organism, characteristic and age-related pathology) is a prerequisite not only with regard to the interpretation of the findings but also for successful imaging. The experience and biases of the radiologist conducting the examination will, and should, influence the choice of the technical procedure. However, there are recomandations of "how to do" things that are generally valid. Professional expertise combined with up-to-date technology allows highly accurate diagnostic imaging even with the simple means of X-ray and ultrasonography. Technically more powerful and sophisticated equipment such as CT and MRI are of great help and may be indispensable in selected cases. There are challenges of differential diagnosis waiting for even the most experienced diagnostician.

## References

1. Cohen MD (1992) Imaging of children with cancer. Mosby, St. Louis
2. Patriquin HB, Lafortune MA (1995) Doppler sonography of the child's abdomen. In: Taylor KJW, Burns PN, Wells PNT (eds) Clinical application of Doppler ultrasound, 2nd edn. Raven, New York
3. Siegel MJ (1995) Pediatric sonography, 2nd edn. Raven, New York
4. Teele RL, Share JC (1991) Abdominal masses. In Teele RL, Share (eds) Ultrasonography of infants and children. Saunders, Philadelphia

# New Interventional Procedures in the Abdomen

J. Lammer

Universität für Radiodiagnostik, Allgemeines Krankenhaus, Wahringer Gürtel 18-20, A-1090 Vienna, Austria

The further development of metal stents in the past years has made a major contribution to interventional radiology in the abdomen. Stents are used for the treatment of oesophageal or upper gastrointestinal stenoses, for transhepatic and endoscopic biliary drainage, for treatment of pancreatic duct stenoses, for transjugular intrahepatic portocaval shunts (TIPS), for distal ureteral stenoses and, in the vascular system for renal ostial stenoses and abdominal aortic aneurysms. In the following the current status of stents for percutaneous trans-hepatic biliary drainage (PTBD), TIPS and abdominal aortic aneurysms (AAA) will be discussed.

## Pecutaneous Transhepatic Biliary Drainage

For palliative decompression of obstructive jaundice transhepatic or endoscopic placement of endoprostheses is the accepted treatment of choice. Initially, plastic endoprostheses made of Teflon, polyethylene or polyurethane were used [1].

However, incrustation and sludge formation cause

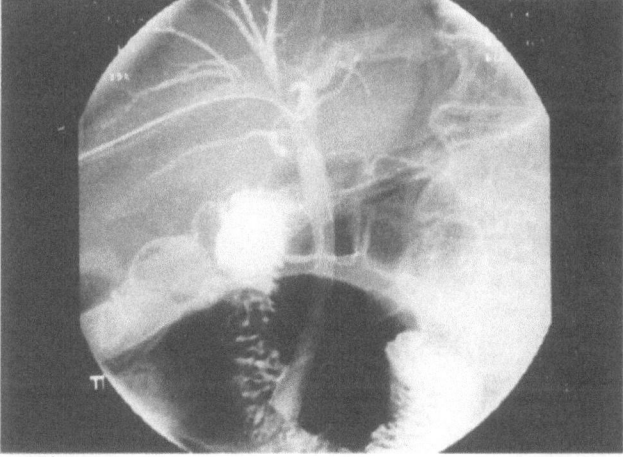

**Fig. 1.** Wallstent endoprosthesis in the common bile duct for treatment of obstructive jaundice due to lymph node metastases

premature blockage of the plastic stents. To overcome early reocclusion large bore stents 10 Fr to 14 Fr in diameter were used. Expandable metallic stents can be inserted less traumatically through a 7-Fr to 10-Fr introducing sheath. Once in place the stent opens to 8 mm or 10 mm in diameter (Fig. 1). Later, metal stents are incorporated into the wall of the common bile duct due to submucosal growth around the stent struts. A complete incorporation of a metal stent can be expected 6 to 12 months after implantation.

A European multicentre trial investigated four different stents for palliative decompression of malignant obstructive jaundice. Significantly higher patency rates with the Wallstent and the nitinol Elastalloy-Strecker stent were found than those with the Gianturco-Rösch Z stent or the tantalum Strecker stent ($p<0.0001$, respectively) [2]. Reobstruction requiring reintervention was observed in 19% with Wallstents and 17% with the nitinol Elastalloy-Strecker stent. The average time between stent placement and reobstruction was 5.9 months for the Wallstent and 8.5 months for the nitinol Strecker stent. Two randomized trials compared independently plastic versus metal stents. In the first trial a 10-Fr polyethylene stent or a 10-mm Wallstent was placed endoscopically [3]. It was reported that the median patency was significantly prolonged in patients with a metal stent compared with those with a polyethylene stent (8.9 vs 4.1 months; $p$ = 0.006). The reobstruction rate was reported as 33% for the Wallstent and 54% for the polyethylene stent. In the second prospective randomized trial in 101 patients a 12-Fr Percuflex endoprosthesis or a 10-mm Wallstent was inserted transhepatically [4]. The average time of patency for the plastic versus metal stent wa 4.3 versus 13.4 months, respectively ($p < 0.005$). The reobstruction rate was 29% versus 19% (Wallstent). Thus, metal stents such as the Wallstent or nitinol Elastalloy-Strecker stent seem to be significantly more advantageous than plastic stents or other metal stent designs for palliative decompression of malignant obstructive jaundice.

Currently, metal stents covered by a plastic membrane such as polyester or polyurethane are being tested clinically. The plastic membrane is expected to prevent

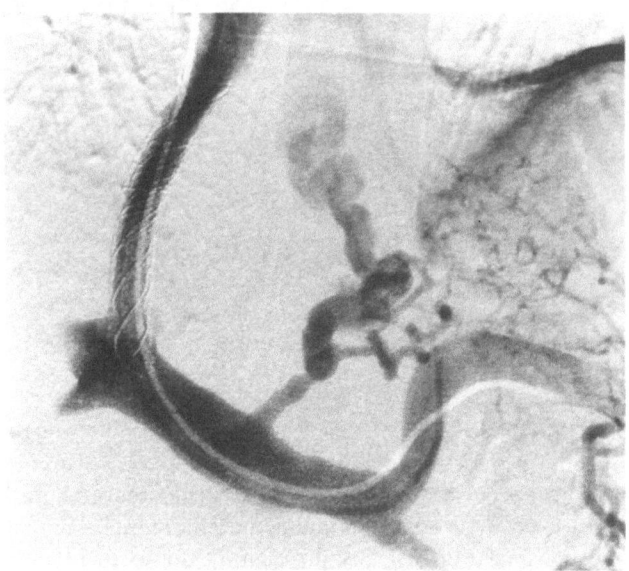

**Fig. 2.** Transjugular intrahepatic portocaval shunt in a patient with esophageal varix bleeding

tumour ingrowth and improve the long-term patency rates [5].

For treatment of benign biliary stenoses metal stents can be used if surgery or balloon dilatation fails. However, in animal studies and in clinical trials a hyperplastic reaction of the bile duct epithelium was observed after stent implantation. Mucosal hypertrophy decreased after 9-12 months in canine studies. In humans, the 3-year patency rate of stents in benign stenoses was 69% [6].

## Transjugular Intrahepatic Portocaval Shunt

Use of TIPS in humans was first described in 1990 [7]. Since that time TIPS has been established for the treatment of recurrent bleeding of oesophageal varices, incurable ascites and in Budd-Chiari syndrome. Patients are usually referred in the clinical stage Child-Pugh B (> 50%) after more than two episodes of variceal bleeding. However, also patients in stages A and C of the Child-Pugh classification and those in whom there is acute bleeding were treated by TIPS. Portal vein thrombosis is a contraindication; an extremely small liver or massive ascites renders the procedure more difficult.

Technically, TIPS can be peformed in 95% of patients (Fig. 2). Ultrasound before or during portal vein puncture turned out to be beneficial. Various stents, such as the Palmaz stent, Wallstent and Cragg-Endopro covered stent were used for establishing the intrahepatic shunt. Shunt diameter is usually 8-10 mm. The shunt is gradually dilated until the portosystemic pressure gradient is reduced to 10 mmHg. Patients are anticoagulated during the procedure by 5000 IU of heparin intravenously. Potential complications are intraperitoneal bleeding, haemobilia and subcapsular haematoma of the liver. After successful establishment of a shunt, a significant improvement of the clinical stage to Child-Pugh A was observed ($p < 0.01$). Ascites was reduced in 89%; patients were free of variceal rebleeding in 82% at 1 year and the 1-year survival rate was 85% [8]. However, the hepatic encephalopathy rate increased from 10% before TIPS to 25% after TIPS.

A relatively high reobstruction rate of the intrahepatic stent shunt is an obvious problem. Restenosis, especially at the site of the hepatic vein, was observed in 20%-25%; a total reobstruction was seen in 10%-15% of patients. Rösch hypothesized that exposure to the lacerated liver parenchyma within the stent tract might increase intimal proliferation. Therefore, covered stents should reduce the reobstruction rate. This hypothesis is currently under clinical investigation. Reobstructed shunts can be reestablished by balloon dilatation or placement of a second stent within the first one. However, control studies by Doppler ultrasound after 1, 3, 6 and 12 months are necessary for early diagnosis of a shunt stenosis.

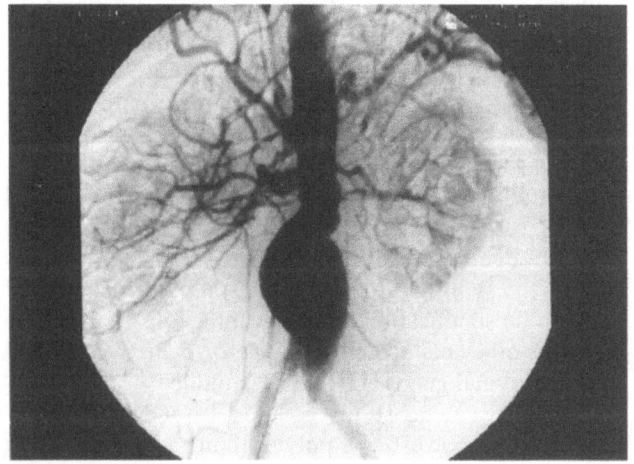
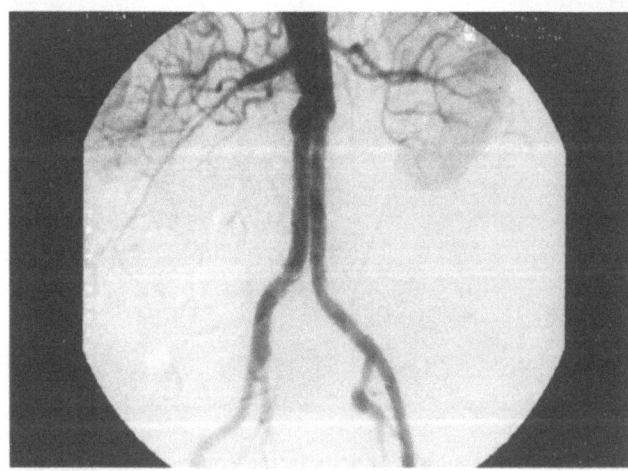

a                                                                                                                                      b

**Fig. 3a, b.** Abdominal aortic aneurysm before (**a**) and after (**b**) implantation of bifurcated stent graft

## Stent Graft in Abdominal Aortic Aneurysm

Treatment of AAA in humans using a covered stent graft was first described by Parodi in 1992 [9]. Since 1994 three stent grafts (Stentor/Mintec, EVT, Corvita) have been under clinical investigation. The most experience to date has been with the Stentor system. The Stentor graft is made of a self-expanding nitinol metal stent. Nitinol is a thermoplastic nickel-titanium alloy which expands at body temperature to a pregiven configuration. The nitinol wire is bent in a zigzag configuration and tied by nylon sutures to a tube. This framework is coated by a polyester fabric. The stent graft is preloaded in an 18-Fr introducer system. A tube graft and a bifurcated graft are available (Fig. 3). For exact infrarenal placement there should be a neck between the renal arteries and the aneurysm of at least 15 mm in length and not more than 26 mm in diameter. Distally the stent graft has to seal off the aneursysm at the aortic bifurcation or at the common iliac artery. The most common problem after successful deployment of the stent graft is leakage into the aneurysm at the proximal or distal end. If the leak does not close spontaneously, additional stent grafts have to be placed to seal it. Long-term follow-up for more than 1 year showed stability of the endoprostheses and permanent exclusion of the aneurysm.

## References

1. Lammer J (1990) Biliary endoprostheses. Plastic versus metal stents. Radiol Clin North Am 28: 1211-1222
2. Rossi P, Bezzi M, Rossi M et al (1994) Metallic stents in malignant biliary obstruction: results of a multicenter European study of 240 patients. JVIR 5: 279-285
3. Davids PH, Groen AK, Rauws EAJ et al (1992) Randomized trial of self-expanding metal stents versus polyethylene stents for distal malignant biliary obstruction. Lancet 304: 1488-1492
4. Lammer J, Hausegger K, Flückiger F et al (1996) Plastic versus metal stents for transhepatic treatment of malignant obstructive jaundice. A prospective randomized trial. Radiology (submitted)
5. Thurnher S, Lammer J, Winkelbauer F et al (1996) Covered self-expandable transhepatic biliary stent: clinical pilot study. Cardiovasc Intervent Radiol 19: 10-14
6. Maccioni F, Rossi M, Salvatori FM et al (1992) Metallic stents in benign biliary strictures: 3 years follow up. Cardiovasc Intervent Radiol 15: 360-366
7. Richter GM, Nöldge G, Palmaz JC et al (1990) Transjugular intrahepatic portocaval stent shunt: preliminary clinical results. Radiology 174: 1027-1030
8. Rössle M, Haag K, Ochs A et al (1994) The transjugular intrahepatic portosystemic stent shunt procedure for variceal bleeding. N Engl J Med 330: 165-171
9. Parodi JC, Barone HD (1992) Transluminal treatment of abdominal aortic aneurysms and peripheral arteriovenous fistulas. 19th Annual Montefiore Medical Center/Albert Einstein College Symposium. New York, NY

# URORADIOLOGY

# New Frontiers in Uroangiographic Contrast Media

F. Stacul

Istituto di Radiologia, Ospedale di Cattinara, Strada di Fiume, 34149 Trieste, Italy

More than 70 years of research on contrast media (CM) had led to the synthesis of effective and extremely well-tolerated compounds. Moreover, we have achieved a deep knowledge of the design principles of CM molecule. We have learned that:

- Nonionic contrast agents display lower toxicity than ionic agents.
- Putting an iodine atom on a carrier molecule renders it more toxic.
- More hydrophilic molecules are less toxic.
- The nature of the carrier molecule substituents, other than iodines, may profoundly affect the overall toxicity.
- Metrizamide has the lowest osmolality of any nonionic monomer commercially produced, but it is far from being the least toxic agent.
- Being nonionic and having the lowest osmolality are still not enough to guarantee the lowest possible toxicity.
- Iso-osmolal formulations of contrast agents still have measurable toxic effects [1].

We are close to synthesizing the ideal CM molecule. Therefore it seems appropriate to evaluate the current status of our knowledge both of agents which have just entered the market (new nonionic monomers, the nonionic dimers) and of possible further developments to see where there is still a margin for improvement.

## Today

The long debate concerning the choice between high osmolar ionic agents and low osmolar nonionic compounds has come to an end, the latter showing definite advantages over the former.

However, at least eight nonionic monomers (iobitridol, iohexol, iomeprol, iopamidol, iopentol, iopromide, ioversol, ioxilan) and two nonionic dimers (iodixanol and iotrolan) are now available. Do we have clinical evidence of any advantage of one of these two classes over the other? Do we have clinical evidence of any advantage of one/some of the compounds within one class?

Concerning comparisons among different nonionic monomers, we know that they differ to some extent by a variety of factors: number of hydroxyl groups, possibility of crystallization, osmolality, viscosity, hydrophilicity, $LD_{50}$ and $EB_{50}$ [2]. However, the existing differences are usually slight and so far there has been no study showing clinical advantages of one of these compounds over another, except concerning $EB_{50}$, which reflects the direct neurotoxicity.

For instance, iopromide has an $EB_{50}$ three times lower than iopamidol and this is probably why iopromide is not suitable for myelography and is associated with a higher incidence of effects on the nervous system when compared to iomeprol [3].

Therefore it appears that the minor differences highlighted by the manufacturers are of very limited clinical relevance [2], but we have to bear in mind that such a conclusion is closely related to the way trials are carried out. In other words, we need well-designed, randomized, double-blind clinical trials in which all possible biases are avoided and in which study populations that are more susceptible to CM toxicity are selected to maximize the differences in safety between the agents. Otherwise we could miss a difference that indeed exists.

Great hope has been set on the nonionic dimers recently placed on the market because of their iso-osmolality with plasma. Many trials have been carried out in the past years testing their efficacy and safety compared to nonionic monomers. There is general agreement that the cardiovascular efficacy is largely the same as that of nonionic monomers [4]. There was some claim that results similar to those obtained with monomers could be achieved with lower doses of dimers, because of studies comparing monomers to dimers with slightly lower iodine concentration. However, it is not scientifically correct to draw such conclusions comparing solutions with small iodine concentration differences following gross methods for efficacy analysis [2]. The higher viscosity of the dimers apparently was not considered to be a problem in cardiovascular procedures [5].

The efficacy of the dimers in urography was the subject of some papers; however, unanimous conclusions were not reached. Some authors [6] showed a higher opacification of the excretory pathway following injection of the dimers as compared to monomers, as could theoretically be expected. Possible advantages, for instance in patients with impaired renal function, can be foreseen. However, poorer distention of the excretory pathway, namely of the bladder, was sometimes recorded, suggesting it would be inappropriate to inject lower doses of the dimer [2].

The analysis of nonionic dimer tolerability compared to nonionic monomers demonstrated a clear advantage of the former: lower frequency and/or intensity of heat sensation were recorded following intravascular administration and less pain was demonstated on peripheral arteriography [4]. However, it should be kept in mind that the tolerability of nonionic monomers has always been judged to be very good in clinical experience.

The effects of the dimers on the heart were not assessed to any great extent as compared to nonionic monomers. However, they turned out to be very well tolerated in preclinical studies and in comparative trials with ionic compounds. Concerning their effects on the microcirculation, it was suggested that a more viscous iso-osmolar CM (the dimer) mixed with blood could cause a transient slowing of blood flow through the microcirculation. As a result, the anoxia time would be prolonged, possibly causing ischaemia. However, clinical evidence shows that clinical symptoms and signs of ischaemia are not recorded. Instead, there is less pain following dimer injection on peripheral arteriography.

How nonionic dimers affect the kidney was a matter of concern: the higher concentration reached by these agents in the tubules and the detection of vacuoles in proximal tubular cells containing the CM with a definite higher incidence than nonionic monomers was perplexing. However, clinical trials carried out so far have not shown lower renal tolerance of the dimers according to either serum creatinine or urinary enzyme excretion [4, 7]. Indeed, some data suggested a better renal tolerance of the dimers, but not enough trials have been conducted yet in patients with risk factors for the onset of acute renal failure.

It is very difficult to compare kind and frequency of adverse events between nonionic monomers and dimers. Comparative trials carried out so far have not shown significant differences [4], but the safety level of all these agents is possibly so high that it may be extremely difficult to detect difference in clinical trials.

However, recently acquired data raised some concern about the safety of one nonionic dimer, namely iotrolan. In fact, in October 1995 the manufacturer of this agent sent a letter to its customers declaring that the sale of iotrolan 280 mgI/ml was being temporarily suspended as a precautionary measure, because following the more widespread use of the CM, there was an increase in the number of reports from physicians of delayed reactions, in particular allergy-like skin reactions. The reason for this is still unclear and requires additional investigations.

## And The Future

"... Because the current agents are so good, it seems unlikely that anything more than modest incremental improvements are possible" stated P. Dawson [1]. But, "despite these caveats", he continues "all the major pharmaceutical companies involved in this field are working on new agents". This means that companies still predict an expansion in the CM market. How? Two different goals and consequently two different research lines are being followed.

Improved efficacy, namely an increased specificity of new agents, is the goal of much ongoing research. The focus of attention has been concentrated on the so-called blood pool agents, namely CM that do not leave the vascular bed and therefore do not distribute into the interstitium. They could be used in contrast-enhanced perfusion studies and as markers of regions of pathologically increased capillary permeability in the body [8]. There are three approaches to developing such compounds [9]: radiopaque macromolecules, micronized particles of insoluble iodinated contrast agents and packaging low-molecular-weight media in liposomes.

The first approach, suggested by Almen 30 years ago already, was recently proposed again, when polymeric carbohydrates grafted with ionic iodinated molecules were patented by Guerbet. These agents are at a very early stage of development and it is impossible to draw any conclusions yet. Some concern has been expressed as to their possible low excretion rate and high viscosity [9]. Sovak et al. [10] elected to develop co-polymers rather than to graft a carrier to predetermine the polymeric composition and to limit the spread of molecular weight to a minimum, but results proved to be unsatisfactory.

The second recent approach is related to the use of micronized particles of insoluble iodinated agents, which are captured by cells of the reticuloendothelial system. Their small size and surface modifications allow a long half-life in blood, which is needed in a good blood-pool agent. However, it does not look like this goal will be easy to achieve at all. These agents are generally rapidly taken up by the liver and have a short blood-pool enhancement phase. The balance between blood-pool and liver-spleen enhancement could be controlled by modifying the surfactant formulation [11].

The third approach is the use of low-molecular-weight iodinated CM packaged in liposomes. No doubt this is the most realistic approach, as testified by the involvement of all the main companies in this research [8, 9, 12]. Again, to render good blood-pool agents, their surfaces must be modified to prolong the presence in blood. The liposomes are taken up mainly by the Kupffer cells of the liver and by macrophages in the spleen. Tumours contain very few of these macrophages and, therefore, following the initial opacification of the entire liver due to persistence of the CM in the vessels, we can expect to detect focal liver lesions after wash-out of the CM: the lesions appear radiolucent while the normal parenchyma remains opacified because the CM is trapped by the macrophages. It means that we would use an agent acting as a blood-pool agent early after the injection and as a marker of the reticuloendothelial system later.

If there is a demand for safety at a level beyond that now achieved, entirely different compounds will have to be developed [8]. Research towards metal complexes as an alternative to iodinated compounds is being carried out by CM manufacturers. These agents could decrease the frequency of CM administration-related side effects and, furthermore, some heavy metal elements easily form stable clusters with a very high content of the attenuating element [12], resulting in a greater attenuation of X-rays compared to iodine. The same efficacy could be obtained at a lower CM dose or the use of radiation with higher energy could reduce the radiation dose for the patients [13]. Encouraging results were achieved with gadolinium-DTPA, which was used for intra-arterial digital substraction angiography [14] and computed tomography [15]. Tungsten is another element that has received investigators' attention [12].

In conclusion, these perspectives show that CM research is far from being over and will provide radiologists with new tools for more accurate diagnoses, possibly improving the already excellent level of safety of CM. In the next few years we will still be involved in discussions on the stimulating features of the new compounds.

# References

1. Dawson P (1995) Design plays major role in new contrast media. Diagn Imaging Eur [Suppl June 1995]: 3-4
2. Stacul F, Thomsen HS (1996) Nonionic monomers and dimers. Eur Radiol (in press)
3. Rosati G, Davies A, Spinazzi A (1996) Predictable and unpredictable adverse reactions to iomeprol and iopromide. Acad Radiol (in press)
4. Grynne BH, Nossen JO, Bolstad B, Borch KW (1996) Main results of the first comparative clinical studies on Visipaque. Acta Radiol (in press)
5. Klow NE, Levorstad K, Berg KJ, Brodhal U, Endressen K, Kistoffersen DT, Laake B, Simonsen S, Tofte AJ, Lundby B (1993) Iodixanol in cardioangiography in patients with coronary artery disease. Acta Radiol 34: 72-77
6. Adolph JMG, Engelkamp H, Herbig W, Peters PE, Wenzel-Hora BI (1995) Iotrolan in urography: efficacy and tolerance in comparison with iohexol and iopamidol. Eur Radiol 5 [Suppl 2]: S63-S68
7. Clauss W, Dinger J, Meissner C (1995) Renal tolerance of iotrolan 280 - a meta-analysis of 14 double-blind studies. Eur Radiol 5 [Suppl 2]: S79-S84
8. Niendorf HP, Fritzsch T, Herrschaft G, Krause W, Muhler A, Schurmann R (1995) Looking into the future: iotrolan and beyond. Eur Radiol 5: S107-S111
9. De Haen C (1995) CT and new contrast media widen diagnostic options. Diagn Imaging Eur [Suppl June 1995]: 32-33
10. Sovak M, Douglas III JG, Terry RC, Brown JW, Bakir F, Shibusawa Wasden T (1994) Blood pool radiopaque polymers. Design considerations. Invest Radiol [Suppl] 29: S271-S274
11. Rubin DL, Desser TS, Qing F, Muller HH, Young SW, McIntire GL, Bacon E, Cooper E, Toner J (1994) Nanoparticulate contrast media. Blood-pool and liver-spleen imaging. Invest Radiol [Suppl] 29: S280-S283
12. Strande P (1994) Nycomed's X-ray contrast media development; Visipaque and beyond. In: Twenty years on nonionic contrast media. Pioneers, Oslo, pp 11-13
13. Fritzsch T, Krause W, Weinmann HJ (1992) Status of contrast media research in MRI, ultrasound and X-ray. Eur Radiol 2: 2-13
14. Schild HH, Weber W, Boeck E, Mildenberger P, Strunk H, Duber C (1994) Gadolinium DTPA (Magnevist) als Konstrastmittel für die arterielle DSA. ROFO 160: 218-221
15. Quinn AD, O'Hare NJ, Wallis FJ, Wilson GF (1994) Gd-DTPA: an alternative contrast medium for CT. J Comput Assist Tomogr 18: 634-636

# Imaging in Renovascular Hypertension

N. Grenier

Service de Radiologie, Groupe Hospitalier Pellegrin - Tripode, Place Amélie Raba Léon, 33076 Bordeaux, France

Renovascular hypertension (RVH) is the result of significant decrease of renal blood flow secondary to a severe arterial lesion (unilateral or bilateral). Renal artery stenosis (RAS) is the most frequent cause of RVH and we will focus on this.

Detection of RVH is important because it is potentially curable by revascularization (percutaneous angioplasty or surgery). Even if medical treatment can be effective in RVH, its cause should be identified so as to avoid having to take such medication for life. Also, if left untreated, RAS is a source of thrombosis with a corresponding loss of renal function.

There is a major upheaval underway concerning the gold standard in the diagnosis of RVH. Partial or total remission of hypertension obtained 2 months after a revascularization procedure is considered as the actual gold standard.

The prevalence of RVH in the general population of hypertensive patients does not exceed O.5%-1% [1]. This is why, to avoid false-positive results, radiological screening of patients must be preceded by a clinical selection. The clinical criteria currently accepted as suggestive of RVH are abrupt onset or worsening of hypertension, severe hypertension in a smoker or in a patient with evidence of occlusive arterial disease elsewhere, onset before 20 years of age or after the age of 50, hypertension refractory to standard therapy, abnormal physical findings such as grade III or grade IV retinopathy or localized systolic/diastolic bruit over the renal artery. The prevalence of RVH in this selected population could reach 47% [2]. The imaging techniques available today can be classified into two groups, the techniques allowing identification of an anatomical RAS and those that recognize secondary renal function impairment (functional RAS). Techniques of the former group are numerous [intravenous (IV) and intraarterial (IA) digital substraction angiography (DSA), helical computed tomography and magnetic resonance (MR) angiography], whereas the latter group is restricted to methods based on angiotensin-converting enzyme (ACE) inhibition testing.

## Detection of RAS

Stenoses reducing internal diameter by more than 60% produce a significant decrease in renal blood flow. They can be atheromatous or dysplastic (fibromuscular dysplasia, FMD), ostial or nonostial, and involve main, accessory or segmental arteries.

### Intraarterial Digital Subtraction Angiography

Considered as the gold standard for the diagnosis of RAS, IADSA should be limited to the confirmation of stenosis and followed by transluminal angioplasty during the same procedure. Small catheters (4-5 Fr) are recommended. Injection in the aorta with posteroanterior and posterior oblique views at the level of renal arteries to avoid superimposition with the coeliac trunk and superior mesenteric artery must be followed by selective injection in each renal artery if a distal stenosis is suspected (FMD).

### Intravenous Digital Subtraction Angiography

IVDSA was proposed in the early 1980s as an alternative to IADSA. With a peripheral brachial injection, the results of 15%-20% of studies were considered inadequate because of insufficient contrast, respiratory movements and gas superimposition. This proportion fell to 9% with the use of a central infusion in the right atrium [3]. Sensitivity of IVDSA is 83%-100% and specificity 90%-93% if technically inadequate studies are excluded. FMD lesions go undetected in 50% of cases. Therefore, although some authors no longer consider IVDSA as the best screening tool [4], it is still performed by many [2].

### Ultrasound

With the advent of colour encoding of the Doppler signal, ultrasonography has gained a major place in the detection of RAS. The procedure must be complete to be valuable, including examination of the kidneys with measurement of their size, spectral sampling of several

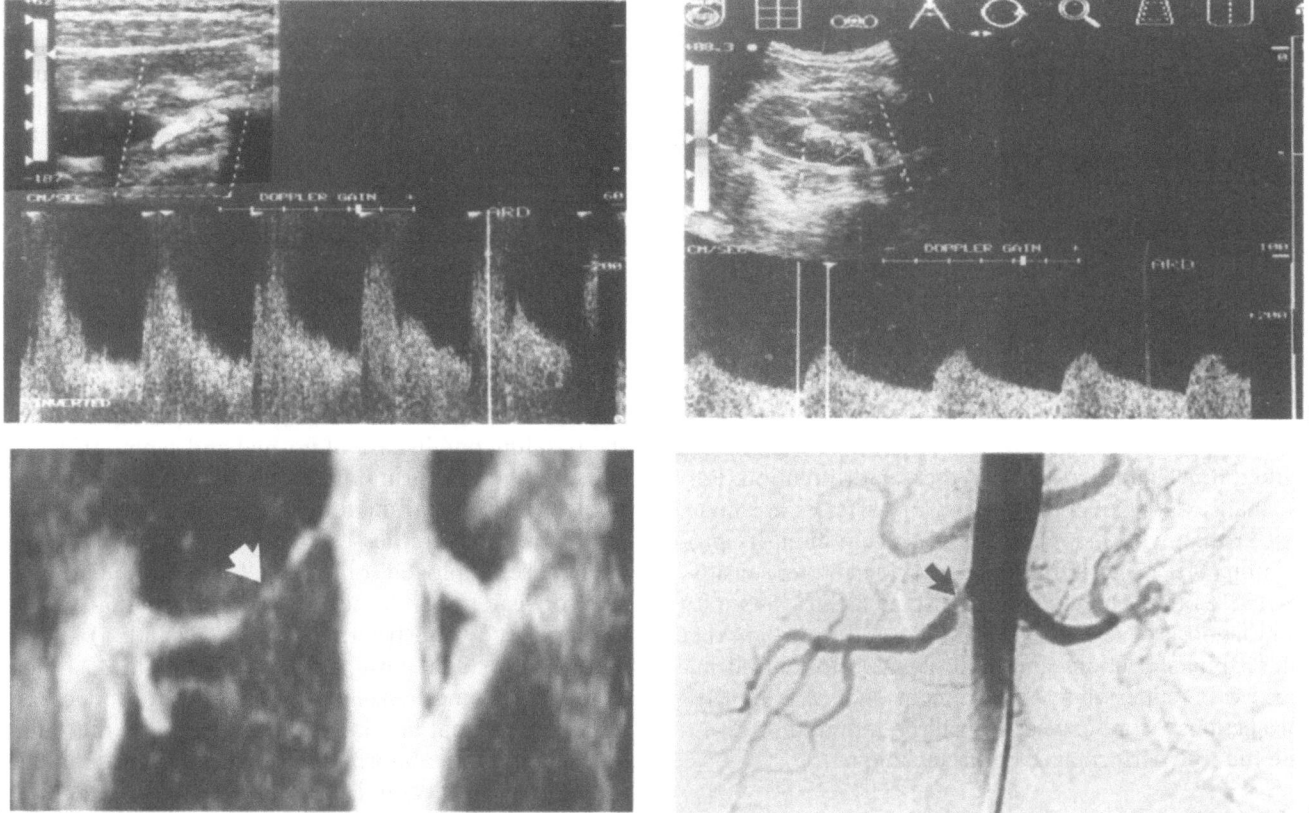

**Fig. 1 a-d.** Fibromuscular dysplasia with stenosis of the right renal artery. On the colour flow sonography , the postostial stenosis produces turbulences with a mosaic of colours (not shown). **a** Spectral sampling at the site of stenosis shows a high peak systolic velocity at 210 cm/s. **b** Intrarenal waveforms are dampered with a decreased systolic acceleration and increased ascension time. **c** Three-dimensional time-of-flight magnetic resonance angiography shows the stenosis (*arrow*), which is overestimated in diameter and in length when compared with the same stenosis shown by arteriography (*arrow*) (**d**)

interlobar or segmental vessels (at the lower and upper pole) of each kidney and spectral sampling under colour guidance for angle correction of both renal arteries allowing peak systolic velocity measurement. The use of phased-array low-frequency probes may be necessary in large patients. The percentages of technical failures of the anterior approach can reach 20%-25%, but those of the lateral approach are much lower. Accessory arteries are undetectable in most cases.

The stenosis may be seen on colour flow images. There are numerous criteria for haemodynamically significant stenosis. At the site of stenosis, a peak systolic velocity higher than 150 cm/s corresponds to a stenosis reducing diameter by more than 50%; one higher than 180 cm/s is evidence for a stenosis reducing diameter more than 60% (Fig. 1a). The renoaortic velocity ratio (RAR) must be higher than 3.5 to consider stenosis significant. In distal intrarenal vessels, the presence of a tardus-parvus phenomenon [5] suggests severe stenoses, decreasing diameter more than 75% (Fig 1b), with the following criteria: acceleration (ascending slope of the systolic peak) must be less than 3 m/s$^2$, the acceleration index > 4, the ascension time of systolic peak > 0.07 s

and the difference of resistivity indexes between both kidneys ($\Delta$RI) > 5%. Absence of the early systolic peak must not be taken into account for diagnosis.

Sensitivity of the technique has been reported to be between 35% and 95% [2, 6, 7]. Administration of captopril, by decreasing intrarenal vascular resistance, increases Doppler sensitivity by enhancing the pulsus tardus distal to significant stenoses [8]. However, the role of Doppler in predicting curability of hypertension after treatment of stenoses remains controversial.

**Helical CT**

The use of slip-ring CT scanners capable of 40 contiguous 1-s tube rotations coupled with continuous table incrementation permits a volumetric acquisition during a single breath-hold [9]. For renal artery studies, a 30-s bolus in an antecubital vein is necessary (between 90 ml of contrast materlal at 3 ml/s and 150 ml at 5 ml/s, depending on the body weight). Delay time ranges between 12 and 25 s. Slice thickness must not exceed 3 mm and table speed is set between 3 and 6 mm/s. Data must be reconstructed at 2-mm intervals in all cases with a 180° algo-

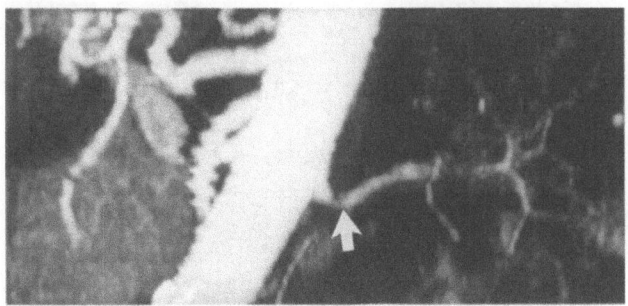

**Fig. 2.** Helical computed tomography of the aorta showing a stenosis of the left renal artery with the maximum intensity projection algorithm (*arrow*).

rithm, if available, to improve the axial resolution. Performances for detection of accessory arteries are much better than with Doppler. The maximum intensity projection (MIP) algorithm (Fig. 2) provided better sensitivity (92%) than shaded surface display (SSD) (59%) [9] for diagnosis of severe (>70%) stenoses. For Galanski et al. [10] axial sections and multiplanar reformatted images were superior to three-dimensional SSD or MIP projections. More experience will be required to evaluate the true performance of this technique.

**MR Angiography**

With time-of-flight or phase-contrast techniques, MR angiography allows visualization of the ostia and the proximal portion (3-3.5 mm) of renal arteries. Under the best conditions, only 50% of accessory arteries are depicted. With the time-of-flight method, the 3D-TONE acquisition decreases saturation effects and venous overlap [11]. Because of turbulence, significant stenoses are seen as a signal loss on MIP images. Distal recovery of flow signal intensity is observed if the stenosis is not too tight. Otherwise, the signal intensity is not recovered distal to the stenosis and a thrombosis cannot be ruled out. Quantification of the degree of stenosis, based on these features, is difficult and overestimation is the rule (Fig. 1c). Sensitivity and specificity for the diagnosis of a significant stenosis are between 53% and 100% and between 65% and 97%, respectively, depending on the technique used [12, 13] . Distal, segmental and accessory artery stenoses are generally missed.

## Detection of Functional Stenoses

### Principles of ACE Inhibition

ACE inhibitors, such as captopril, decrease the synthesis of angiotensin II, blocking its vasoconstrictor-stimulating effect, mostly on the efferent arterioles. This blockage produces a decrease in hydrostatic pressure within the glomerulus and a drop in filtration on the

side of stenosis. The principle of the test is to image the renal elimination of a tracer before and after administration of captopril to detect captopril-induced functional changes. When the test is positive, improvement or cure of hypertension is obtained in most cases following treatment of stenosis. This test has been coupled with scintigraphy [14] and, more recently, with dynamic MR [15].

### ACE Inhibition Scintigraphy [14]

$99_m T_c$-MAG3 (tubular agent) is now preferred to $99_m T_c$-DTPA (glomerular agent) by many. Some centres begin with an ACE-sensitized study first, obviating the baseline one in case of normal and symmetrical results. Others perform both in all cases with an interval of 24 h. Several parameters are considered on the side of stenosis during the sensitized study. When tubular agents are employed, one looks for a prolongation of the cortical transit time compared with that of the baseline study (obstruction must be excluded) and an increased residual cortical activity at 20 min postinjection. With glomerular agents, one looks for a decrease in the early renal uptake of the tracer and a flattening of the graph. An abnormal postcaptopril renogram has a mean sensitivity and specificity of 86% and 82%, respectively.

### ACE Inhibition Dynamic MR [14]

Gadolinium chelates behave as glomerular tracers in the same manner as iodine contrast media. After infusion of a bolus of 0.1 mmol/kg, it is possible to follow the intrarenal transit of this chelate with a series of coronal gradient echo images obtained during breath holding. This transit begins with a vasculointerstitial phase with a cortical and then a medullary enhancement of signal intensity (T1 shortening effect), a tubular phase characterized by a drop in signal intensity (T2 shortening effect) within the external medulla that extends centripetally towards the papilla and, finally, a ductal phase characterized by a late, low signal intensity within the internal medulla and the renal collecting system. In RVH, normal kinetics are altered by captopril on the side of stenosis, inducing a delay or disappearance of the tubular and ductal phases or a late T2 effect extending across the whole kidney [15] (Fig. 3).

### Strategy

The best strategy for diagnosis of RVH remains unclear and controversial. There is controversy, first of all, concerning the type of stenosis that warrants detecting: anatomical or only functional stenoses? A second question is which technique to use in either of these choices.

The diagnosis of functional stenoses must continue to be based upon ACE inhibition scintigraphy [4] because

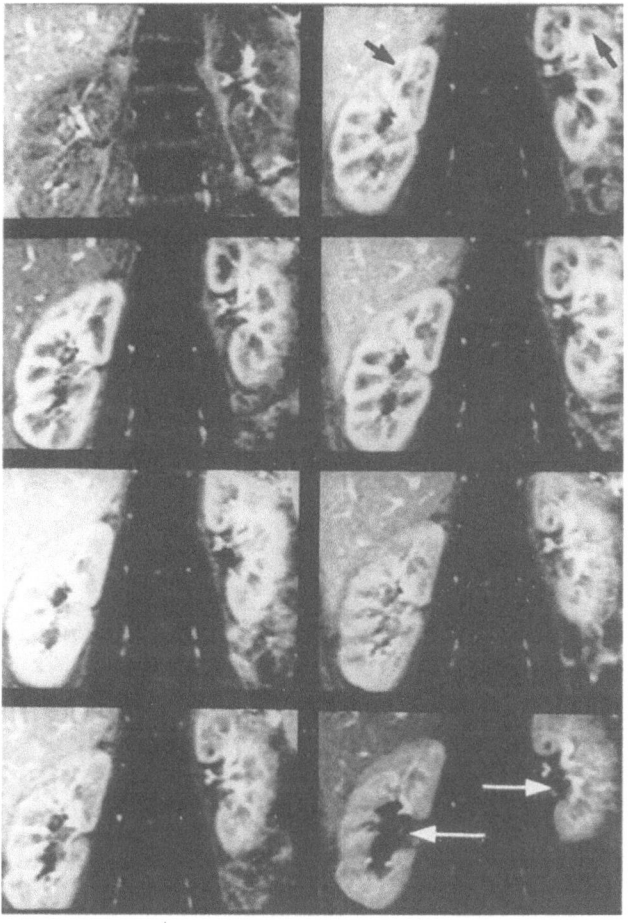
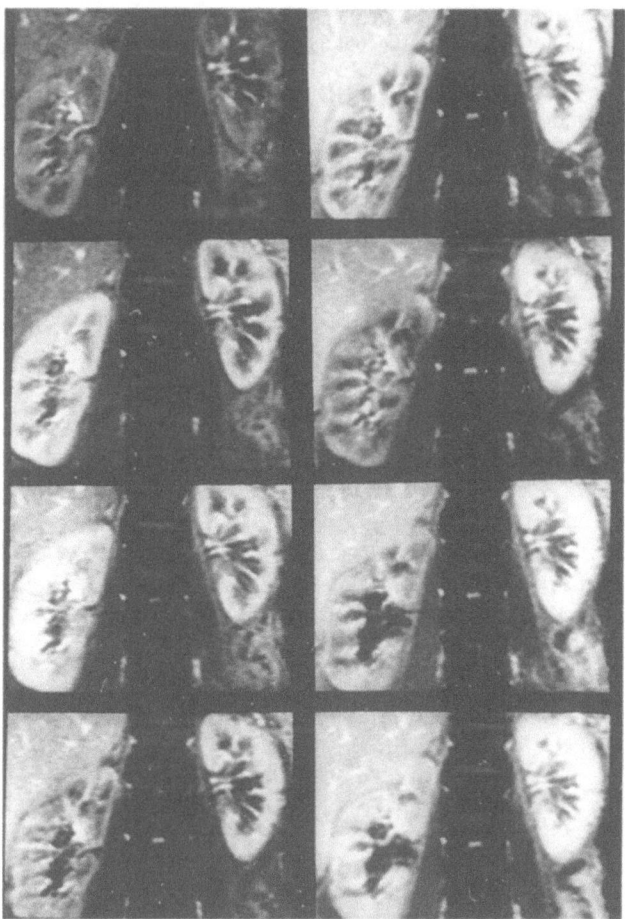

a                                                                                                                                                                                                b

**Fig. 3 a, b.** Dynamic gadolinium-enhanced magnetic resonance imaging of the kidneys before (**a**) and after (**b**) captopril administration in a patient with stenosis of the left renal artery (from *top to bottom*, then *left to right*). Before captopril, the tubular phase (*black arrows*) and excretion of contrast medium within renal collecting system (*white arrows*) are symmetrical. **b** After captopril, neither the tubular phase nor excretion are visible in the left kidney

ACE inhibition MR imaging is still in the process of being evaluated and compared with radionuclide methods. If performance appears to be equivalent, cost-effectiveness of these tests will have to be compared, taking into account the potential offered by MR of showing the anatomical stenosis simultaneously on MR angiographic sequences. For the diagnosis of anatomical stenoses, the choice of the best noninvasive test to perform currently depends on the investigators' experience.

# References

1. Working Group on Renovascular Hypertension (1987) Detection, evaluation and treatment of renovascular hypertension. Arch Intern Med 147: 820-829
2. Davidson RA, Wilcox CS (1992) Newer tests for the diagnosis of renovascular disease. JAMA 268: 3353-3358
3. Dunnick NR, Svetkey LP, Cohan RH, Newman GE, Braun SD, Himmelstein SI, Bollinger RR, McCann- RL, Wilkinson RH, Klotman PE (1989) Intravenous digital substraction renal angiography: use in screening for renovascular hypertension. Radiology 171: 219-222
4. Mann SJ, Pickering TG (1992) Detection of renovascular hypertension. State of the art. Ann Intern Med 117: 845-853
5. Lafortune M, Patriquin H, Demeule H et al (1992) Renal arterial stenosis: slowed systole in the downstream circulation. Experimental study in dogs. Radiology 184: 475-478
6. Middleton WD (1992) Doppler US evaluation of renal artery stenosis: past, present, and future. Radiology 184: 307-308
7. Olin JW, Piedmonte MR, Young JR, DeAnna S, Grub M, Childs MB (1995) The utility of duplex ultrasound scanning of the renal arteries for diagnosing significant renal artery stenosis. Ann Intern Med 122: 833-838
8. René PC, Oliva VL, Bui BT, Froment D, Harel C, Nicolet Vfi Courteau M, Carignan L (1995) Renal artery stenosis: evaluation of Doppler US after inhibition of angiotensin-converting enzyme with captopril. Radiology 196: 675-679
9. Rubin GD, Dake MD, Napel S, Jeffrey RB, McDonnel CH, Sommer FG, Wexler L, Williams DM (1994) Spiral CT of renal artery stenosis: comparison of three-dimensional rendering techniques. Radiology 190: 181-189
10. Galanski M, Prokop M, Chavan A, Schaefer CM, Jandeleit K, Nischelsky JE (1993) Renal artery stenoses: spiral CT angiography. Radiology 189:185-192
11. Fellner C, Strotzer M, Geissler-A, Kohler SM, Kramer BK, Spies V, Held P, Gmeinwieser J (1995) Renal arteries: eval-

uation with optimized 2D and 3D time-of-flight MR angiography. Radiology 196: 651-687

12. Debatin JF, Spritzer CE, Grist TM, Beam C, Svetkey LP, Newman GE, Sostman HD (1991) Imaging of the renal arteries: value of MR angiography. AJR 157: 981-990

13. Loubeyre P, Revel D, Garcia P, Delignette A, Canet E, Chirossel P, Genin G, Amiel M (1995) Screening patients for renal artery stenosis: value of three-dimensional time-of-flight MR angiography. AJR 162: 847-852

14. Sfiakanakis GN, Bourgoignie JJ, Georgiou M, Guerra JJ (1993) Diagnosis of renovascular hypertension with ACE inhibition scintigraphy. Radiol Clin North Am 31: 831 -848

15. Grenier N, Trillaud H, Combe C, Douws C, Jeandot J, Gosse P (1996) Diagnosis of renovascular hypertension with captopril sensitized dynamic MR of the kidney: feasability and comparison with scintigraphy. AJR (in press)

# Urinary Tract Infection in Children

H. Carty

Department of Radiology, Alder Hey Children's Hospital, Eaton Road, Liverpool L12 2AP, UK

There is a large body of literature on the subject of urinary tract infection in children and its investigation. The fact that so much has been written is an index of the controversy. Investigation is influenced by the cohort of children presenting to a unit and the facilities available.

## Aim of Investigations

The aim of investigation is twofold:
1. To identify those children with a structural anomaly of the urinary tract which requires surgical correction, with cure of symptoms and prevention of renal damage.
2. Identification of children with vesico-ureteric reflux (VUR) with and without renal scarring, to prevent damage to the upper tracts by sterilization of the urine, and to control symptoms of infection. The presumption is that scarred upper tracts due to reflux nephropathy may lead to renal failure or render the patient more susceptible to hypertension with its consequences.

As urinary tract infection is a very common clinical presentation in children, the dilemma for the clinician is to decide who, when and to what level to investigate children radiologically, as most children presenting with a first infection will have normal investigation results.

## Symptoms

Urinary tract infection may present with systemic or local symptoms. Systemic symptoms include fever, rigors, loin pain, vomiting, smelly urine, and general malaise. These indicate upper tract infection. Local symptoms, which are mainly those of cystitis, include frequency, nocturia, urgency, secondary enuresis, suprapubic pain and dysuria, and smelly urine. It is generally acknowledged that presentation with systemic illness requires investigation at all ages, even with a single infection. Feverish children presenting with lower tract signs only may require limited investigation for a first infection, when over 2 years of age.

Before embarking on investigation, a radiologist should ensure that urinary tract infection is proven bacteriologically. A bacterial count of 100 000 colony forming organisms/ml of urine is regarded as proof of urinary tract infection.

## Investigations

The available investigations include: plain films of the abdomen, ultrasound, micturating cystourethrography (MCU), scintigraphy, radionuclide cystography, intravenous urogram, and magnetic resonance imaging (MRI). The advantages and disadvantages of each investigation require comment.

### Plain Films

The abdominal X-ray is of limited value, but has the advantage of occasionally detecting renal stones missed by ultrasound and ureteric stones in those patients who do not have upper tract dilatation and ensuring there is no spinal anomaly which might be associated with renal anomalies. It is inexpensive and freely available.

Faecal loading or gaseous distension of the bowel often means that the renal tracts are obscured.

### Ultrasound of the Renal Tracts

The obvious advantage of ultrasound is that it is a noninvasive, radiation-free method of identifying the presence and location of both kidneys and structural anomalies of the collecting systems and the urinary bladder (Fig. 1). Accurate measurements of renal size and volume may be done and these compared with normal growth charts. It is also inexpensive and freely available. Its limitations are well known. It is operator dependent, and renal scarring may be missed. Ultrasound is not a sensitive method of detecting scars. It is not sensitive for the detection of vesicoureteric reflux (VUR). No functional information is obtained. Overdistension of the bladder may lead to dilatation of the renal pelvis, leading to overdiagnosis of

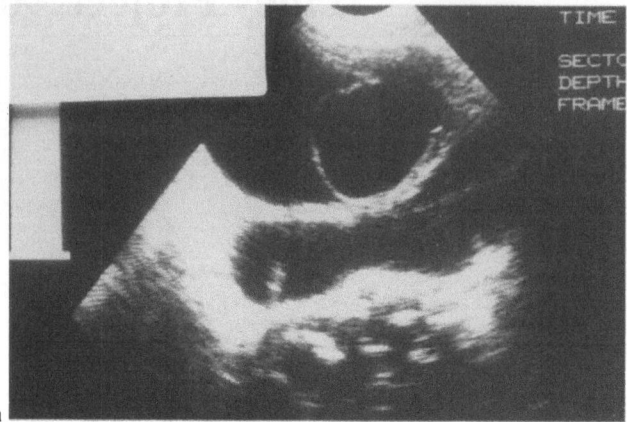

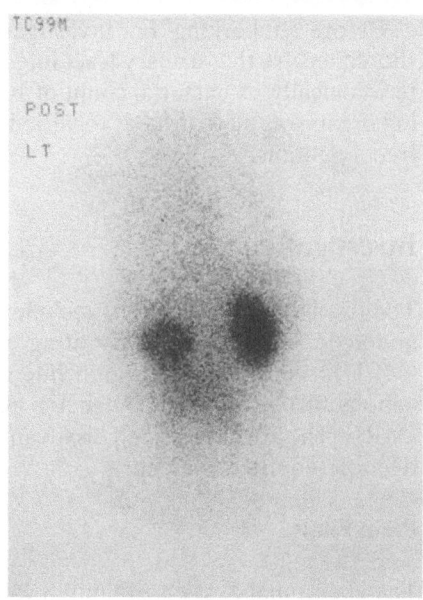

**Fig. 1 a, b.** Boy age 2 months. **a** Ultrasound of bladder. Typical appearance of ureterocoele in the bladder, with a dilated distal ureter. **b** Dimercaptosuccinic acid scintigraphy, same child. Note normal right kidney. There is a nonfunctioning upper moiety of the left kidney

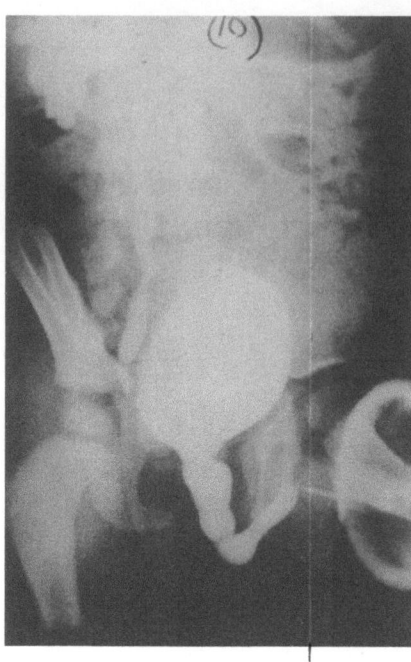

**Fig. 2.** Boy age 2 years with urinary tract infection. Micturating cystourethrography demonstrating mild posterior urethral valves with dilatation of the proximal urethra and right-sided reflux

catheterisation, which in unskilled hands is often traumatic, a variable though often high radiation dose to the gonads, and the possibility of missing reflux as fluoroscopy is intermittent, although severe reflux is not likely to be missed. It is also an undignified procedure for children unless a micturating seat is available.

In all children in whom reflux is demonstrated, therapeutic levels of antibiotics should be instituted before leaving the Radiology Department. Prophylactic antibiotics prior to cystography or for those in whom reflux is not demonstrated is more controversial.

## Scintigraphy

Renal scintigraphy in urinary tract infection is carried out with $^{99m}$Tc-labelled dimercaptosuccinic acid (DMSA), a radiopharmaceutical bound in the renal cortex, with

VUR. Renal pelvic dilatation of 1 cm or less without calyceal dilatation is a normal finding in children with overdistended bladders. A repeat examination with an empty bladder will usually show resolution of the pelvic dilatation.

In acute pyelonephritis, focal areas of increased echogenicity may be seen in the kidneys and should not be misinterpreted as tumours.

## Micturating Cystourethrography

MCU is the single most unpleasant radiological examination to perform in children once they are beyond about 1 year old, even when well done. Its purpose is to demonstrate VUR, grade it and demonstrate urethral anomalies, such as valves (Fig. 2) which may be associated with reflux. Its advantage is the excellent anatomical demonstration of any problem. Reflux may only be present during active infection, but cystography during infection may lead to a recurrence of infection and is therefore best left until the infection has been successfully treated. The disadvantages are self-evident;

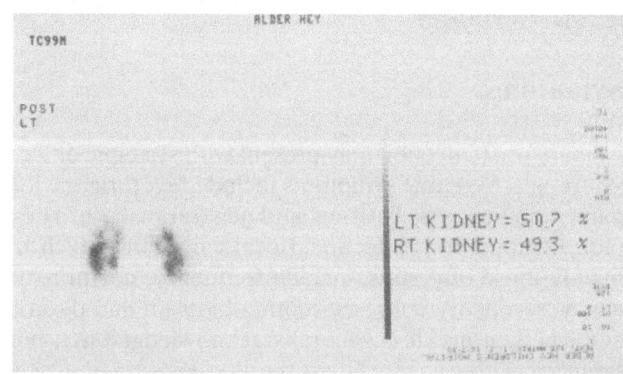

**Fig. 3.** Dimercaptosuccinic acid scintigram. Girl age 3. There are multiple photopenic areas in both kidneys due to scarring. Note the differential uptakes, indicating that both kidneys are equally affected

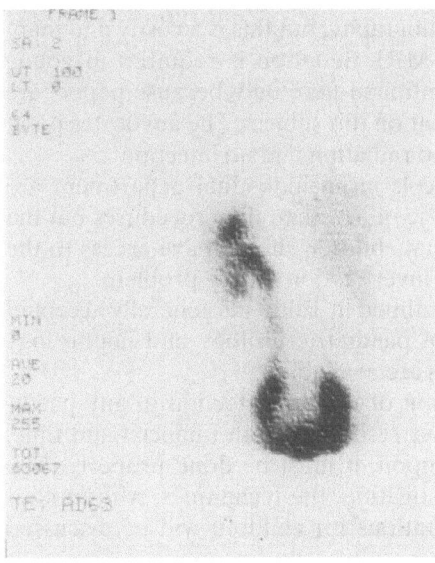

**Fig. 4.** Direct radionuclide cystography with reflux to the left kidney

limited excretion. It is accepted as the gold standard for the demonstration of renal scars (Fig. 3). Scars appear as photopenic areas with interruption of the smooth renographic outline. Three views, a posterior and both oblique views, are taken. The relative uptake of the isotope by the kidneys is calculated and provides a reliable estimate of the contribution of each kidney to renal function. A second manifestation of reflux is the overall failure of growth of a kidney which remains smooth. A discrepancy of greater than 10% in uptakes between the kidneys is regarded as indicating impaired function.

*Pitfalls.* If scanning is done early after infection, areas of photopenia due to the infection may be shown which do not progress to demonstrable scarring. Scars present just after infection may not be permanent. A unilateral duplex though normal kidney may show a relative increased uptake of greater than 10%, leading to an erro-

neous diagnosis of damage to the contralateral kidney. This is avoidable if the scan is reviewed in conjunction with ultrasound images. Symmetrical smooth kidneys with growth failure but no scarring may be interpreted as normal. If the examination is reviewed with ultrasonic measurement of renal volume, this is an avoidable pitfall. It is not easily available in most paediatric departments and is underused.

### Radionuclide Cystography

Radionuclide cystography may be direct or indirect. Direct cystography involves catheterisation as for an MCU and filling the bladder with saline which has had a small amount of $^{99m}$Tc (25 MBq) added to it. It therefore carries the same risk of infection and potential trauma as an MCU. The advantages claimed for this are continuous monitoring during filling and micturition, as there is no increased radiation dose. Trivial reflux is less likely to be missed. A lower radiation dose is claimed than with a fluoroscopic MCU. This is quoted in older literature. Modern screening techniques with coning, grid removal and intermittent fluoroscopy have significantly reduced doses. The anatomical detail is poor and no urethral information is obtained (Fig. 4).

Indirect radionuclide cystography is performed by first doing a $^{99m}$Tc Mag 3 renogram, which is performed continuously over 16 min. Mag 3 is rapidly excreted from the upper tracts but, to clear any residue that might still be present, the child is given copious amounts of cordial to drink. When the child is ready, micturition takes place in front of the gamma camera. Acquisition should start just before the child starts to micturate, as reflux can occur as the child strains To perform this technique the child must be co-operative. The renogram is performed with the child supine. The voiding cystogram is performed with the child sitting in front of the camera (Fig. 5).

a

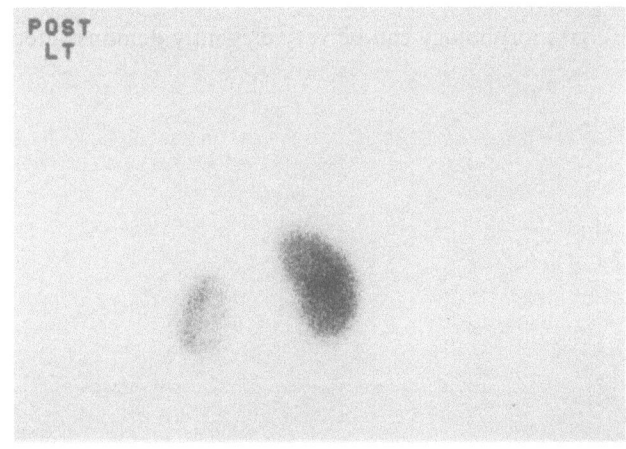

b

**Fig. 5. a** Indirect cystography: reflux to the left kidney is present during micturition. **b** Dimercaptosuccinic acid scintigram in same child. Note small left kidney

**Table 1.** Imaging protocol

| | |
|---|---|
| 0-1 years | Ultrasound of urinary tract |
| | + |
| | Contrast cystourethrography |
| | DMSA |
| | Structural anomalies and hydronephrosis to be investigated further, as appropriate |
| 1-5 years | Plain films of the abdomen |
| | Ultrasound of urinary tract |
| | DMSA |
| | MCU if scarring on DMSA |
| |     Signs or symtoms of upper tract involvement |
| |     Recurrent infections |
| |     Family history of reflux |
| Over 5 years | Plain Films of the abdomen |
| | Ultrasound |
| | Proceed to DMSA if above abnormal |
| |     Upper tract signs |
| |     Repetitive infection |

DMSA, dimercaptosuccinic acid; MCU, micturating cystourethography

The obvious advantage is that there is no catheterisation. The limitation on anatomical information is the same as for direct cystography. Children must have bladder control before this is a suitable method. There is also concern about its sensitivity.

### Intravenous Urography

Intravenous urography is now considered inappropriate for the primary investigation of urinary tract infection. It is not sensitive in detecting early changes of infection, is often badly done, has an inherent radiation dose and, if ionic contrast is used, has unpleasant side effects of vomiting. It may still have an occasional role in demonstrating anatomical details in difficult cases.

### Magnetic Resonance Imaging

Renal morphology can be very elegantly demonstrated on abdominal angiography, but this is a costly and inappropriate use of MRI. Sedation is required in young children. It is mentioned here only because papers are beginning to appear on this subject. The advocates point out that there is no radiation and no injection!

Imaging protocols in an individual department are dictated by the ease of access to the procedures but the ideal should be that children should have access to the most appropriate investigation for the problem.

The protocol outlined in Table 1 is generally accepted in departments of paediatric urology and nephrology where all facilities are available.

The investigation of urinary infection in any paediatric unit consumes resources, both financial and time. Once embarked upon, it must be done properly. The pathways of investigation, the techniques, with modifications and adaptations for children will be discussed during the lecture.

### Further Reading

1. Dickinson JA (1979) Incidence and outcome of symptomatic urinary infection in children. BMJ 1: 1330-1332
2. Gleeson FV, Gordon I (1991) Imaging in urinary tract infection. Arch Dis Child 66: 1282-1283
3. Hanbury DC, Whitaker RH, Sherwood T, Farman P (1989) Ultrasound and plain X-ray screening in childhood urinary tract infection. Br J Urol 64: 638-640
4. Haycock G (1986) Investigation of urinary tract infection. Arch Dis Child. 61: 55-58
5. McKerrow W, Davidson-Lamb N, Jones PF (1984) Urinary tract infection in children. BMJ 289: 299-303
6. Rickwood AMK, Carty HM, McKendrick T, Williams MPL, Jackson M, Pilling DW, Sprigg A (1992) Current imaging of childhood urinary infections: prospective survey. BMJ 304: 663-665
7. Sherwood T, Whitaker RH (1984) Initial screening of children with urinary tract infection: is plain film radiography and ultrasonography enough? BMJ 288: 827
8. White RHR (1987) Management of urinary tract infection. Arch Dis Child 62: 421-427
9. Whitear P, Shaw P, Gordon I (1990) Comparison of $^{99m}$Tc dimercaptosuccinic acid scans and intravenous urography in children. Br J Radiol 63: 438-443

# Acute Renal Infections in Adults

L. Dalla Palma

Istituto di Radiologia, Ospedale di Cattinara, Strada di Fiume, 34149 Trieste, Italy

## Terminology

The term "acute renal infection" encompasses a spectrum of pathologic processes involving the renal parenchyma that vary in severity from acute pyelonephritis to a renal abscess which can progress to the peri- and pararenal spaces.

The literature on imaging in patients with aute renal infection has been plagued for a long time by inconsistency and ambiguity in terminology. The terms acute pyelonephritis, acute bacterial nephritis, acute interstitial nephritis, focal pyelonephritis, lobar nephronia, preabscess state, pseudoabscess, carbuncle, phlegmon are encountered but there is no consensus among radiologists and the experts on their use. The Society of Uroradiology has recommended a simplified nomenclature that is based on the traditional and widely understood term **acute pyelonephritis** which can be focal or diffuse, unilateral or bilateral [1]. The acute infection may regress or progress to renal and/or extrarenal **abscess or emphysematous pyelonephritis**; if obstruction is present we may observe **pyonephrosis**. Abscesses may form either from the progression of acute pyelonephritis or from hematogeneous spread of infection.

## Spread of Infection and Pathology

### Ascending Bacterial Infection

The natural history of pyelonephritis is determined by a complex relationship of microbiological virulence factors and host defense factors. The gastrointestinal tract provides the reservoir for bacteria, *Escherichia coli* in over 80% of the cases, producing urinary tract infection by the ascending route. Recent clinical studies demonstrate reflux in only 38%-57% of children with clear-cut parenchymal involvement shown by cortical scintigraphy [2, 3]. Reflux in adults with pyelonephritis is uncommon except in the presence of neuropathic bladder.

In the absence of reflux certain virulent strains of bacteria, such as *E. coli*, ascend the ureter against the ante-grade flow of urine, colonize the upper urinary tract and then penetrate the parenchyma via the collecting ducts and tubules. There are infiltrates of inflammatory cells in both the tubules and interstitial tissues: it is a true tubulointerstitial nephritis [4].

Distribution of the inflammatory lesions is characteristically patchy and sometimes lobar. Macroscopically, infected parenchyma appears as radiating yellow-white stripes or wedges extending through the full thickness of the renal parenchyma from the papillary tip to the cortical surface, following the distribution of the medullary rays just as in experimental animals. In severe cases, the entire kidney parenchyma can be involved: there is an overlapping spectrum of the parenchymal response to infection from acute pyelonephritis to renal abscess. The renal infection is a pathological continuum from bacterial and leucocytic infiltration of the interstitium to abscess formation.

It is difficult for pathologists to trace the evolution of acute parenchyma infection in humans. In this respect computed tomography (CT) offers a unique advantage, since it shows sequentially the various stages of acute renal infection.

Renal scarring, as a late sequela to severe bacterial pyelonephritis, occurs in children but less commonly in adults. Macroscopic parenchymal loss may be in the form of focal, full-thickness scarring in the growing kidneys of infants and children or focal or global atrophy that includes papillary retraction or necrosis in older patients. There is strong experimental evidence that the prompt administration of antibiotics minimizes the parenchymal loss.

### Haematogeneous Bacterial Infection

In humans haematogeneous infection is thought to be less common than the ascending variety and is usually encountered in patients known to abuse intravenous drugs, to be immunocompromised, or to have an extrarenal source of infection such as skin, teeth, heart valve, etc. *Staphylococcus aureus* is the most common pathogen.

The classic example of haematogeneous spread is a

unique or multiple abscess as a result of bacterial dissemination.

## Clinical Features

The syndrome consists of loin pain, tenderness and pyrexia accompanied by bacteriuria, bacteraemia, and sometimes haematuria. The clinical pattern of all the pathological variants is quite similar: therefore if it is easy to diagnose a renal infection, it is impossible to recognize the pathological variant, i.e. the complicated acute pyelonephritis. The imaging modalities may solve this problem.

Most risk factors of acute renal infection can be elicited by a good clinical history and physical examination. Such factors include diabetes mellitus, previous stone disease, previous renal infection, vescicoureteral reflux, obstruction, prolonged catheterization, analgesic abuse, immunodeficiency, surgical complications, pregnancy.

## Imaging Modalities

### Acute Pyelonephritis

**Intravenous urography (IVU)** had a role in the diagnosis of acute renal infections for many years until the appearance of ultrasonography (US) and CT. The results of IVU were reported to be abnormal in 25% of the patients [5]; in our experience the positive rate was higher when nephrotomography (NT) was performed [6].

Renal infection is shown by diffuse or focal kidney enlargement, diffuse or patchy or focal attenuation of the nephrogram, delayed, decreased or absent opacification of the collecting system, mild dilatation and, more frequently, narrowing of the calices. When acute pyelonephritis is complicated NT demonstrates the *abscess* cavity as a hypodense area of different shape, round or triangular, with blurred margins, displacing the collecting system; if the abscess extends to the perirenal space the renal fascia may be thickened.

The value of normal IVU is that it rules out the presence of destructing stones, pyonephrosis and the most serious complications.

**Ultrasonography** is more sensitive than IVU but less sensitive than CT or $^{99m}$Tc – labelled DMSA cortical scintigraphy [6]. It may show a focal or a diffuse enlargement of the kidney with increased parenchymal thickness and reduction or disappearance of the renal sinus. The echogenicity is decreased with focal, almost anechoic, areas. Very rarely US shows hyperechoic areas which correspond to haemorrhagic inflammation [7].

The renal parenchyma may appear normal on US despite the presence of inflammation shown at CT. If the infected parenchyma evolves into an *abscess*, US shows a hypoechoic mass with low level echoes: the intensity of the echoes is related to the debris as well as to the gas

produced by bacteria. The mass can be liquid with possible fluid-fluid levels or with enhanced sound transmission. The borders are usually ill defined and may become visible when the abscess encapsulates. When the complication involves the pararenal spaces, US can demonstrate the extrarenal collection; the technique has poor sensitivity in showing increased thickness of the septa.

**Computed tomography** is more sensitive than the previous modalities. The spectrum of CT findings in acute infection has been thoroughly summarized and illustrated [8].

The kidney can be normal if the renal infection is mild and uncomplicated. On precontrast CT scans the kidney may show one or more areas of low attenuation and may be swollen; in a few cases an increased parenchymal density on precontrast scans has been observed, suggesting that the infection may, at times, cause haemorrhage.

After contrast material injection, CT shows a diffuse or focal enlargement of the kidney, diffuse or focal or multifocal areas of low attenuation, streaky, round or

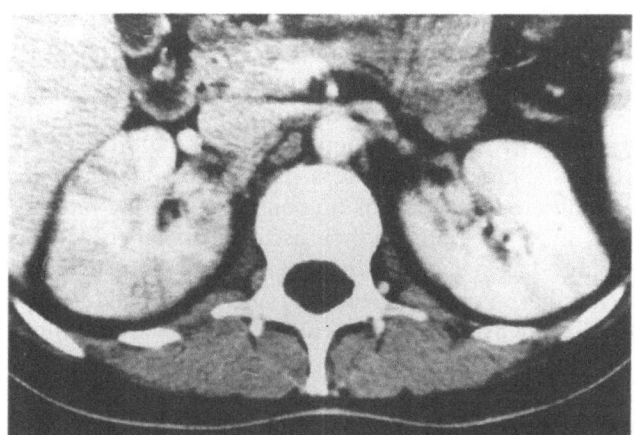

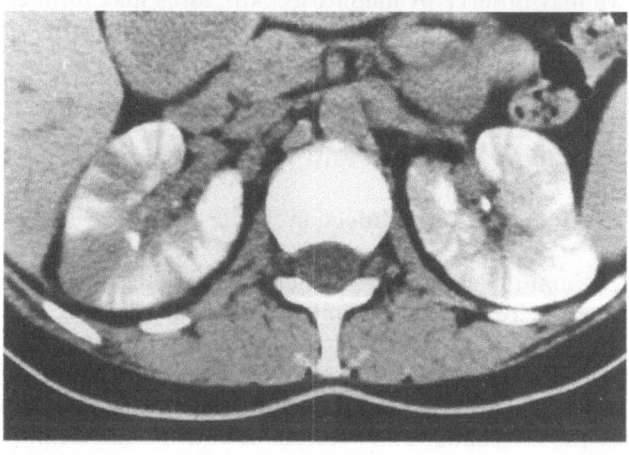

**Fig. 1 a, b.** Bilateral acute pyelonephritis. Contrast-enhanced computed tomography (CT). **a** Early phase: multiple areas of low attenuation which are wedge - and shaped streaky on the right kidney; minimal changes involve the left kidney. **b** Delayed CT shows contrast enhancement in some of the previous areas of low attenuation, indicating therefore the real extension of the infection and the oedema

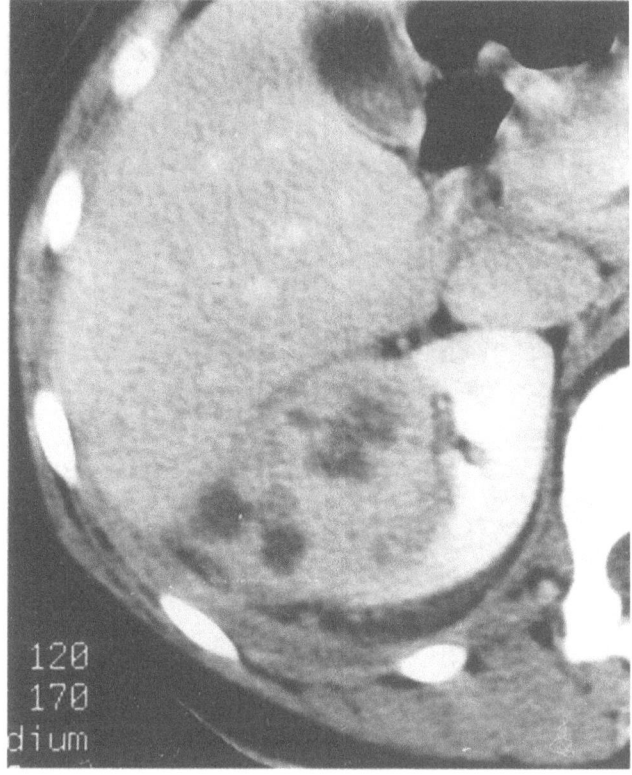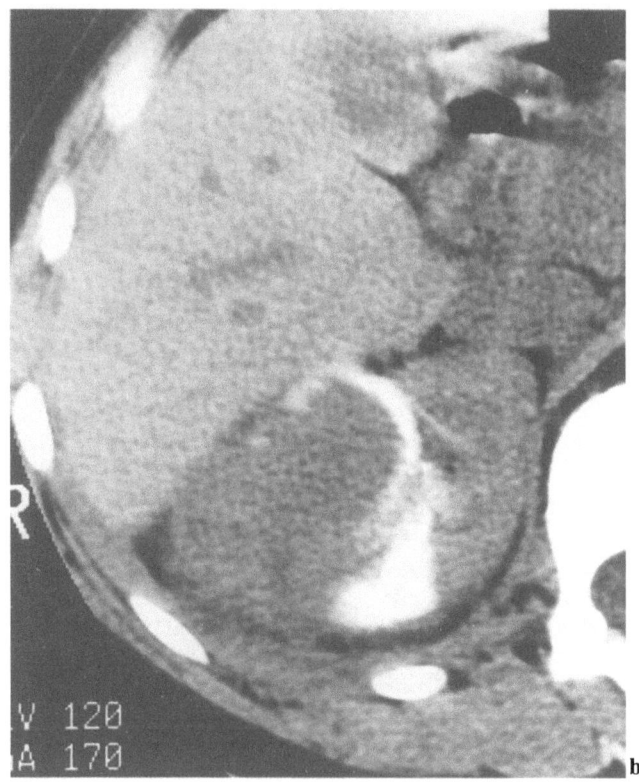

**Fig. 2 a, b.** Right acute focal pyelonephritis. Contrast-enhanced computed tomography (CT). **a** The early phase shows huge, focal non-homogeneous round area of low attenuation. **b** Delayed CT shows contrast enhancement surrounding the focal pyonephritis

wedge-shaped with a cortical base (Fig. 1). They are usually sharp at the edges in the acute phase but become indistinct during the healing process. The septae of the perirenal space can be thickened.

If the acute pyelonephritis cavitates, one or more small cavities can be recognized in the attenuated areas; very rapidly these cavities can coalesce to form a *macroabscess*. In such a case CT demonstrates round or triangular areas with density values between 15-30 HU (Fig. 2).

The abscess has a thick wall which is well enhanced after the injection of the contrast agent. When acute pyelonephritis spreads outside the kidney a collection of fluid can be observed in the peri- and pararenal spaces and, later on, in the posterior abdominal wall. Such a collection can complicate the renal infection even in the absence of a renal abscess.

On the postcontrast delayed (at 3-6 h) CT scans, dense contrast staining of the previously attenuated areas has been described (Fig. 1, 2) [9, 10]. In our material the delayed, 3-h scans have shown such staining with three different patterns [11]:

1. A late, dense, inhomogeneous nephrogram on the previously attenuated nephrogram.
2. A staining surrounding the abscess with different shape.
3. Focal densities localized far away from the hypodense areas of the early scan.

These features are due to the slow progression of contrast medium down the tubules because they are partly obstructed by the inflammatory debris and narrowed by the oedema. The delayed filling of the tubules may also be explained by the arteriolar vasospasm and then ischaemia.

The spectrum of the CT findings in acute pyelonephritis (a) depends on the time at which imaging is performed relative to the onset of infection, (b) may change rapidly (i.e. within hours) and (c) can be modified and regress by antibiotics. Therefore invasive therapy can be avoided or postponed.

CT studies have demonstrated that, despite the clinical improvement, abnormal findings may persist for weeks to months after clinical signs of infection resolve and that scarring in adults occurs more frequently than was previously realized [12].

The cortical agents ([99m]Tc-labelled DMSA and glucoheptonate) are sensitive and specific in the diagnosis and follow-up of acute pyelonephritis [2, 3]. Fraser et al. found **Renal scintigraphy** to be slightly more sensitive than CT for detecting focal abnormalities in patients with the clinical signs of acute renal infection but normal IVU. Scintigraphy cannot distinguish the pathological patterns which are well shown with CT.

**Magnetic resonance imaging** (MRI) in the routine evaluation of renal infections is presently limited and therefore it does not play a role.

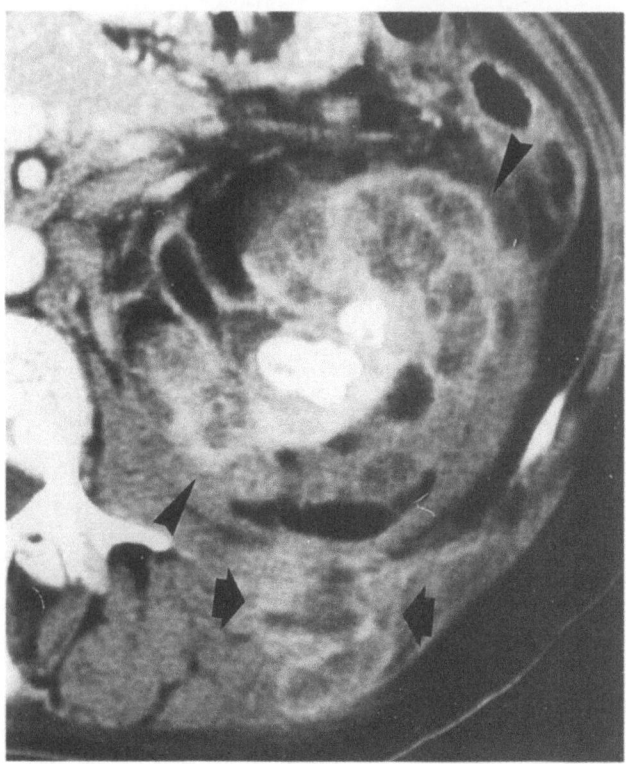
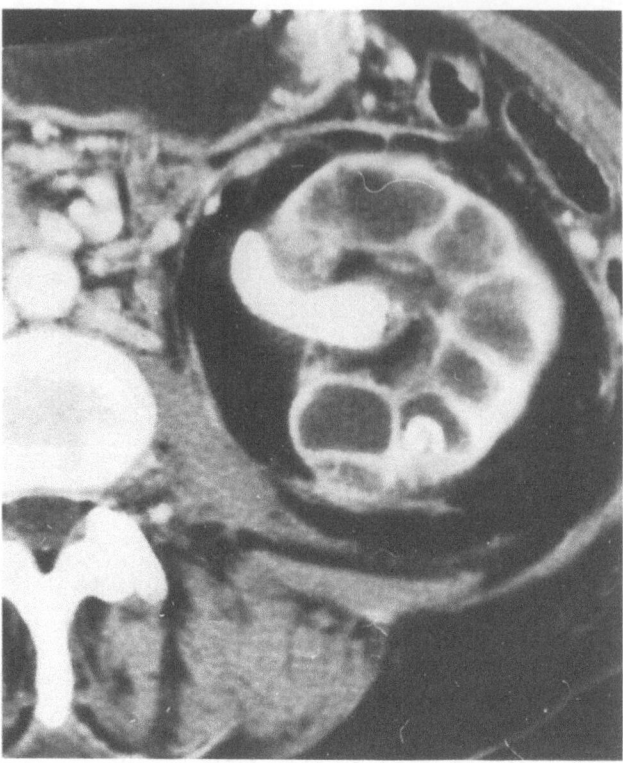

**Fig. 3 a, b.** Pyonephrosis. Contrast-enhanced computed tomography (CT). Staghorn stones and multiple pyonephrotic cavities complicated with abscess extend to the extrarenal spaces (*arrowheads*) and involving the paravertebral muscles (*arrows*)

### Emphysematous Pyelonephritis

Emphysematous pyelonephritis is a rare, severe, life-threatening infection of the kidney characterized by intraparenchymal gas formation and found most exclusively in diabetic patients [13]. Pathologically, widespread abscess formation and necrosis are present. Early diagnosis and prompt percutaneous drainage can lower the mortality rate from 75% to 9% [14].

**The plain film** demonstrates gas within the renal parenchyma; CT is the best modality to differentiate gas within the collecting system and also defines the extent of the disease. Michalei et al. [14] have described three radiological stages: in stage 1 gas is within the renal parenchyma in a diffuse mottled pattern; in stage 2, the gas extends into the perirenal space; and in stage 3 a retroperitoneal extension is present. The use of contrast agents is risky.

### Pyonephrosis

Pyonephrosis consists of infection with pus in the upper collecting system which is dilated because of acute, or more frequently, chronic obstruction.

It is different from infected hydronephrosis because it causes disruption of the wall of the pelvis and of contiguous renal parenchyma and it can progress to peri-pararenal fluid collections.

IVU findings include renal stones (on the plain film), frequently staghorn, nonfunctioning or poorly functioning enlarged kidney.

US is very informative, showing stones, the dilatation of the collecting system, and the presence of fluid and debris and extrarenal collections.

CT is the modality of choice, given its ability to define the renal enlargement, the site and morphology of the stones, the layering of the opaque urine above the pus in the dilated collecting system, and the anatomical extension of the extrarenal collection [13] (Fig. 3).

Common CT findings suggesting pyonephrosis include increased pelvic wall thickness and more severe perirenal fat changes than are seen in uninfected hydronephrosis.

### Haematogeneous Renal Infection

The haematogeneous infection of the kidney is much less common than the ascending variety and is usually encountered in patients with IV drug abuse, who are immunocompromised or have an extrarenal source of infection, e.g. teeth, skin, colonic diverticulae, etc. This infection is usually a result of *Staphylococcus aureus* dissemination and is characterized by single or multiple abscesses localized in the cortex in the early phase. In a late stage it can involve the remaining kidney.

**CT** is the imaging modality of choice, given its ability

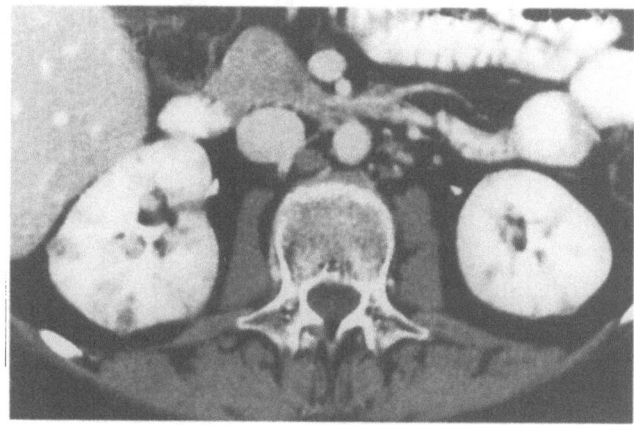

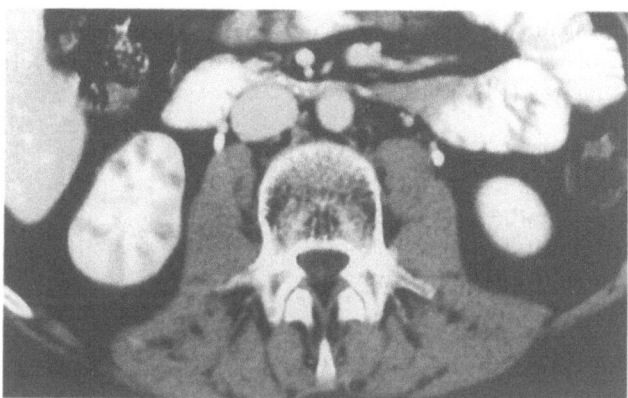

**Fig. 4 a, b.** Bilateral renal abscesses. Contrast-enhanced computed tomography (CT). Multiple, round areas of attenuation on both kidneys in a child with acute lymphatic leukaemia treated with immunosuppressive therapy

to detect early lesions as small, round, peripheral hypodense areas (Fig. 4). In the advanced stage these areas become larger and polymorphous.

## Conclusion

Diagnostic imaging modalities, mainly US and CT, are very important in the management of renal infections since they detect and evaluate the renal and extrarenal infection. Different lesions may have similar clinical patterns: the imaging modalities may define the severity of the renal infection. They are indicated:

1. If the disease is resistant to medical treatment
2. If predisposing factors are present (old age, urinary tract stones, indwelling urinary catether, vesicoureter-

al reflux, neurogenic bladder, diabetes and immunodeficiency)
3. For follow-up under medical treatment
4. To guide drainage in complicated cases which do not respond to antibiotic therapy

Due to the low sensitivity of IVU, renal scintigraphy ($^{99m}$Tc-labelled DMSA) and US should be the first examinations to be performed. Their limitations are due to the incomplete evaluation of the process, mainly in cases of extrarenal extension.

CT is the study of choice to define the pattern of renal involvement and extrarenal extension, intra- or extrafascial. CT is also useful in understanding the pathophysiology of the infection using precontrast and postcontrast, early and delayed scans.

## References

1. Talner L, Davidson A, Lebowitz R, Dalla Palma L, Goldman S (1994) Acute pyelonephritis: can we agree on terminology? Radiology 192: 297-305
2. Melis K, Vandevivere J, Hoskens C et al (1992) Involvement of the renal parenchyma in acute urinary tract infection: the contribution of $^{99m}$TC dimercaptosuccinic acid scan. Eur J Pediatr 151: 536-539
3. Kass EJ, Fink-Bennett D, Cacciarelli AA et al (1992) The sensitivity of renal scintigraphy and sonography in detecting non obstructive acute pyelonephritis. J Urol 148: 606-608
4. Roberts JA (1991) Etiology and pathophysiology of pyelonephritis. Am J Kidney Dis 17: 1-9
5. Fiegler W (1983) Ultrasound in acute renal inflammatory lesions. Eur J Radiol 3: 354-357
6. Dalla Palma L, Pozzi-Mucelli RS, Pozzi-Mucelli F, Magnaldi S (1988) Diagnostica per immagini delle infezioni renali acute. Acta Urol Ital 4: 277-284
7. Rigsby CM, Rosenfield AT, Glickman MG, Hodson J (1986) Haemorrhagic focal bacterial nephritis: findings on gray scale sonography and CT. AJR 146: 1173-1177
8. Gold RP, McClennan BL (1990) Acute infections of the renal parenchyma. In: Pollack HM (ed) Clinical urography. Saunders, Philadelphia, pp 799-821
9. Ishikawa L, Saito Y, Onouchi Z et al (1985) Delayed contrast enhancement in acute focal bacterial nephritis: CT features. J Comput Assisted Tomogr 3: 894-897
10. Lemaitre L, Cotten A, Robert Y et al (1991) Infections aigues du parenchyme renal de l'adulte. Rev Im Med 3: 295-303
11. Dalla Palma L, Pozzi-Mucelli F, Pozzi-Mucelli RS (1995) Delayed CT findings in acute renal infection. Clin Radiol 50: 364-370
12. Soulen MC, Fishman EK, Goldman SM (1989) Sequelae of acute renal infections: CT evaluation. Radiology 173: 423-426
13. Merenich WM, Popky GL (1991) Radiology of renal infection. Med Clin North Am 75: 425-469
14. Michaeli J, Mogle P, Sperlberg S et al (1984) Emphysematous pyelonephritis. J Urol 131: 203-208

# Imaging of Urinary Tract Obstruction

J.A.W. Webb

Diagnostic Radiology Department, St Bartholomew's Hospital, West Smithfield, London EC1A 7BE, UK

The diagnosis of urinary tract obstruction depends on showing increased resistance to flow along the urinary tract. Such increased resistance causes proximal dilatation (obstructive uropathy) and secondary functional effects on the kidney (obstructive nephropathy) with associated nephron damage and parenchymal atrophy (obstructive atrophy) [1]. Ultrasonography (US), intravenous urography (IVU), computed tomography (CT) and magnetic resonance imaging (MR) diagnose obstruction largely by showing the anatomical consequences of obstruction, namely the dilatation of the pelvicalyceal system and ureter proximal to the obstructing lesion. Some limited functional information may be obtained from the pattern of contrast medium excretion with IVU, CT and MR and from Doppler US examination. Scintigraphy, however, provides direct functional evidence of obstruction.

Pelvicalyceal dilatation is often described as "hydronephrosis" and this term may be used as if it is synonymous with obstruction. It is very important to recognise that pelvicalyceal and ureteric dilatation do not always indicate obstruction. Nonobstructive causes of pelvicalyceal dilatation include vesicoureteric reflux, normal anatomical variants (e.g. large extrarenal pelvis) and congenital anomalies (e.g. megacalyces). Also, following relief of obstruction, mild dilatation of the pelvicalyceal system and ureter may persist. Once dilatation has been shown by an "anatomical" method, its significance may need to be assessed either by scintigraphy or by other anatomical methods which give a more detailed assessment.

Another important concept is that the functional severity of obstruction is unrelated to the degree of dilatation of the pelvicalyceal system and ureter. Mild dilatation occurs in some types of severe obstruction, particularly obstruction caused by ureteric stones, retroperitoneal fibrosis and retroperitoneal malignancy.

## Acute Obstruction

Acute ureteric obstruction is most commonly caused by a calculus. Less common causes of obstruction are blood clots, sloughed papillae, or acute idiopathic pelviureteric junction (PUJ) obstruction.

### Intravenous Urography

IVU is the investigation of choice in most suspected acute ureteric obstruction [2]. It should be performed while the patient is in pain.

*Technique*

A full-length plain film on inspiration and a coned renal area view on expiration are used to check for renal and ureteric calculi. They may need to be supplemented by oblique films or plain tomography to check for intrarenal calcification.

After intravenous contrast medium administration a limited series of films is used, with the first film being a full-length film at 15 min. A full-length film following bladder emptying may be necessary to show hold-up at the vesicoureteric junction. Delayed films will be necessary in acute obstruction to show ureteric filling to the level of obstruction.

*Findings*

In complete ureteric obstruction there is an immediate nephrogram which becomes denser with time (Fig. 1). There is delayed filling of the pelvicalyceal system and ureter on the affected side, and they are usually mildly dilated to the level of obstruction. Where obstruction is incomplete, the typical nephrogram pattern does not occur but delayed pelvicalyceal filling with dilatation to the level of obstruction is seen. If the urogram is normal when the patient has pain, ureteric colic can be confidently excluded.

Clot colic is suspected if the patient has heavy haematuria. The clot is seen as a lucent filling defect which has usually resolved by 10-14 days. A sloughed papilla is suspected when the changes of papillary necrosis are seen in the kidneys. In acute PUJ obstruction the rounded, soft tissue density of dilated pelvis may be appreciated on the plain film and will fill with contrast medium on delayed films.

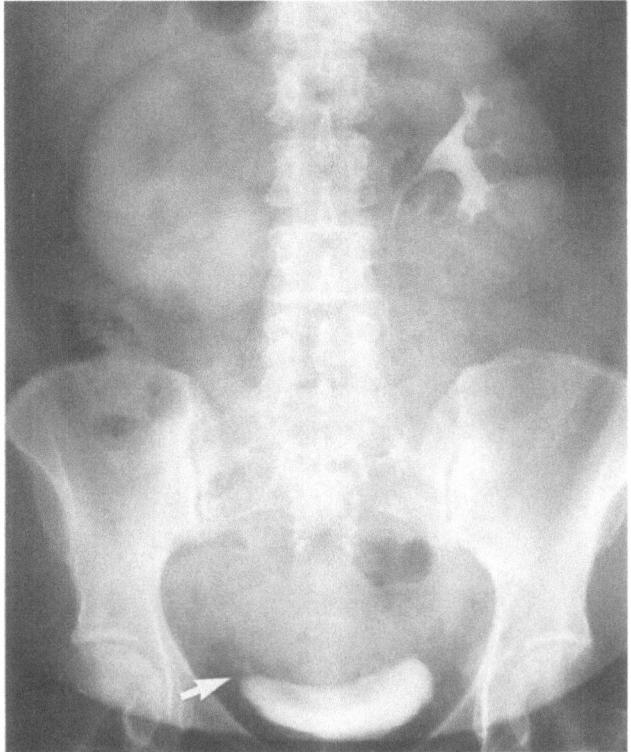

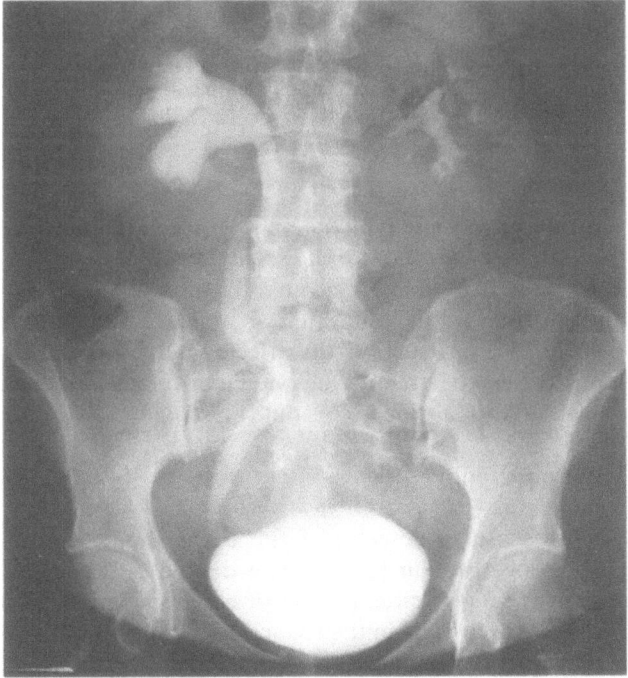

**Fig. 1 a, b.** Acute obstruction of the right ureter by a calculus at the vesicoureteric junction. **a** Note increasingly dense right nephrogram, delayed pelvicalyceal filling, and opacity at right vesicoureteric junction (*arrow*). **b** Delayed film shows pelvicalyceal system and ureter filled to the level of the calculus

## Ultrasonography

US is generally considered less satisfactory than IVU in the diagnosis of ureteric colic [3]. It may fail to demonstrate the mild pelvicalyceal dilatation which occurs. It does not show most of the ureter and cannot assess ureteric drainage. It may be used if IVU is contraindicated (e.g. by pregnancy or allergy to contrast medium).

### Technique

The patient must be hydrated (at least 500 ml orally or IV) [4]. Mild pelvicalyceal dilatation is the expected finding in ureteric obstruction. Attempts should be made to visualise the upper ureter and the lower ureter through the bladder. US is good at showing calculi at the vesicoureteric junction. US must always be combined with plain films to check for opaque calculi.

Supplementary techniques include Doppler US:

1. Colour or pulsed Doppler US can differentiate dilated renal vessels, particularly veins, from a dilated pelvicalyceal system [5].
2. Ureteric jets are seen with colour Doppler in the bladder of normally hydrated subjects. They may be absent or reduced in ureteric obstruction [6].
3. Measurement of the resistance index (RI) in the intrarenal vessels

$$RI = \frac{\text{Systolic velocity - diastolic velocity}}{\text{Systolic velocity}}$$

RI is elevated (>0.7) in obstruction. An inter-renal RI greater than 0.08 is a particularly helpful sign [7].

## Chronic Obstruction

### Anatomical Investigation

The first investigation of choice depends on the clinical setting. If there is pain, and stone disease or pelviureteric junction (PUJ) obstruction are possible, IVU is best. If there is impaired renal function, prostatism, or pelvic or retroperitoneal neoplasm, US and plain radiography should be used first.

Rare cases are recognised in which obstruction is present without pelvicalyceal dilatation [8, 9]. If this is suspected, the diagnosis may only be achieved when renal function improves after either antegrade or retrograde renal drainage.

### Intravenous Urography

On the IVU films obtained immediately after administration of contrast medium, the dilated pelvicalyceal sys-

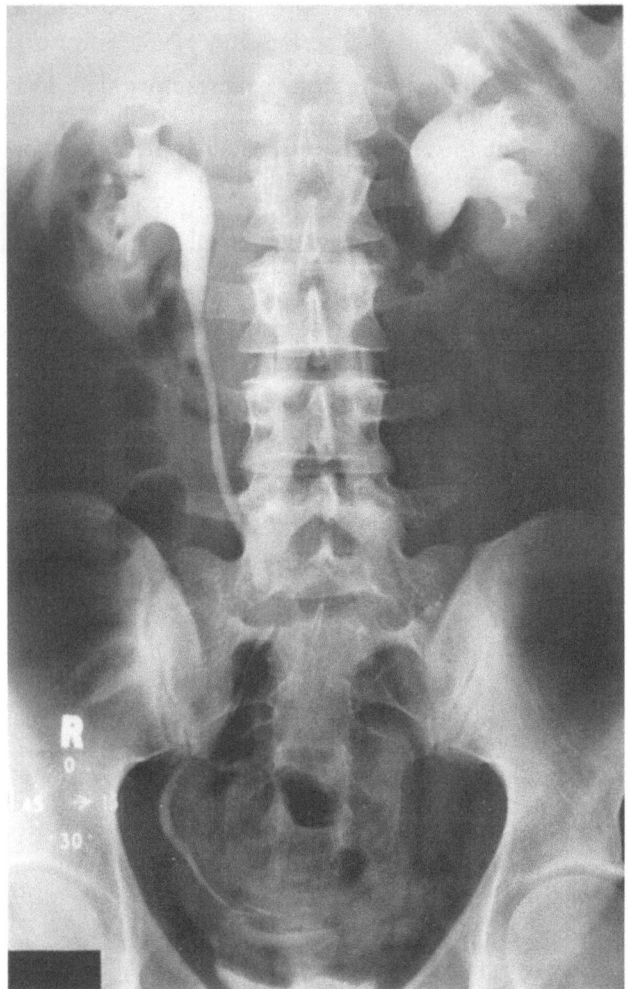

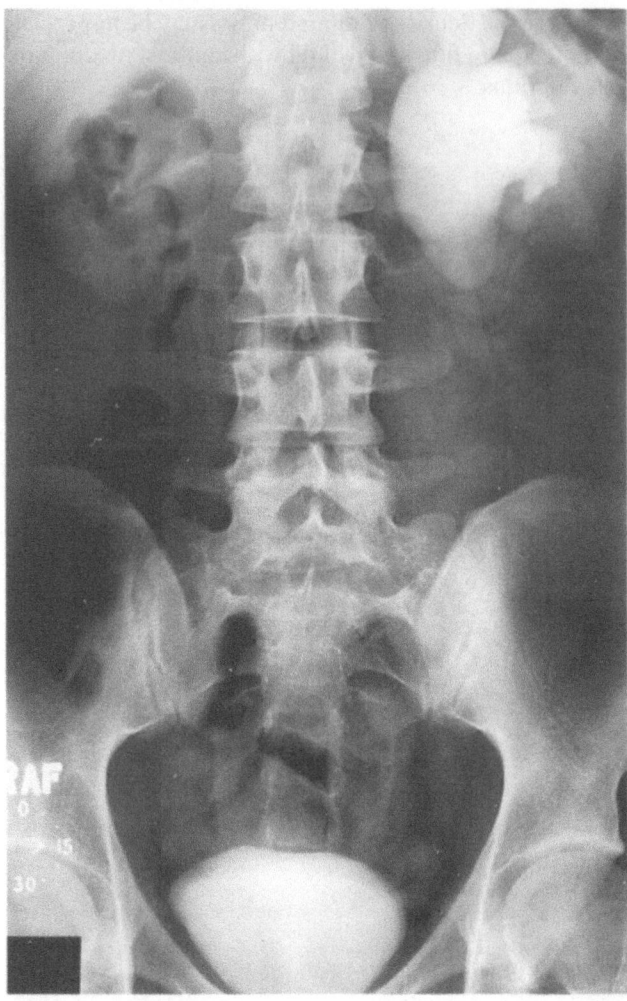

**Fig. 2 a, b.** Frusemide urogram in left pelviureteric junction obstruction. **a** Note mild left pelvicalyceal dilatation with no filling of left ureter. **b** Fifteen minutes after frusemide: the left pelvicalyceal system is larger; the right has drained

tem may be seen as a central lucent "negative pyelo-gram" surrounded by the "rim nephrogram" of opaci-fied parenchyma. The dilated pelvicalyceal system fills on delayed films but contrast medium concentration may be poor and it may be difficult to define the level of

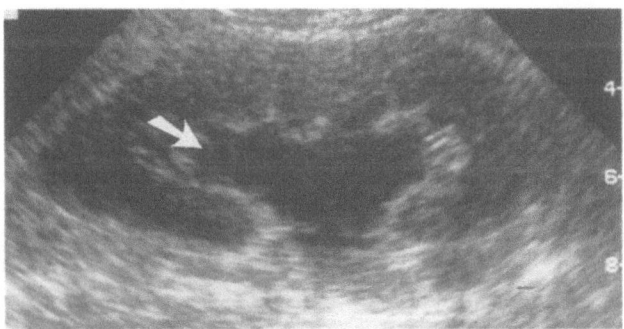

**Fig. 3.** Longitudinal ultrasound scan of an obstructed kidney showing moderate pelvicalyceal dilatation (*arrow*)

obstruction in some patients. In suspected PUJ obstruc-tion, frusemide urography may be helpful [10]. Frusemide (40 mg IV) is given after the full-length film and a further full-length film is obtained 15 min later. If there is PUJ obstruction, the affected pelvicalyceal sys-tem increases in size and the patient develops loin pain, while the normal side drains out (Fig. 2).

## Ultrasonography

US is a sensitive detector of pelvicalyceal dilatation in chronic obstruction [11,12]. The dilated pelvicalyceal system is seen as a collection of communicating fluid collections centrally in the renal sinus (Fig. 3) and there is parenchymal thinning if there is obstructive atrophy. Since minor dilatation can occur in severe obstruction (Fig. 4) any degree of dilatation must be investigated further. With US, however, there will be a significant number of false positive scans caused by nonobstructive pelvicalyceal dilatation [13].

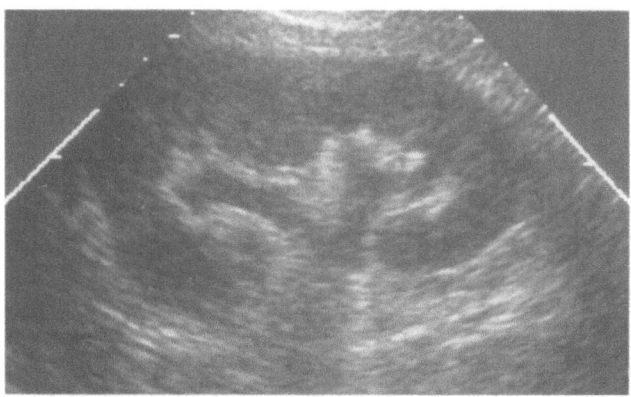

**Fig. 4.** Longitudinal ultrasound scan of kidney in severe obstructive renal failure caused by retroperitoneal fibrosis. Both kidneys showed similar, mild pelvicalyceal dilatation

### Computed Tomography

CT is also sensitive to pelvicalyceal dilatation [12], which is seen as a central collection of communicating structures of fluid density (Fig. 5). With CT, unlike US, the dilated ureter can be followed through the retroperitoneum on contiguous sections to the level of obstruction. After contrast medium administration, opacification of the pelvicalyceal system and ureter is delayed.

## Functional Investigation

⁹⁹ᵐTc-labelled MAG3 (mercaptoacetyl tryglycine) or DTPA (diethylene triamene pentacetic acid) scintigraphy in an obstructed kidney shows that parenchymal clearance of the tracer is delayed (evidence of obstructive nephropathy) as is outflow from the collecting sys-

tem. The renogram shows renal tracer activity rising to a plateau or continuing to rise. After IV administration of frusemide there is continued, retained activity in obstruction, but non-obstructed dilated systems wash out normally.

The Whitaker test (pressure- flow) study involves antegrade puncture of the dilated collecting system and infusion of contrast medium at a rate of 10 ml/min for 10-20 min while pressure measurements are taken from the renal pelvis. It is particularly helpful in suspected PUJ obstruction; in the presence of obstruction, renal pelvis pressure rises.

## Cause of Obstruction

The cause of obstruction may be shown on the initial investigation:
1. IVU may show features such as smooth ureteric tapering, indicating extrinsic obstruction, or a filling defect, indicating intrinsic obstruction at the level of ureteric holdup.
2. US may show the cause of obstruction if it lies in the pelvis (e.g. pelvic mass, urinary retention). It commonly has difficulty in showing retroperitoneal causes of obstruction.

Further investigation usually involves CT, antegrade or retrograde pyelography: **CT** is an excellent method of showing retroperitoneal causes of obstruction (e.g. enlarged nodes, tumours, retroperitoneal fibrosis (Fig. 5) [14]. It is also a sensitive detector of calculi including "nonopaque" stones (e.g. uric acid) [15] which it can distinguish from other filling defects which appear lucent on the IVU (e.g. blood clot, tumour).

**Antegrade pyelography** is used to outline the collecting system and ureter to the level of obstruction and can usually show whether the obstrucing lesion is intrisic or extrinsic (Fig. 6). It is also a preliminary to percutaneous renal drainage.

**Retrograde pyelography** may be used to outline the ureter and collecting system with contrast medium if pelvicalyceal dilatation is mild and antegrade puncture is likely to be difficult. Rarely, it may be used when obstruction is suspected in the absence of pelvicalyceal dilatation [8, 9]. It has the disadvantage of the potential to introduce infection into the obstructed system.

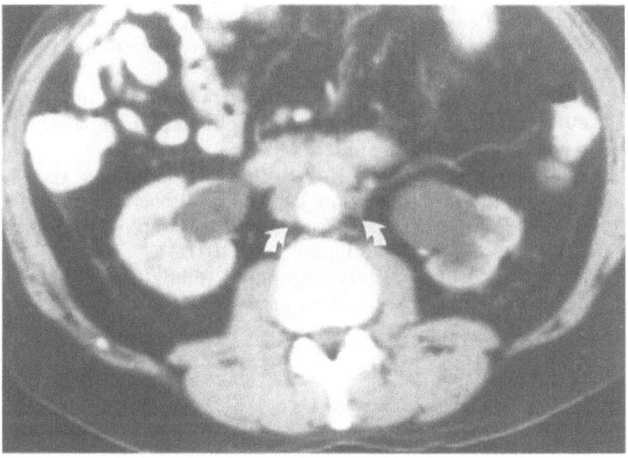

**Fig. 5.** Enhanced computed tomographic scan showing bilateral pelvicalyceal dilatation in obstructed kidneys. Note the soft tissue density around the aorta (*arrow*) caused by retroperitoneal fibrosis which was obstructing the ureters

146                                                    J.A.W. Webb

**Fig. 6 a, b.** Ante-
grade pyelogram of
obstructed right kid-
ney via a nephrosto-
my catheter (**a**). The
lucent intrinsic filling
defect in the ureter
(*arrow*) was a urate
stone (**b**)

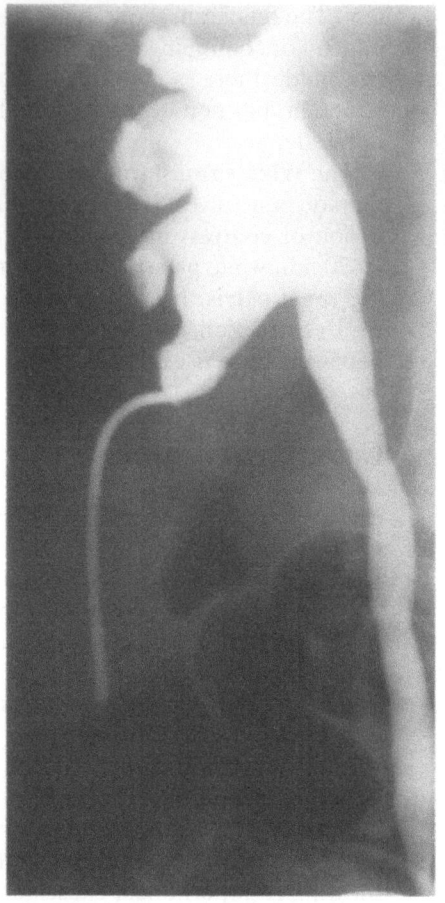 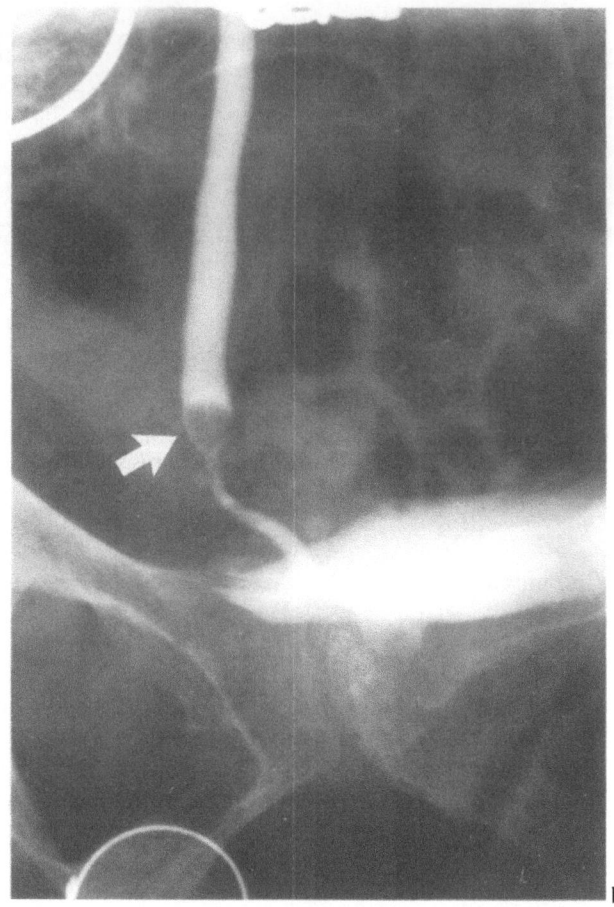

a                                                          b

## References

1. Talner LB (1992) Urinary obstruction. In: Grainger RG, Allison DJ (eds) Diagnostic radiology, 2nd edn. Churchill Livingstone, Edinburgh
2. Svedstrom E et al (1990) Radiologic diagnosis of renal colic: the role of plain films, excretory urography and sonography. Eur J Radiol 11: 180-183
3. Laing FC et al (1985) Ultrasound versus excretory urography in evaluating acute flank pain. Radiology 134: 613-616
4. Dalla Palma L et al (1993) Ultrasonography and plain film versus intravenous urography in ureteric colic. Clin Radiol 47: 333-336
5. Scola FH et al (1989) Grade hydronephrosis: pulsed doppler US evaluation. Radiology 171: 519-520
6. Burge HJ et al (1991) Ureteral jets in healthy subjects and in patients with unilateral ureteral calculi: comparison with colour Doppler US. Radiology 180: 437-442
7. Rodgers PM et al (1992) Intrarenal Doppler ultrasound studies in normal and acutely obstructed kidneys. Br J Radiol 65: 207-212
8. Naidich JB et al (1986) Non-dilated obstructive uropathy: percutaneous nephrostomy performed to reverse renal failure. Radiology 160: 653-659
9. Maillet PJ et al (1986) Non-dilated obstructive acute renal failure: diagnostic procedures and therapeutic management. Radiology 160: 659-662
10. Whitfield HN et al (1979) Frusemide intravenous urography in the diagnosis of the pelviureteric junction obstruction. Br J Urol 51: 445-448
11. Talner LB et al (1981) How accurate is ultrasonography in detecting hydronephrosis in azotaemic patients? Urol Radiol 3: 1-6
12. Webb JAW et al (1984) Can ultrasound and computed tomography replace high dose urography in patients with impaired renal function? Quart J Med 53: 411-425
13. Webb JAW et al (1990) Review: ultrasonography in the diagnosis of renal obstruction. Br Med J 301: 944-946
14. Bosniak MA et al (1982) Computed tomography of ureteral obstruction. Am J Roentgenol 138: 1107-1113
15. Pollack HM et al (1981) Computed tomography of renal pelvic filling defects. Radiology 138: 645-651

# Malignant Renal Tumours

J.F. Moreau and O. Hélénon

Department of Radiology, Necker Hospital, 161 Rue de Sèvres, 75743 Paris, France

Renal cell carcinoma (RCC) is the most common malignant renal parenchymal tumour, accounting for about 86% of all primary malignant renal neoplasms [1, 2].

## Anatomoclinical Aspects

### Pathology

Typical RCCs are seen as a solid renal mass with irregular lobulated margins, yellow-orange in colour and heterogeneous in appearance at gross pathological examination because of the presence of necrotic and/or haemorrhagic intratumoural areas [2].

Histologically, RCCs are of the clear-cell type in most cases. Among other categories, tubulopapillary RCCs, which represent about 15% of RCCs, are characterized by their architectural arrangement (tubulopapillary or papillary arrangement of cells) and poor vascularity, whatever their macroscopic appearance: solid or pseudocystic due to massive necrosis.

Cystic RCCs are not uncommon and frequently raise diagnostic problems. Three types of cystic RCCs can be differentiated: unilocular cystic RCC due to extensive necrosis or less frequently intrinsic cystic growth, presenting as fluid-filled nodules often containing old blood delineated by thick vascularized septa; and finally RCC which has developed in a preexisting cyst as a mural nodule, which represents a very unusual and controversial entity.

### Clinical Aspects

Incidence rates are closely related to age, with a minimal incidence before the age of 30 and a progressive increase in frequency between 40 and 70 years old. The incidence of RCC is also influenced by some other factors, including sex, with a male-to-female incidence rate of 2.5; environmental, since incidence is higher in industrialized countries; and hereditary, particularly in von Hippel-Lindau's disease, which is associated with an extremely high incidence of multiple and bilateral RCCs.

Clinical symptoms which can reveal RCCs include haematuria (40%), lumbar pain (10%) or mass (5%) and rare nonurological symptoms such as fever, hypertension, polycytaemia, endocrine manifestations and those related to bone and lung metastases. However, most RCCs are clinically silent and incidentally diagnosed, in 45% of cases because of the wide use of abdominal ultrasonography (US) and computed tomography (CT). As a matter of fact, the discovery of small (<3 cm) RCCs has dramatically increased during the past decade [3]. Such small incidentally detected renal tumours pose diagnostic problems because of their nonspecific appearance and the relatively high proportion of small benign tumours (about 20%).

## Radiological Diagnosis

The radiological diagnosis of a malignant renal tumour involves three steps: (1) to recognize a tumoural syndrome; (2) to assess its malignancy; and (3) to stage the extent of spread.

### Classical Approach Based on Intravenous Urography and Arteriography

The classical approach is based on preliminary intravenous urography (IVU) [4]. The diagnosis of a renal mass is made in association with: (a) deformity of the renal contour (bulging, swelling, diffuse enlargement); (b) spheric nephrographic defect; and (c) deformity of the pelvicalyceal system (displacement, compression, elongation).

The diagnosis of renal cancer is suggested when [4] the mass is calcified, there is a blush at the early nephrographic stage, filling defects are present, indicating invasion of the pelvicaliceal system, and the kidney is silent.

In fact, most of the time, IVU signs of malignancy are absent or difficult to assess. Moreover, IVU is insensitive and particularly small or exophytic anterior/posterior RCCs may be misdiagnosed owing to the absence of deformity. In any case, it is possible to assess the benignity of a mass by IVU.

Renal arteriography using the Seldinger technique is now rarely performed except preoperatively when conservative surgery is being considered. It should always consist in a preliminary, nonselective aortogram followed by selective renal arteriograms. Typically, it exhibits a vascularized, heterogeneous mass, with irregular neovessels and arteriovenous shunts.

This classical approach is rather obsolete because:

- Most of the malignant renal tumours are clinically silent or revealed by atypical clinical patterns (fever, pain, abdominal mass, metastases).
- Conventional IVU is neither sensitive nor specific for the diagnosis of small masses; it cannot assess safely the benignity of a tumoural syndrome (benign tumour or pseudo tumour).
- US has become the most common screening imaging test in uronephrology and therefore detects most of the renal masses, followed by CT, the commonest complementary examination.
- Malignant renal tumours can present as an avascular mass because of minimal nondetectable intratumoural vascularization or extensive necrosis. In contrast, benign nontumoural masses can be vascularized.

## Ultrasound: First and/or Only Approach

Using high-resolution, conventional US, it is now possible to detect solid masses, even smaller than 1 cm in diameter. Most of the masses are echogenic (Fig. 1), more or less heterogeneous and poorly delineated, depending on their size. When large enough, they often present with scattered intratumoural calcification, acoustic shadowing and echolucent necrotic areas.

False negatives may result from cystic carcinomas, homogeneous hypoechogenic solid carcinomas (often but not always related to incorrect setting of the beam, mimicking haemorrhagic or superinfected cyst), or egg-shell calcified rim (mimicking hydatic cyst or complex calcified cyst). False positives may result from

pseudotumoural Bertin's column hypertrophy, subacute or chronic renal abscesses, comple cysts, and nonfatty benign tumours such as anococytomas (refer to "Differential Diagnosis"). Fine-needle US-guided puncture can be used to obtain histological data, but there are many pitfalls and so physicians are usually reluctant to use it because of the risk, though rare, of neoplastic spread induced by the capsular rupture in malignant tumours.

If colour Doppler US (CDUS) is available the sensitivity for the diagnosis of a vascularized mass improves; the specificity is also better because of the obviously normal vascularity of the Bertin's columns, which may help to characterize such pseudotumours. But, it is not possible to differentiate malignant from benign masses using spectral analysis obtained with pulsed Doppler. CDUS is diagnostic when it shows neoplastic thrombus in the renocaval venous system.

## CT: First and/or Only Approach

The basic technical rule for successful CT of the kidney is to consistently perform a noncontrast CT scan first, with an excellent control of breathing. This important stage is often lacking when a renal mass is discovered incidently during an abdominal contrast-enhanced CT prescribed for other reasons. A second scan is urged systematically after a large IV bolus injection, with subsequent infusion of iodinated contrast medium using 5-mm-thick contiguous sections.

A renal carcinoma is usually isodense before infection and sometimes calcified. The degree of enhancement obtained after injection reflects the ratio of vascularity to necrosis of the tumour. The enhancement is usually heterogeneous and centripetal and occurs early after injection [1, 5]. Small RCCs (<3 cm) often show a homogeneous pattern, sometimes with delayed and/or slight postcontrast enhancement and especially in tubulopapillary RCC (Fig. 2).

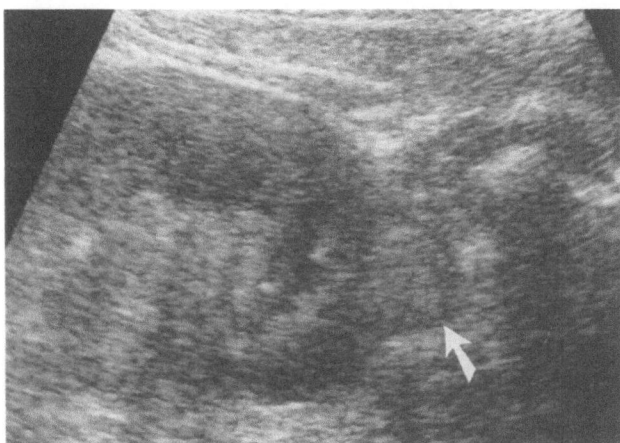

**Fig. 1.** Ultrasonography of a small renal cell carcinoma (*arrow*) with homogeneous, slightly hyperattenuating appearance

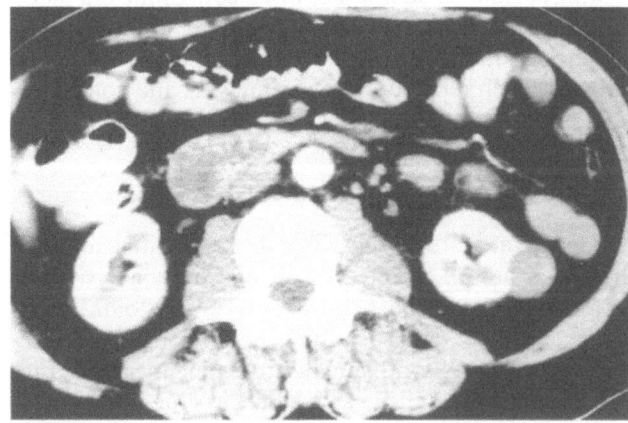

**Fig. 2.** Postcontrast computed tomographic scan shows a small homogeneous tumour of the left kidney (tubulopapillary renal cell carcinoma at pathology)

Many pitfalls, whether false-positive or false-negative diagnoses, result from technical inadequacies, mostly from inadequate breathing control and/or from poor injection of contrast medium. One of the weaknesses of the CT technique is the difficulty to perform multiplanar scanning. Thus, false negatives should result only from very small (< 1.5 cm) masses, since the Hounsfield scale may not be precise enough to distinguish small serous masses from tumours because of partial volume effect. Unfortunately, because of technical failures, false negatives too often involve larger tumours. The risk is higher at the poles of the kidney, especially in cases of exophytic small masses.

False positives are more common. They mainly result from benign nonfatty tumours and inflammatory pseudotumours, e.g. inflammatory complex cyst, chronic abscess, xantho-granulomatous pyelonephritis, or hydatic cyst. The partial volume effect may also induce erroneous diagnoses in cases of small cysts, from which attenuation values may be overestimated.

## Magnetic Resonance Imaging

At the beginning, magnetic resonance imaging (MRI) only appeared to be helpful for the evaluation of the local venous extent of a previously detected renal cancer (refer to "Staging of RCC"). At present - and this trend should increase in the future because of the progress in technology and in contrast enhancement - MRI is also useful in the differential diagnosis of solid tumours and complex haemorrhagic cysts [6, 7] (refer to "Differential Diagnosis").

## Fine-Needle US/CT-Guided Biopsy

Fine-needle biopsy is not indicated in most cases of solitary renal masses, more because of a high risk of false-negative results than the small risk of local neoplastic postbiopsy spread, which remains debated. The current indications for fine-needle US- or CT-guided biopsies are multiple and/or bilateral tumours or infiltrative renal tumours associated with extrarenal manifestations that suggest renal metastases or lymphoma.

## Risks and Problems

Formerly, the major risk resulted from false-negative diagnoses of renal cancer, because it was difficult to diagnose the renal mass itself, whether solid or fluid. At present, problems are chiefly related to false positives, because we can diagnose more easily renal serous cysts and more and more small solid renal masses. Tissular characterization of a renal mass by any kind of imaging technique remains a dream but the radiologist now possesses many more tools which are helpful in a specific clinical situation.

The rate of malignancy of a renal cancer is either high or low. When the cancer is severe, it will evolve quickly and it will be likely discovered when there are signs of general metastatic extent; whatever the size of the cancer, the prognosis is very bad.

Clear-cell carcinomas often grow slowly and only locally. Then, the most important step in the therapeutic discussion is to know whether the cancer has trespassed the renal capsule and whether the renal vein and/or the caval vein are thrombotic. If not, doctors have time to discuss the best diagnostic approach of a mass and its treatment. This is especially important when a small solid mass is discovered in a still rather young adult. Both the frequency of benign angiomyolipoma (AML) and the difficulty of its diagnosis when it is small are too high to promote the concept of total nephrectomy without deep discussion, chiefly based upon the CT findings. The trend toward conservative focal surgical treatment of small solid, even malignant tumours should grow up very rapidly if imaging techniques become really accurate.

## Differential Diagnosis of RCC

### Pseudotumoural Hypertrophy

Pseudotumoural hypertrophy (Bertin's column hypertrophy, focal parenchymal hypertrophy accompanying parenchymal scarring) is accurately diagnosed at CT on the following criteria: isodense mass on the precontrast CT scan with postcontrast enhancement comparable to surrounding parenchyma at both early and delayed CT nephrographic stages.

### Solid and Fluid-Filled Inflammatory Lesions

Lesions such as pseudotumoural, focal, acute pyelonephritis, chronic abscesses and xanthogranulomatous pyelonephritis are suspected in the clinical context and according to CT findings, including inflammatory perinephric changes and follow-up improvement. However, surgery is often required.

### Complex Cysts

According to the Bosniak classification of complex cystic masses (Table 1) [8], those in category 3 often pose difficult differential diagnostic problems with cystic neoplasms, whereas categories 2 and 4 are without doubt benign, minimally complicated cysts and cystic (Fig. 3) or necrotic RCCs (Fig. 4), respectively.

Category 3 complex cysts result mostly from intracystic haemorrhage or infection, which can exhibit a thick peripheral wall, irregularity, septations and calcifications with or without postcontrast enhancement. High attenuation values within a cyst suggest haemorrhage in a benign cyst when the mass is rather small in size with

**Table 1.** Bosniak classification of cystic renal masses [3]

|  | Precontrast CT | Postcontrast CT | Diagnosis |
|---|---|---|---|
| **Category I** | Water density (<20 HU)<br>Homogeneous, smooth<br>Sharply marginated<br>Nonvisible, thin wall | No enhancement (<10 HU) | Simple cyst |
| **Category II** | Thin, regular septa<br>Minimally calcified cyst<br>Hyperdense cyst (<50 HU)[a] | No enhancement (<10 HU) | Minimally complicated cyst |
| **Category III**<br>*Indeterminate lesions* | Irregular margins<br>Thick, uniform wall or septa<br>Thick, irregular calcification<br>Isodense lesion[b] | Enhancing wall or septa | Complicated cyts or "cystic" neoplasm |
| **Category IV** | Irregular, thick wall<br>Solid nodular component<br>Sharply marginated | Enhancing solid elements | "Cystic" neoplasm |

[a] Hyperattenuating (50-90 HU), homogeneous, (<3 cm) small round lesion extending ouside of the kidney, perfectly smooth and sharply marginated, with no enhancement on postcontrast scan.
[b] Isodense mass (20-50 HU) or any other hyperdense lesion not fulfilling all the criteria mentioned above.

CT values higher than 50 HU, homogeneous, and sharply marginated either on pre- or post-contrast scans with no change after contrast enhancement (lack of enhancement). Spontaneously hyperdense RCCs are rare, mimicking a hyperdense complex cyst. Particular attention should be paid to the postcontrast behaviour of such a hyperdense mass in order not to overlook a slight enhancement of the mass. Small hypovascularized tumours (mostly tubulopapillary RCCs) may also mimic a spontaneously hyperattenuating cyst, owing to the fact that postcontrast enhancement might render it undetectable. Such pitfalls should be avoided using strict CT scanning technique and diagnostic criteria. A spontaneously isodense (20-50 HU) avascular mass should be viewed as a possible small hypovascularized tumour, es-

pecially when CT scanning technique is inadequate, and should prompt US examination or repeat CT examination. On US, hyperdense cysts are typically anechoic in about 30%-50% cases [3]. When US or technically appropriate CT scan are not conclusive, MRI may be indicated to demonstrate a homogeneously bright signal or fluid-iron level pattern within the lesion on both T1- and T2-weighted images [7]. Such a typical pattern is encountered in about 50% of haemorrhagic cysts.

**Benign Renal Tumours**

*AML versus RCC.* The presence of intratumoural areas of fat density (lower than -20 HU; Fig. 5), which may require narrowly collimated (≤5 mm) precontrast CT

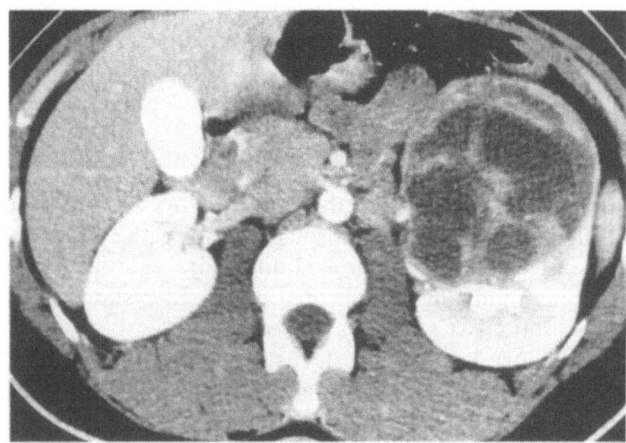

**Fig. 3.** Postcontrast computed tomographic scan shows a multilocular, cystic tumour of the left kidney (cystic renal cell carcinoma at pathology)

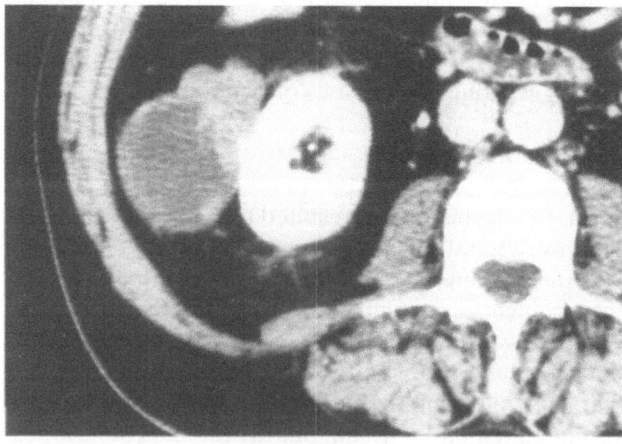

**Fig. 4.** Pseudocystic renal cell carcinoma due to extensive necrosis with obvious peripheral solid tumour component (postcontrast computed tomography scan)

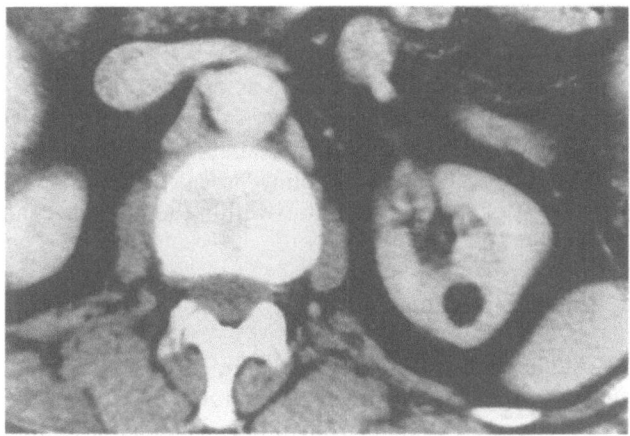

**Fig. 5.** Typical small angiomyolipoma of the left kidney almost exclusively made of fat. Computed tomographic scan shows low attenuation values (-80 HU) indicating fat

scanning, is the key diagnostic component of an AML [9]. Typically, AML shows a well-defined, hyperechoic lesion on US. Although a markedly hyperechoic (as hyperechoic as the renal sinus) lesion is highly suggestive of AML, it is not specific - about 30% of small RCCs appear as a markedly hyperchoic mass [10] and therefore require CT with appropriate technique.

In a patient presenting with a renal mass, evidence of fat within the lesion on CT helps to rule out a RCC, avoiding surgery in most cases. However, this attitude has been countered by isolated observations reporting the presence of fat in RCC [11, 14], including large RCCs invading perirenal fat, large RCCs with lipid-producing necrosis and RCCs containing areas of osseous metaplasia. Thus, with the exception of renal tumours containing calcifications, large necrotic tumours and large infiltrative tumours which rarely entrap fat while invading sinusal or perirenal fat tissues, it can be stated that when CT demonstrates islands of fat within a renal mass, RCC can be excluded.

*Renal Oncocytoma versus RCC.* Renal oncocytoma (RO) is a rare (about 5% of renal cell tumours), benign epithelial tumour defined as a well-differentiated neoplasm made of large cuboidal cells with finely granular eosinophilic cytoplasm and uniform round nuclei. On gross inspection, the cut surface is typically tan-brown and uniform or slightly lobulated. Large ROs frequently exhibit a central fibrous scar.

There is controversy on the potential for malignancy and metastasis of some oncocytomas, resulting from the presence of the so-called "oncocytic cells" in addition to more typical malignant elements in some renal carcinomas with distant metastases. Further confusion is caused by the similarity between ROs and chromophobe carcinomas. If the oncocytoma is restricted to tumours composed of purely well-differentiated oncocytic cells, in the absence of cellular anaplasia, then RO can be considered

a nonaggressive benign tumour in which renal-sparing surgery should be preferred to enlarged nephrectomy.

RO contributes to the differential diagnosis of non-fat-containing solid renal tumours, which are RCCs in about 85% of the cases. Up to now, preoperative imaging features allowing a confident diagnosis of RO have been lacking, although classically, it may be suggested in some typical cases on CT or angiography.

For large ROs, the most reliable diagnostic criterion is currently provided by CT. A "spoke-wheel" pattern of enhancement on early postcontrast sections and a sharply defined central stellate area of low attenuation (indicating the presence of a central myxoid-fibrotic scar) within an otherwise homogeneous tumour on more delayed scans strongly suggest the diagnosis of RO, although it is not specific [16].

Reported CT criteria for small ROs (solid tumour with marked postcontrast enhancement and homogeneous pattern) are of poor value in the diagnosis of small ROs [17]. Tumours with the above-mentioned imaging features on CT should be intraoperatively evaluated by means of frozen sections in order to avoid radical nephrectomy.

### Multiple Renal Tumours

Multiple, bilateral solid tumours suggest phacomatosis with multiple AMLs, chiefly Bourneville's disease; von Hipple-Lindau's disease, with solid tumours which are either malignant (adenocarcinoma) or benign (adenoma) associated with cysts, lymphomas (Fig. 6); multiple metastases; or, in infants, nephroblastomatosis.

## Local Staging of RCC

CT remains the method of choice to assess local extent of RCC and lymph node involevement even though US

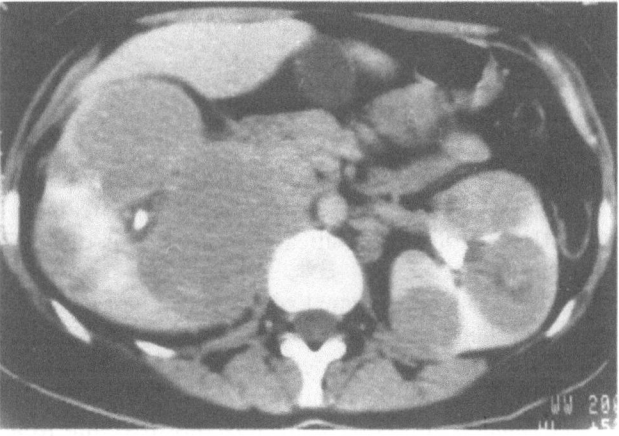

**Fig. 6.** Lymphoma with renal involvement. Computed tomographic scan shows multiple, bilateral, renal solid masses associated with enlarged retroperitoneal lymph nodes

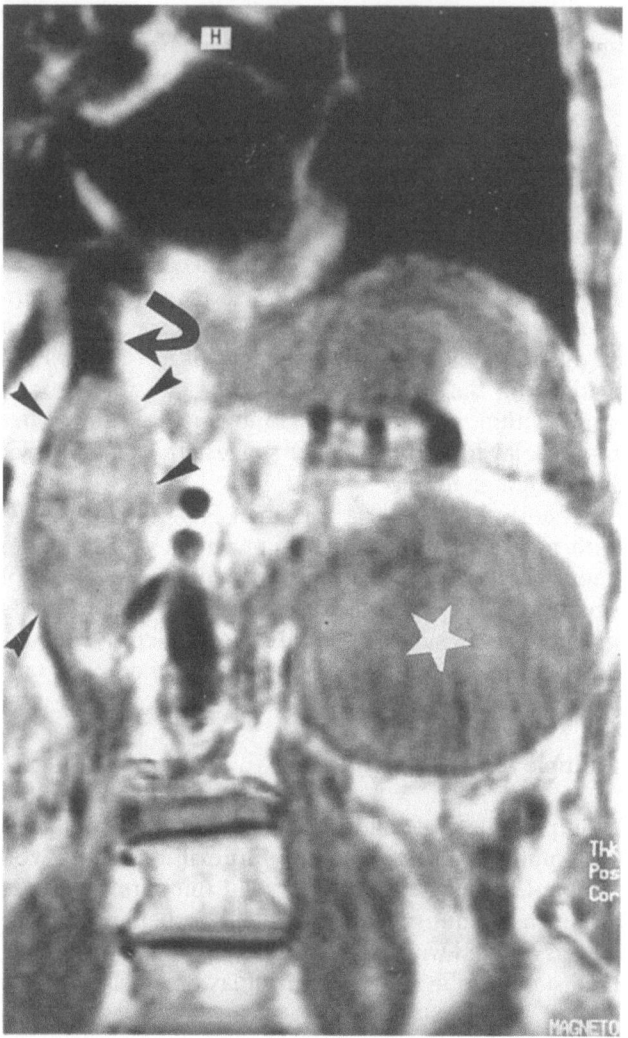

**Fig. 7.** Coronal T1-weighted magnetic resonance image shows a large tumour of the left kidney (*star*) that extends within the inferior vena cava. Tumour thrombus (*arrowheads*) is well delineated. Distal portion of the inferior vena cava remains patent (*curved arrow*)

and/or MRI may be indicated alone or as a complementary study.

### Venous Spread

Intraluminal defects within an enlarged renal vein on postcontrast CT scans indicate venous involvement (stage III of Robson classification), usually associated with a large RCC.

Pitfalls in diagnosing renal vein involvement include: renal vein enlargement due to intratumoural arteriovenous shunting; markedly arterialized tumour thrombus which can be overlooked; multiple renal veins with accessory renal vein involvement; false positive due to a renal vein compressed by the tumour; or misinterpretation of distal tumour extent within the inferior vena cava. In most cases, such pitfalls can be avoided by obtain-

ing dynamic CT scanning at the level of the renal vein after bolus injection.

When colour Doppler fails to assess the tumour's venous thrombous extent, an inferior cavogram or MRI using longitudinal scans, when available, are useful complementary techniques enabling precise assessment of the extent of tumour thrombus within the inferior vena cava (Fig. 7).

### Capsular Effraction

Capsular effraction (stage II of the Robson classification) is suggested by irregular margins of the tumour and obliteration and blurring of the perirenal fat related to tumour infiltration (Fig. 8).

### Neighbouring Organ Involvement

Adjacent organ and abdominal wall involvement (stage IV of the Robson classification) are suggested when the tumour extends into the adjacent structure with an irregular interface (Fig. 8) and postcontrast alteration of attenuation values compared with surrounding normal parenchyma.

### Contralateral or Ipsilateral Synchronous Secondary Lesions

Multiple tumours should be accurately diagnosed preoperatively in order to avoid incomplete surgery and to prompt renal sparing surgery in case of bilateral RCCs.

## Malignant Renal Tumours in Children

Most of malignant tumours discovered in children are Wilms tumours. The clinical symptomatology is usually summarized by an abdominal mass without haematuria.

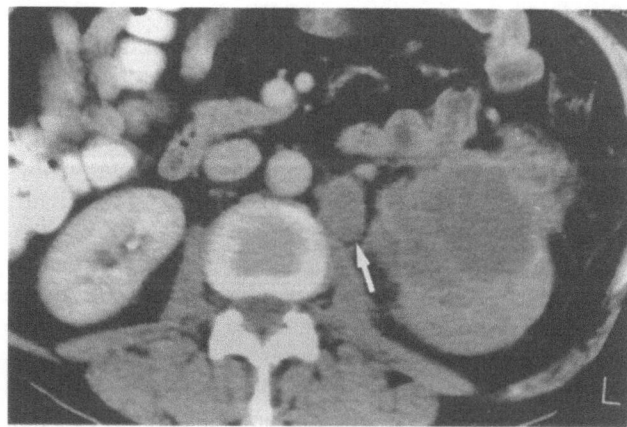

**Fig. 8.** Renal cell carcinoma of the left kidney with capsular effraction. Note irregular margins of the tumour with perirenal fat infiltration and lymph node involvement (*arrow*)

The imaging patterns are rather similar to those of vascularized renal carcinoma. Cystic components are common and there is a pseudocystic form. Calcifications are seen in 15% of the cases. The venous spread must be carefully studied. Metastases are discovered most often in the lungs, the lymph nodes and the liver. For this reason, CT or MRI scanning should systematically include the thorax and the abdomen when the mass has been discoverd on US.

# References

1. Barbaric ZI (1994) Principles of genitourinary radiology, 2nd edn. Thieme, New York
2. Bennington JL, Beckwith JB (1975) Tumours of the kidney, renal pelvis and ureter. In: Atlas of tumor pathology. Second series, fascicle 12. Armed Forces Institute of Pathology
3. Bosniak MA (1991) The small (<3.0 cm) renal parenchymal tumour: detection, diagnosis, and controversies. Radiology 179: 307-317
4. Moreau JF, Affre J (1979) L'urographie intra-veineuse. Flammarion médecine, Paris, pp 50-66
5. Dalla Palma L, Pozzi-Mucelli R (1991) Malignant renal neoplasm. In: Lang EK (ed) Radiology of the upper urinary tract. Springer, Berlin Heidelberg New York, pp 251-274
6. Denys A, Hélénon O, Gilles R et al (1993) MR detection and characterization of small renal masses: value of T2-weighted and Gd-DOTA-enhanced images. Eur Radiol 3: 447-452
7. Levy P, Hélénon O, Melki Ph, Paraf P, Chauveau D, Chretien Y, Moreau JF (1994) Kystes atypiques bénins du rein: aspects IRM J Radiol 75: 543-552
8. Bosniak MA (1986) The current radiological approach to renal cyst. Radiology 158: 1-10
9. Bosniak MA, Megibow AJ, Hunick DH, Horii S, Raghavendra BN (1988) CT diagnosis of renal angiomyolipoma: the importance of detecting small amounts of fat. AJR 151: 497-501
10. Forman HP, Middleton WD, Melson GL, McLennan (1993) Hyperechoic renal cell carcinomas: increase in detection at US. Radiology 188: 431-434
11. Hélénon O, Chrétien Y, Paraf F, Melki P, Denys A, Moreau JF (1993) Renal cell carcinoma containing fat: demonstration with CT. Radiology 188: 429-430
12. Prando A (1991) Intratumoural fat in a renal cell carcinoma. AJR 156: 871
13. Strotzer M, Lehner KB, Becker K (1993) Detection of fat in a renal cell carcinoma mimicking angiomyolipoma. Radiology 188: 427-428
14. Radin DR, Charndrasoma P (1992) CT demonstration of fat density in renal cell carcinoma. Acta Radiol 33: 365-367
15. Morra MN, Das S (1993) Renal oncocytoma: a review of histogenesis, histopathology, diagnosis and treatment. J Urol 150: 295-302
16. Neisius D, Braedel HU, Schindler E et al (1988) Computed tomographic and angiographic findings in renal oncocytoma. Br J Radiol 61: 1019-1025
17. Davidson AJ, Hayes WS, Harman DS, McCarthy WF, Davis CJ Jr (1993) Renal oncocytoma and carcinoma: failure of differentiation with CT. Radiology 186: 693-696

# Imaging of the Lower Urinary Tract

S. Dorph

Dept. of Radiology, Herlev Hospital, Herlev Ringvej, 2730 Herlev, Denmark

## Anatomy and Clinical Symptoms

The lower urinary tract includes the urinary bladder and the urethra.

The normal bladder holds 200-500 ml urine and should preferably be full for visualization. The wall thickness decreases from 2 cm to 2 mm during expansion. Only the dome of the bladder is covered by peritoneum. It is important to remember the close relation between the prostate and seminal vesicles and the bladder base and posterior urethra in men and between the urethra and the anterior vaginal wall in women.

Haematuria is a main symptom in a large variety of urinary tract diseases. When due to lower tract disease, the haematuria is most often gross. Terminal or initial haematuria points towards disease in the bladder trigone and/or urethra, whereas diffuse haematuria more likely indicates disease in other parts of the bladder or in the kidney and upper tract.

Various disturbances of normal micturition such as dysuria, pollakisuria, urgency, incontinence and retention are characteristic symptoms of disease involving the lower urinary tract. However, many diseases may be asymptomatic for a long period of time.

## Imaging Modalities Used

The lower urinary tract is imaged mainly by conventional X-ray (plain films, the indirect urographic cystogram, direct cystogram, micturition cystourethrography and retrograde urethrogram) and ultrasound (US) (transabdominal, transrectal and transurethral). Computed tomography (CT) is indicated in case of major pelvic trauma, and both CT and magnetic resonance imaging (MRI) are useful in tumour staging. Nuclear medical studies are used primarily to establish whether disease in the lower urinary tract affects kidney function. Arteriography of the bladder is very rarely indicated, mostly prior to or combined with embolization for intractable pelvic bleeding.

## Pathology

Bladder diverticula are congenital or acquired, due to a variety of conditions. The most common is bladder outlet obstruction. Large diverticula may cause compression of the bladder and dislocation of neighboring organs. The smooth inner surface contrasts to the more irregular bladder surface. Twenty-five per cent of diverticula contain stones. Abdominal US is well suited for the study of diverticula. The neck of the diverticulum should be located so as not to mistake it for a perivesical fluid collection (Fig. 1). Tumours occur with a higher frequency than in the true bladder (3%). They may be difficult to diagnose by cystography and are best detected by US or CT. Urography demonstrates the contrast-filled diverticulum, which may increase or first appear after voiding, but urography may miss anterior and posterior diverticula.

Urethral diverticula are more common in women

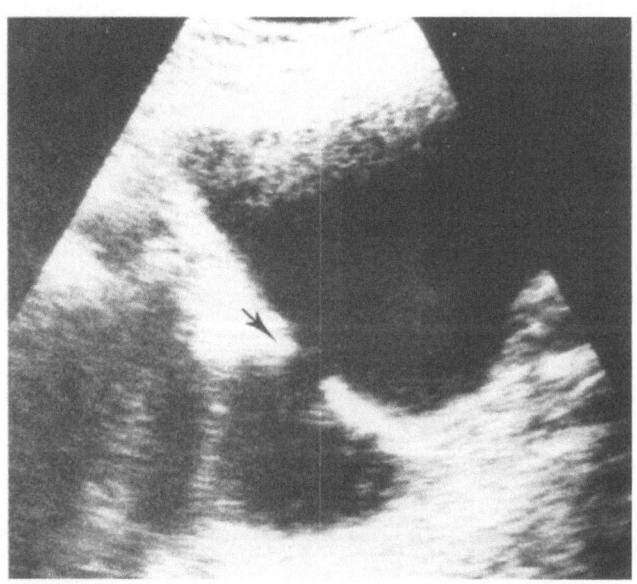

**Fig. 1.** Abdominal ultrasound of bladder with diverticulum. The neck of the diverticulum is demonstrated (*arrow*)

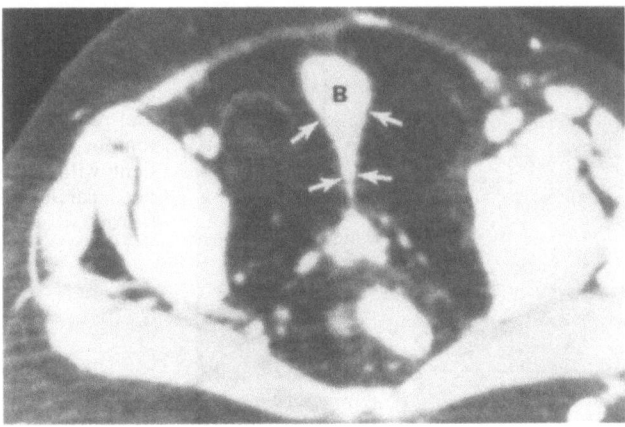

Fig. 2. Computed tomography of pelvic lipomatosis compressing and dislocating the bladder (*B*) (*arrows*)

than in men. Large diverticula may lift the bladder base. Some diverticula are difficult to fill by antegrade or retrograde contrast administration and are best demonstrated by US during micturition.

Urachal remnants can be seen in every degree from slight tapering of the upper anterior bladder wall to a fistula to the umbilicus. Tumour may occur, which is best demonstrated by CT or US. Urachal tumours may contain characteristic calcifications.

The "tear drop" bladder is a bladder compressed and dislocated by perivesical processes. US, CT and MRI may reveal and partly differentiate the underlying process. A prostatic tumour invading or dislocating the bladder base may be difficult to differentiate from intrinsic tumour and also from benign prostatic hyperplasia, which can cause a quite irregular and asymmetrical filling defect. Rectal and cervical carcinoma may also impress

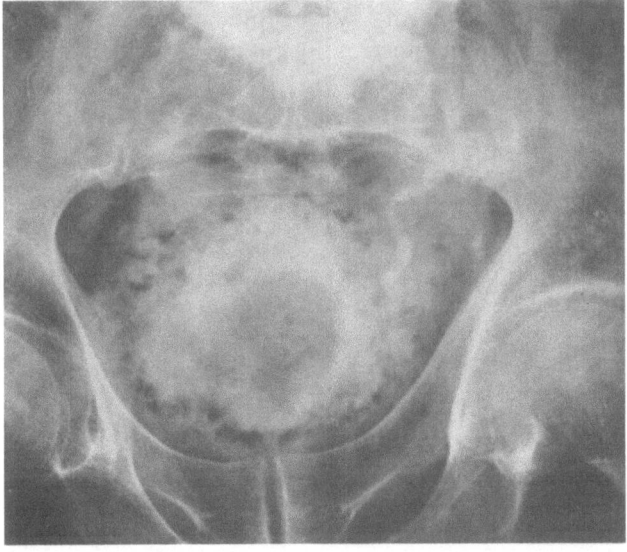

Fig. 3. Intravenous cystogram demonstrating air in the bladder wall in a diabetic patient; emphysematous cystitis

or even invade the bladder. Other causes of bladder compression and dislocation are ovarian tumour, mesenchymal pelvic tumour, haematoma, abscess, urinoma, lymphoma, hypertrophic ileopsoas muscle, fibrosis and lipomatosis. Lipomatosis is characterized by excessive fatty tissue deposition in the pelvis. It typically causes symmetrical lifting and compression of both the bladder and rectum. CT is diagnostic by demonstrating the excessive amount of fat as well as the compression (Fig. 2).

Simple acute cystitis is rarely detectable by any imaging modality, while severe cystitis may cause wall oedema detectable by US, CT or MRI. Urography rarely demonstrates affected mucosa unless the bladder wall contains air as in emphysematous cystitis, typically occurring in diabetic patients (Fig. 3).

Chronic cystitis may result in bladder contraction. Bilharzia often causes calcification of the bladder wall while tuberculous calcifications are more frequent in the neighbouring seminal vesicles.

Stones in the bladder often arise from passed ureteral calculi. Most stones leave the bladder, but may remain in case of urinary retention or infection and act as a nidus for further growth. Most bladder calcifications are radiopaque, but uric acid stones may be radiolucent and therefore best demonstrated by US.

Urinary retention is best demonstrated and quantified by US or nuclear medical cystography. It is seen in neurogenic bladder disturbances, prostatic enlargement and other causes of urethral obstruction.

Neurogenic bladder dysfunction, such as bladder instability, hyperreflexia or areflexia occurs in various degrees and may be due to lesions or congenital defects in the central nervous system, the spinal cord or in peripheral sacral nerves. There are distinctive X-ray pictures of the neurogenic or, better, neuropathic bladder, depending on the level of the neuronal lesion. In its simplest form it points to the thick-walled, trabeculated bladder of a typical upper motor neuronal lesion contrasted with the thin-walled flaccid bladder in lower motor neuronal lesions. However, in practice the picture is often mixed, and the infravesically obstructed bladder can have a typical "neurogenic shape".

Micturition cystourethrography is done in children (and adults) for vesicoureteric reflux. Nuclear medical cystography may be just as sensitive. However, the initial study to demonstrate or exclude the condition in children with recurrent infection or evidence of reflux nephropathy may reasonably be a radiological examination since it would be advisable to exclude anatomical abnormalities in these patients. Follow-up, on the other hand, may well be scintigraphic studies.

Trauma to the pelvis may result in ruptures of the bladder and the male urethra. Traumatic bladder rupture is relatively uncommon. It almost exclusively occurs when the bladder is full. The diagnosis is confirmed by cystography, which is also helpful to categorize the lesion. CT, which is often the first examination in severe

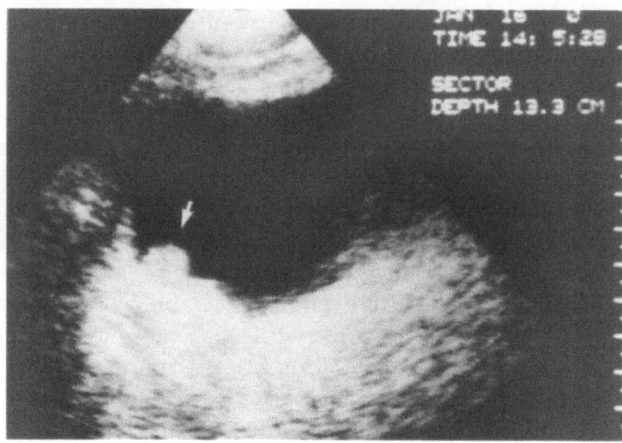

**Fig. 4.** Abdominal ultrasound can demonstrate bladder tumours 1 cm or less in size (*arrow*) and can replace cystoscopy for control of recurrence of noninvasive tumour

pelvic trauma, may miss small bladder ruptures. When urethral rupture is suspected, the cystogram should be obtained by retrograde urethral or suprapubic contrast injection, since urethral catheterization may turn a partial urethral rupture into a complete one.

Traumatic urethral injury may involve the anterior and posterior male urethra or both. Female injury is extremely rare. Anterior lesions are typically straddle injuries while posterior injuries are usually crush injuries from car accidents. The retrograde urethrogram is the examination of choice both for diagnosis and categorization. The immediate operative repair has been replaced by a more conservative approach with suprapubic catheterization and secondary delayed repair. This has brought a marked reduction in the rate of recurrent stricture, incontinence and impotence [1].

Bladder herniation can be demonstrated by US or simple cystography. Dynamic colpocystourethrography for female genital descent has been widely used as a guide for operative treatment, but is now considered less important.

Urethral stenosis is seen almost exclusively in men. Strictures in adult men are always acquired (trauma, infection). They are best demonstrated by retrograde urethrography. The posterior urethral valve, seen in male infants, is best demonstrated by micturition cystourethrography, while it may be missed on the retrograde urethrogram.

Functional stenosis of the bladder neck is typically seen in men below the prostatic age and is best demonstrated by micturition cystourethrography combined with urodynamic studies.

Severe urinary incontinence, seen in many patients with neuropathic bladder disease and as a result of urethral lesions, can now be treated effectively by an artificial urethral sphincter. Radiography is directed against the integrity of the contrast-filled system, consisting of cuff, reservoir and tubings [2].

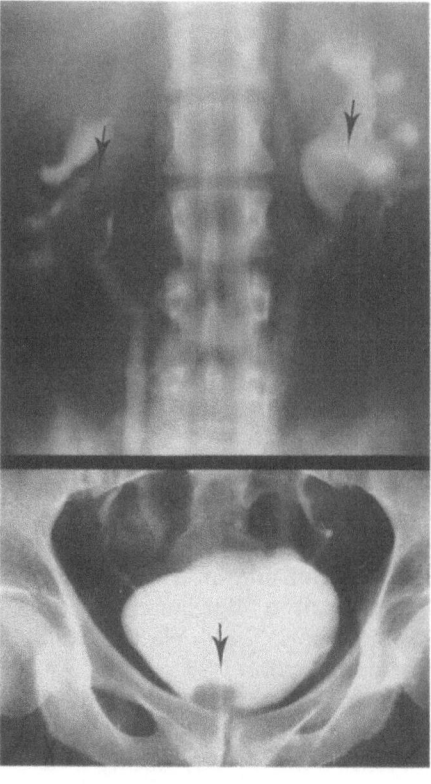

**Fig. 5.** Intravenous urogram showing synchronous bilateral renal pelvic tumour in a patient with bladder carcinoma (*arrows*)

Bladder tumours are urothelial in 90% of cases. Benign neoplasias make up less than 5% and include lymphangioma, haemangioma, neurofibroma and muscular tumours. US is the primary imaging modality for the detection, but cannot replace cystoscopy for the safe exclusion of tumour. Abdominal or transrectal US demonstrates local expansion and protrusion into the lumen and the relation to the ureteral orifices and may reveal tumour in diverticula (Fig. 4). However, US makes no contribution to the staging of the disease. Transurethral US performed during cystoscopy can detect tumours down to a few millimetres [3], but its reliability in distin-

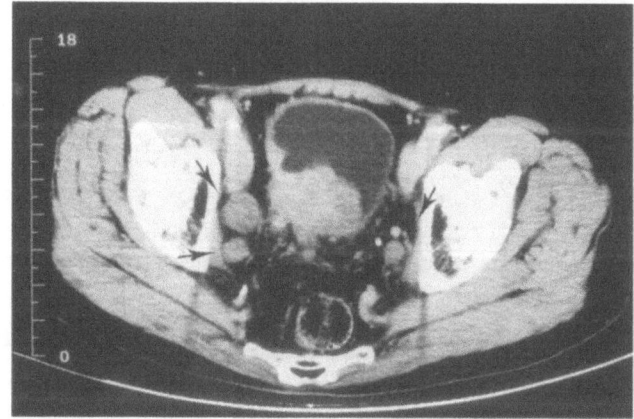

**Fig. 6.** Computed tomography of bladder tumour with perivesical extension and lymph node metastases (*arrows*)

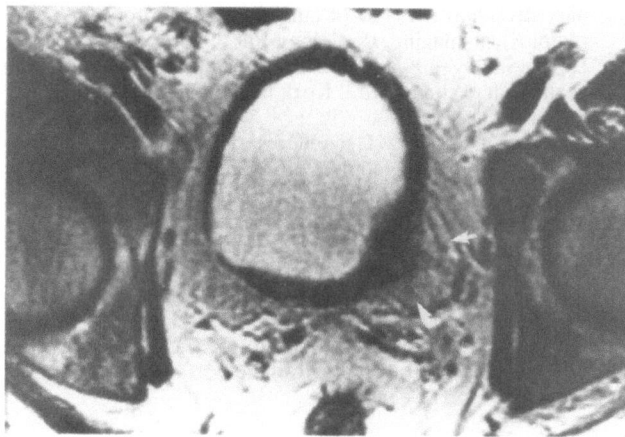

**Fig. 7.** T2-weighted magnetic resonance imaging of bladder carcinoma, stage T3. The tumour is breaking through the entire bladder wall (*arrow*), represented by the *black ring*. (Courtesy of HM Pollack, Philadelphia)

guishing superficial from invasive tumour is not high enough. Abdominal US seems capable of replacing cystoscopy for control of recurrence in patients with noninvasive tumours [4]. Intravenous urography is only used to exclude synchronous urothelial tumours in the upper tract, occurring in a few per cent of cases (Fig. 5). CT is currently the imaging modality of choice for the staging of invasive bladder carcinoma in spite of some limitations. It can demonstrate perivesical extension, pelvic wall involvement, lymphadenopathy and distant metastases with reasonable accuracy (Fig. 6) but is inaccurate in assessing the depth of tumour invasion and cannot distinguish inflammatory or postoperative changes from tumour. MRI offers a partly still unexplored potential for staging and shows possibilities in evaluating the degree of wall invasion (Fig. 7) [5, 6].

Cystectomy is indicated in muscular invasion of a urothelial tumour. Former urinary diversions such as ureterosigmoidostomy and Bricker bladder have been replaced by new techniques for bladder substitution, using detubularized bowel segments with intussusceptions, which secure continence and prevent reflux. Imaging by pyelography, cystography and intravenous urography is directed against capacity, leakage, obstruction, stone formation and reflux (Fig. 8) [7, 8].

## Intervention

Interventional techniques in the lower urinary tract include biopsy of tumours and drainage of fluid collections, guided by US or CT. Transcatheter embolization of otherwise intractable bleeding from bladder, prostate or uterus (tumour, irradiation) may occasionally be indicated. There are surprisingly few complications, even when superselective catheterization is not possible [9].

Balloon dilatation of prostatic urethral obstruction or urethral stricture is used with varying results [10, 11].

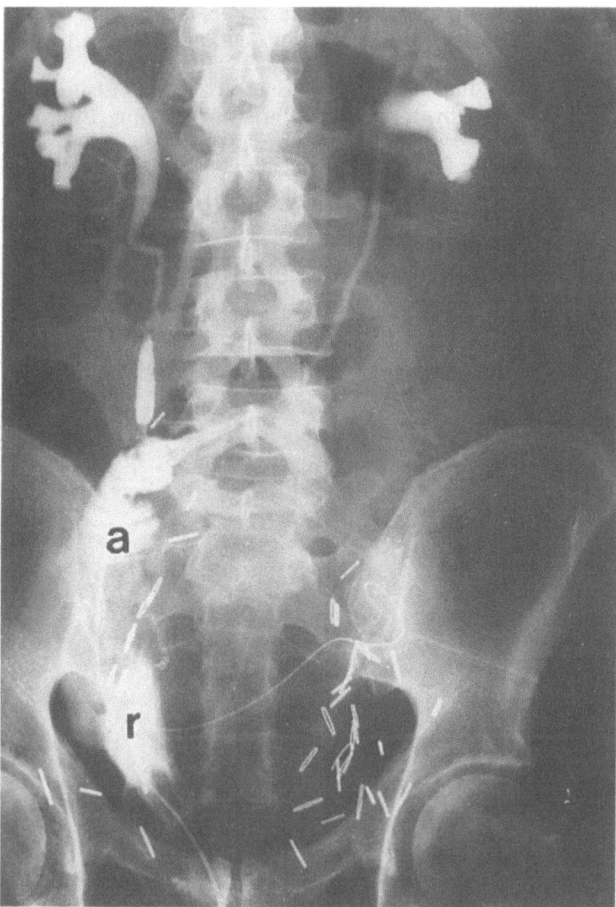

**Fig. 8.** Hemikock bladder substitution formed from isolated ileum. Ureters in common anastomosis with afferent ileal segment (*a*) intussuscepted into reservoir (*r*), which is anastomosed with posterior urethra. Bilateral retrograde pyelogram via indwelling catheters in each ureter

Self-expandable stents can be inserted to secure patency [12].

## Conclusion

Conventional radiographic techniques are still most useful to solve a large variety of diagnostic problems in the lower urinary tract. However, US has significantly broadened the scope of lower urinary tract imaging and intervention, and both CT and MRI have been shown to be extremely useful in solving specific problems, especially in tumour staging. There will undoubtedly be more diagnostic information to gain from these modalities along with their further technical refinement.

## References

1. Morehouse DD, Mac Kinnon KJ (1980) Management of prostatomembranous urethral disruption: 13 years experience. J Urol 123:173

2. Lorentzen T, Dorph S, Hald T (1987) Artificial urinary sphincters. Radiographic evaluation. Acta Radiol 28 63

3. Holm HH, Juul N, Torp-Pedersen S et al (1988) Bladder tumour staging by transurethral ultrasonic scanning. Eur Urol 15: 31

4. Juul N, Torp-Pedersen S, Larsen S et al (1986) Bladder tumour control by abdominal ultrasound and urine cytology. Scand J Urol Nephrol 20: 275

5. Amendola MA, Glazer SGM, Grossman HB et al (1986) Staging of bladder carcinoma: MRI - CT - surgical correlation. AJR 146: 1179

6. Namura Y, Indue EK (1991) MR staging of bladder tumours with gd-DTPA-enhanced oblique imaging. Radiology 181: 96

7. Amis ES Jr, Newhouse JH, Olsson CA (1988) Continent urinary diversions: review of current surgical procedures and radiological imaging. Radiology 168: 395

8. Dorph S, Steven K, Mygind T, Horn T (1993) Radiographic evaluation of the urethral Kock ileal bladder substitute. Acta Radiol 34: 133

9. Appleton DS, Silbey GNA, Doyle PT (1988) Internal iliac embolization for the control of severe bladder and prostatic haemorrhage. Br J Urol 61: 45

10. Reddy PK, Wasserman N, Castaneda F et al (1988) Balloon dilatation of prostate for the treatment of benign hyperplasia. Urol Clin North Am 15: 529

11. Jordan GH, Devine PC (1988) Management of urethral stricture disease. Urol J North Am 15: 277

12. Donald JJ, Rickards D, Milroy EJC (1991) Stricture disease: radiology of urethral stents. Radiology 180: 447

# Imaging of Prostate Cancer

R.H. Oyen

Department of Radiology, University Hospitals K.U.L., Herestraat 49, 3000 Leuven, Belgium

## Introduction

The popularity of imaging techniques to detect and to stage prostatic carcinomas has increased tremendously in the past decade. Nevertheless, most of the imaging techniques still have to compete with the digital rectal examination (DRE) and the serum concentration of prostate-specific antigen (PSA). There are two important reasons: the first is that the sensitivity of the imaging techniques now commonly used (i.e. transrectal ultrasonography, TRUS, and magnetic resonance imaging, MRI) lack sensitivity (a) to detect all cancers which originate in the prostate and (b) to stage the detected cancers accurately at a microscopic level. The second is that the imaging techniques lack specificity: many benign lesions closely resemble prostate carcinomas. For both reasons, biopsies are still required to obtain the final histological diagnosis.

The advantages and disadvantages of TRUS and MRI are discussed for the diagnosis and the staging of prostatic carcinoma.

## The Diagnosis of Prostate Cancer with Imaging

### Transrectal Ultrasonography

*Techniques*

A very convenient probe design is an endfiring, end-viewing transducer which allows multiplanar imaging in oblique coronal and sagittal projections by simply tilting the transducer 90°. Other transducers allow biplanar imaging (axial and sagittal) by simply switching the direction of the crystals. Most of the electronic transducers offer the ability for transrectal colour Doppler and duplex Doppler US as well. The patients are preferably scanned in left lateral position. Needle guidance systems are available for the probes with guides that clamp onto the side of the probe and place electronic guide lines showing the needle path on the monitor. A common needle device for transrectal prostate biopsies is the automatic spring-driven biopsy gun supplied with an 18-gauge needle. This device allows precise needle localization and performs a core type of biopsy (17-mm length) with minimal manipulation and with remarkable safety due to the speed at which the biopsy is performed.

TRUS guidance for transrectal biopsy is a safe and relatively painless procedure for the patient and is more accurate than digitally guided biopsy, even for palpable lesions. It can be performed without significant complications on an outpatient basis with little or no prior warning. The use of a cleansing enema is sometimes recommended but is not mandatory. It has become standard practice to administer a rapidly absorbed antibiotic just prior to the biopsy. One of the newer broad-spectrum antibiotics (such as fluoroquinolone) will almost completely eliminate the risk of major complications.

*Prostatic Carcinoma*

In the typical case (≥T2), prostate cancer is a hypoechoic lesion that originates subcapsularly in the peripheral zone of the prostate gland (Figs. 1-3). Many other benign lesions, though, are hypoechoic as well. Therefore biopsies are necessary to obtain a histological diagnosis (Fig. 3). In most series approximately 50% of hypoechoic lesions in the peripheral zone are cancerous. Biopsy sensitivity is superior with US guidance for all categories of tumours, with an overall sensitivity of 88% compared to 74% with digital guidance [1].

Many cancers (as much as 40%-60%) are isoechoic, because of too small a volume (microfoci) and/or because of an infiltrative growth pattern. Isoechogenicity is the likely explanation that some of these cancers are palpable but not visible at TRUS. When an isoechoic cancer is present, it can be detected only when secondary signs of malignancy are appreciated. These include glandular asymmetry, which is most often obviated on transverse scans. Other secondary signs are capsular bulging and areas of attenuation. Nevertheless, none of them is specific for malignant disease. It is therefore

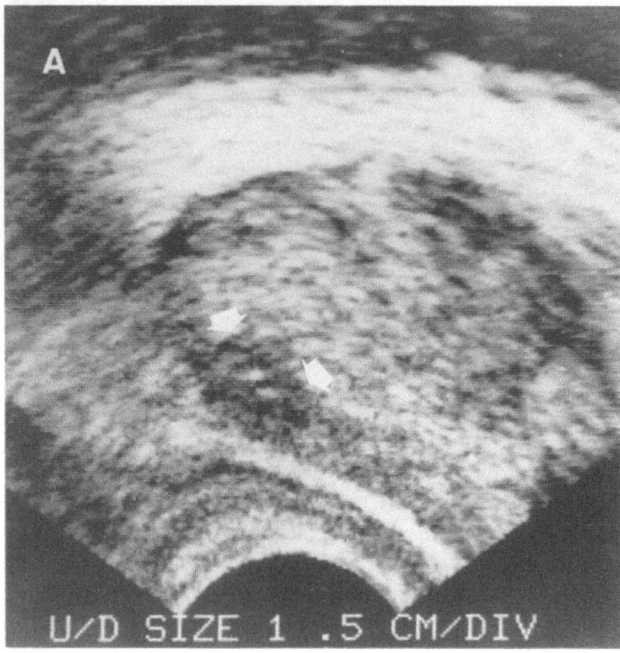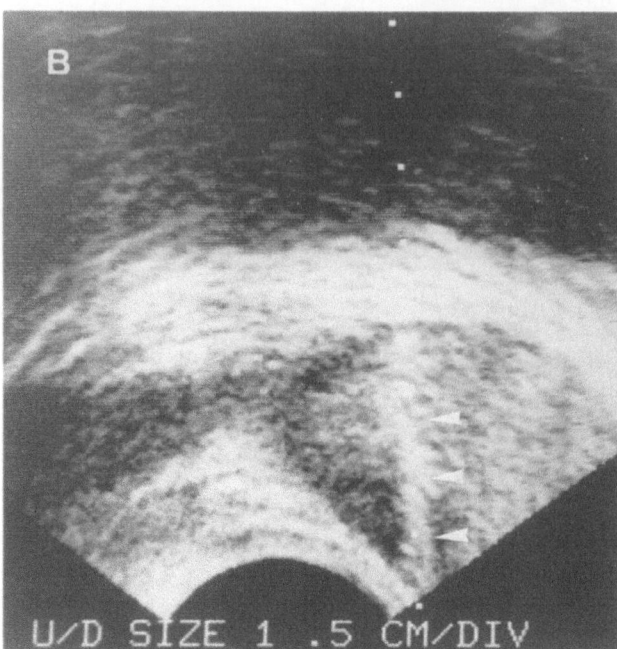

**Fig. 1. A, B.** Transrectal ultrasonography (TRUS); parasagittal scan of the right peripheral zone. Hypoechoic nodule (*arrow*) subcapsularly in the peripheral zone (**A**). Since differentiation from benign lesions is impossible, TRUS-guided biopsy is required (**B**). The needle course is clearly visible as it produces a white line throughout the lesion (*arrowheads*). Note that even in this particular case it is difficult provide objective criteria to stage this cancer accurately (confined or not; T2a at digital rectal examination and TRUS; proven pT2a at radical prostatectomy)

important to be aware of this pitfall and, if there is strong clinical suspicion of prostate cancer and a palpable nodule, to urge that a biopsy be performed even in the face of a negative TRUS examination.

Often, prostate cancer is bilateral or, perhaps better, multifocal. The sonographer may not appreciate the multiple foci when encountering a well-defined hypoechoic lesion. This has been demonstrated in a multi-

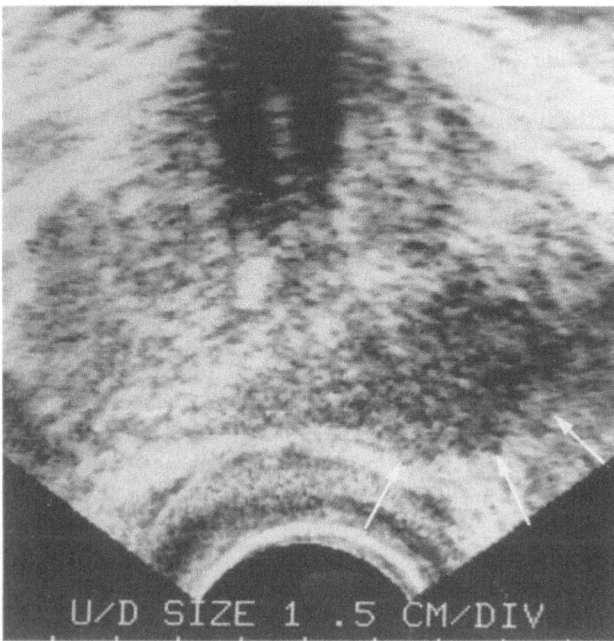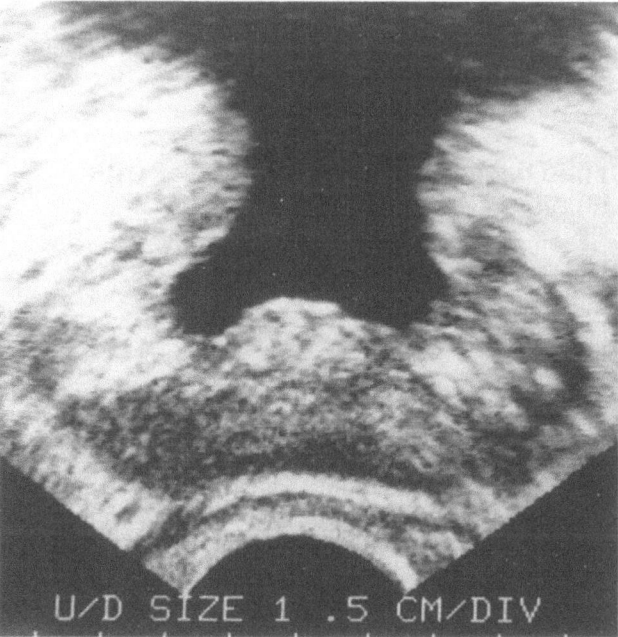

**Fig. 2.** Transrectal ultrasonography (TRUS); transverse scan. Large hypoechoic cancer in the left peripheral zone clearly extending beyond the confines of the capsule (*arrow*) (T3a both at digital rectal examination and TRUS, proven pT3a at radical prostatectomy)

**Fig. 3.** Transrectal ultrasonography; transverse scan after transurethral resection. Infiltrating hypoechoic cancer in the peripheral zone, probably not confined (T3a). Proven pT3a at staging biopsies

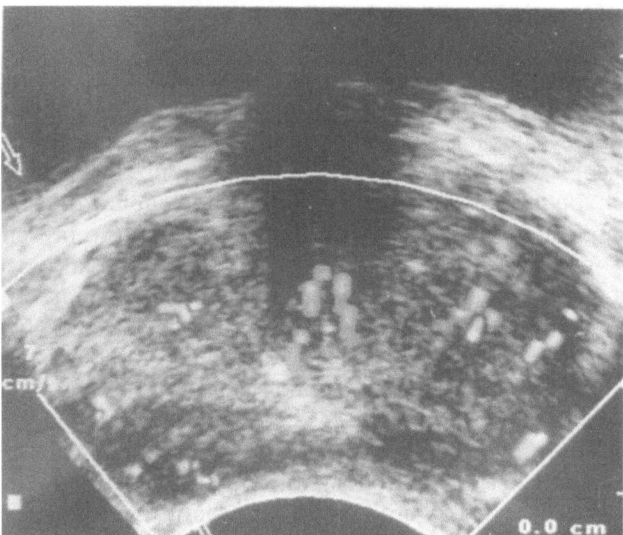

**Fig. 4.** Colour Doppler transrectal ultrasonography; transverse scan. Diffusely hypoechoic and hypervascular peripheral zone. Firm gland at digital rectal examination; prostate-specific antigen 14 hg/ml. Bioptically proven granulomatous prostatitis

institutional trial in which TRUS was only able to correctly identify 59% of all lesions and 72% of lesions larger than 1 cm [2].

Colour Doppler US increases the sensitivity for the detection of subtle and still isoechoic lesions in the peripheral zone of the prostate gland, but does not increase the specificity since considerable overlap exists between the vascularity of benign and malignant lesions (Fig. 4) [3]. The addition of objective, measurable flow-related criteria, such as the resistive index, is not found to be a specific discriminator either: spectral waveform analysis of the area of potential concern shows no statistical difference in the mean resistive indices in any patient with focal hypoechoic lesions in the peripheral zone.

Tumours originating in the transitional zone of the prostate gland remain virtually invisible (T1). The reason is that the carcinoma arises in or in between hyperplastic tissue or nodules in men with associated benign prostatic hyperplasia (i.e. isoechoic). Such tumours can only be detected by any set of systematics at random biopsies indicated by abnormal DRE, increased serum PSA, increased age-related PSA or increased PSA index (T1c) [4].

With growing experience of radical prostatectomy and histological examination of whole mount specimens, it has become clear that these stage T1 tumours in fact closely resemble palpable prostate cancers (T2) [5]. The mean tumour volume of stage T1c tumours is about 2.0 ml. Only about 20-25% of T1c tumours have a tumour volume < 0.5 ml; tumours > 0.5 ml are generally considered to have significant biological potential. Possible reasons for nonpalpability (and nonvisibility) of T1c tumours include (a) tumour location in the central and/or

anterior areas of the prostate, (b) increased gland volume due to nodular benign prostatic hyperplasia, (c) and infiltrative growth pattern, making T1c tumours more difficult to palpate and differentiate from other nodules.

## Magnetic Resonance Imaging

### Techniques

As compare with the body coil, the advent of the pelvic or phased-array coils has improved the overall resolution of MR images of the prostate. Endorectal coils in combination with phased-array coils have brought the imaging resolution of the prostate to new heights, with excellent depiction of the zonal anatomy, capsule, and neurovascular bundles [6]. Consensus has not been reached on whether one of these two approaches is clearly better.

If only occasional studies are performed, external phased-array coils are the better choice, as they are superior to the body coil and less dependent on the operator and result in fewer mistakes than are made with the inexpertly used endorectal coil [7].

### Prostatic Carcinoma

The prostate gland has a homogeneous low signal intensity on T1-weighted images. Peripheral zone cancers (≥T2) are hypointense on predominantly T2-weighted or T2-like images (Fig. 5). The hyperplastic tissue of the transitional zone displays heterogeneous signal intensities, depending on the degree of glandular and/or stromal

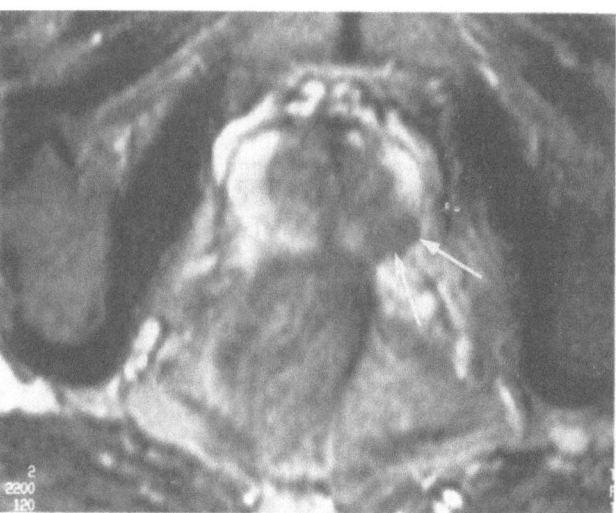

**Fig. 5.** Magnetic resonance imaging (MRI); axial T2-weighted image. Carcinoma the left peripheral zone (*arrow*), hypointense compared to the normal hyperintense glandular tissue of the peripheral zone. Note that the cancer is isointense compared to the hyperplastic transitional zone. This lesion was accurately staged as T3a (digital rectal examination, transrectal ultrasonography, MRI) and was confirmed by radical prostatectomy (pT3a)

hyperplasia. Again, this is the main reason why cancers originating in this particular area cannot be distinguished. Haemorrhage from previous biopsies may interfere with the diagnosis of prostate cancer as well. If artefacts from biopsy are absolutely to be avoided, a delay of 4-6 weeks between the biopsy and the MRI is necessary [8].

No advantages in detecting prostate cancer, in differentiating cancer from benign prostatic hyperplasia or normal prostatic tissue, or in assessing extraprostatic spread of cancer are observed for routine contrast-enhanced studies compared to T2-weighted (fast) SE imaging [9].

## Staging of Prostate Cancer

Assurance of confinement of the disease to the prostate would make the morbidity of each treatment more acceptable to the man contemplating therapeutic options. Therefore, if imaging were more accurate than clinical staging, it would have enormous potential in therapy planning.

### Transrectal Ultrasonography

A lesion greater than 1.5 cm (> 3 ml) suggests nonconfined cancer. It is accepted that nonconfined cancer is overdiagnosed in 9.1% of cases and missed in 31.3%. Problems of staging occur both for gross and microscopic extension (Figs. 1-3) [10]. However, it is not yet clear whether microscopically unconfined cancer is unfavourable for patient prognosis and affects the therapy [11]. In many cases it is difficult to distinguish the tumour from the prostatic capsule, the ejaculatory ducts, the bladder neck, the seminal vesicles, the anterior fibromuscular stroma, the apex and the neurovascular bundles. Because of the difficulty to accurately stage the tumours, TRUS-guided biopsies of areas potentially involved are suggested. Thus, seminal vesicle biopsies are recommended in patients with stage T2b or greater disease and with a lower clinical stage when the PSA level is 20 ng/ml or greater and the Gleason score is 7 or above. Others recommend staging biopsies of the seminal vesicles in patients with a Gleason score of more than 4 and a PSA of more than 10 ng/ml [12, 13].

Of T1c tumours 30%-50% have penetrated the prostatic capsule, 20%-30% demonstrate positive surgical margins, and 5%-10% demonstrate seminal vesicle invasion and/or positive pelvic lymph nodes. A combination of PSA density (index) <0.1 and favourable needle biopsy pathology (no Gleason 4 or 5 pattern in any core, <3 cores positive for cancer, and <50% involvement of any single core) will identify about 75% of men with tumours <0.5 ml who might be followed without immediate treatment. However, most T1c tumours are significant cancers >0.5 ml that warrant aggressive treatment in accordance with age and other health considerations.

### Magnetic Resonance Imaging

Periprostatic extension is readily detectable, and the overall accuracy of separating confined from nonconfined cancer is approximately 90%, excluding microscopic extension which cannot be recognized. Tumours involving the prostatic apex and those not within the high signal intensity peripheral zone still represent somewhat of a problem. In expert hands, the accuracy of endorectal coil MRI is as high as 90%, compared to only 50%-70% when no endorectal coils are used (Fig. 5) [6]. The accuracy of less experienced radiologists is higher when no endorectal coil is used (80% vs 50%). MRI is found to have a 54% specificity with a high degree of interobserver agreement. The accuracy in staging advanced disease is significantly affected by the diagnostic criterion used for extraprostatic extension.

One of the greatest advantages of MRI is the potential to noninvasively prove or exclude cancer spread into the seminal vesicles. The overall staging accuracy is 68%, with a 74% accuracy rate in staging advanced disease and a 91% accuracy rate for depiction of seminal vesicle involvement.

The value of MRI in assessing the nodal involvement (N-staging) in men with prostate cancer has been the subject of several studies. Metastatic and reactive, enlarged lymph nodes cannot be differentiated based on their signal intensities. For practical purposes, clusters of nodes >1 cm in diameter are considered pathologic. Recently, a sensitivity of 25% and a specificity of 97% was reported.

### Computed Tomography

The presence or absence of lymph node metastases is an important prognostic factor. When considering treatment for localized disease, the lymph node status should be ascertained with reasonable certainty. In general, a relationship exists between tumour (Gleason) grade, concentration of PSA in the serum, and lymph node status. Screening for lymph node metastases with CT (or staging lymphadenectomy) may no longer be justified on a routine basis in patients undergoing radical retropubic prostatectomy [15].

Lymph node involvement correlates significantly with elevated serum PSA values, high Gleason score, and advanced clinical stage. Lymph node metastases are particularly uncommon in patients with nonpalpable tumours (1.5%), PSA values less than 10 ng/ml (1.3%), and Gleason scores less than 6 (3.8%). Only 2.2% of the patients with at least one of these favourable characteristics will have lymph node involvement [16].

A staging procedure such as CT or (laparoscopic) pelvic lymph node dissection should be considered in patients with high risk features, especially those with a positive seminal vesicle biopsy where the likelihood of encountering positive nodes is 48%, or when the Gleason

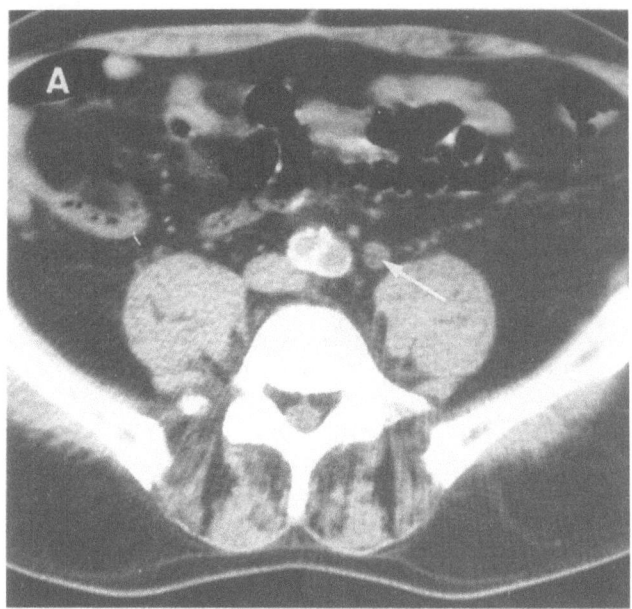
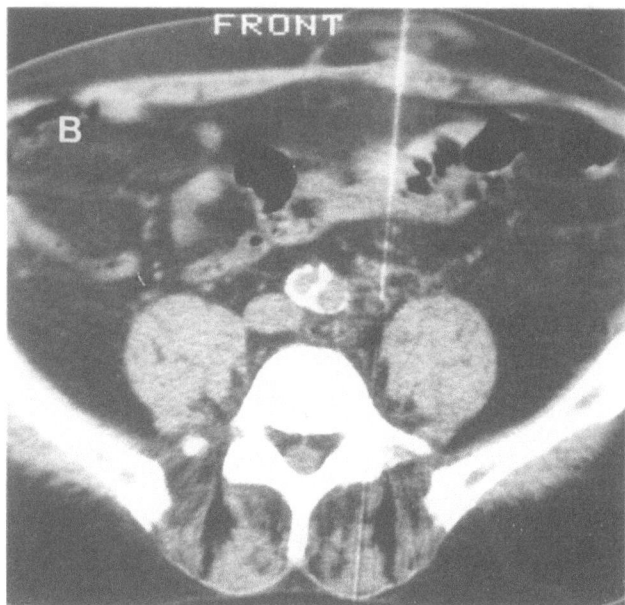

**Fig. 6 A, B.** Computed tomography. **A** Lymph node (*arrow*) at the level of the aortic bifurcation in a patient with clinically confined prostatic carcinoma. **B** Metastasis from prostate carcinoma at cytological examination of material obtained by transperitoneal fine-needle aspiration biopsy

score is 7 or more or PSA is over 20 ng/ml. These minimally invasive staging techniques can accurately identify the subgroup of stages T1 and T2 cancer patients who in reality have stage T3c or N+ disease initiating therapy. CT-guided fine-needle aspiration biopsy is a valuable alternative to surgical lymph node exploration to clarify the nature of lymph node enlargement (Fig. 6) [17].

## Conclusion

As the twenty-first century approaches, it is necessary to diagnose and stage prostatic malignancies in a cost-effective manner. With the recent advances in the use PSA, it is now possible to avoid many time-consuming, expensive, and invasive procedures that have been commonplace in the past. PSA thus has replaced TRUS as a firstline diagnostic test for evaluating men for early, curable prostate cancer. In older men, the use of age-specific antigen reference ranges for serum PSA can significantly decrease the number of prostate biopsies that are routinely performed.

With regard to the staging procedures, PSA can now be used successfully to eliminate the bilateral pelvic lymphadenectomy in 30% of men with clinically localized disease and the radionuclide bone scan in 40% of patients with newly diagnosed prostate cancer.

## References

1. Renfer LG, Schow D, Thompson IM, Optenberg S (1995) Is ultrasound guidance necessary for transrectal prostate biopsy? J Urol 154: 1390-1391
2. Rifkin MD, Zerhouni EA, Gatsonis CA et al (1990) Comparison of MR imaging and US staging in staging early prostate cancer: results of a multi-institutional cooperative trial. N Engl J Med 323: 621-626
3. Kelly IMG, Lees WR, Rickards D (1993) Prostate cancer and the role of color Doppler US. Radiology 189: 153-156
4. Terris MK, McNeal JE, W Stamey TA (1992) Detection of clinically significant prostate cancer by transrectal ultrasound-guided systematic biopsies. J Urol 148: 829-832
5. Brendler CB (1995) Characteristics of prostate cancer found with early detection regimens. Urology [suppl 3A]: 71-76
6. Tempany CM, Zhou X, Zerhouni A et al (1994) Staging of prostate cancer: results of Radiology Diagnostic Oncology Group project: comparison of three MR imaging techniques. Radiology 192: 47-54
7. Hricak H, White S, Vigneron D et al (1994) Carcinoma of the prostate: MR imaging with pelvic phased array coils versus integrated endorectal-pelvic phased array coils. Radiology 193: 703-709
8. Schnall MD, Imai Y, Tomaszewski J, Pollack HM; Lenkinski RE, Kressel HY (1991) Prostate cancer: local staging with endorectal surface coil MR imaging. Radiology 178: 797-802
9. Schiebler ML, Schnall MD, Pollack HM et al (1993) Current role of MR imaging in staging of adenocarcinoma of the prostate. Radiology 189: 339-352
10. Hamper UM, Sheth S, Walsh PC, Holtz PM, Epstein JI (1991) Capsular transgression of prostatic carcinoma: evaluation with transrectal US with pathologic correlation. Radiology 178 (3): 791-795
11. Hering F, Rist M, Roth J et al (1990) Does microinvasion of the capsule and/or micrometastases in regional lymph nodes influence disease-free survival after radical prostatectomy? Br J Urol 66: 177-181
12. Vallancien G, Prapotnich D, Veillon B, Brisset JM, Andre-Bougaran J (1991) Seminal vesicle biopsies in the preoperative staging of prostatic cancer. Eur Urol 19: 196-200
13. Stone NN, Stock RG, Unger P (1995) Indications for seminal vesicle biopsy and laparoscopic pelvic lymph node dis-

section in men with-localized carcinoma of the prostate. J Urol 154: 1392-1396

14. Wolf JS, Cher M, Dall'era M, Presti JC, Hricak H, Carroll PR (1995) The use and accuracy of cross-sectional imaging and fine needle aspiration cytology for detection of pelvic lymph node metastases before radical prostatectomy. J Urol 153: 993-999

15. Oesterling JE (1995) Using prostate-specific antigen to eliminate unnecessary diagnostic tests: significant worldwide economic implications. Urology 46: 26-33

16. Campbell SC, Klein EA, Levin HS, Piedmonte MR (1995) Open pelvic lymph node dissection for prostate cancer: a reassessment. Urology 46(3): 352-355

17. Oyen RH, Van Poppel HP, Ameye FE, Van de Voorde WA, Baert AL, Baert LV (1994) Lymph node staging of localized prostatic carcinoma with CT and CT-guided fine needle aspiration biopsy: prospective study of 285 patients. Radiology 190: 315-321

# Interventional Uroradiology

M.J. Kellett

Department of Uroradiology, St Peter's Hospital, the Middlesex Hospital, Mortimer Street, London, W1N8AA, UK

## Introduction

There are many percutaneous manipulations which can be performed in the upper urinary tract using the basic needle nephrostomy access. This paper will cover the method of needle nephrostomy for drainage of obstructed and diversion of nonobstructed kidneys. The different percutaneous manipulations will then be covered.

## Percutaneous Nephrostomy

A needle nephrostomy can be performed using local anaesthetic to the skin and around the capsule of the kidney. Sedation in the adult is very rarely needed, provided that a full explanation is given to the patient and adequate local anaesthesia is injected into the puncture site. Children may require sedation or occasionally general anaesthesia.

Ultrasound is the preferred imaging modality when puncturing an obstructed kidney. Fluoroscopy is required to position the catheter in the renal pelvis in patients with a complicated anatomy such as caliceal neck stenosis. It is advisable therefore to have both imaging modalities to hand.

Intravenous contrast may be given to outline the dilated collecting system. However, with the patient prone (which is the preferred position for a needle nephrostomy) the denser contrast medium will only outline the anterior calices. A needle puncture of these will lead to difficulty negotiating a guide wire and catheter back into the renal pelvis. The ideal puncture passes into a posterior calix, causing potentially less damage to the kidney as it passes through the least depth of parenchyma and allows the guidewire and catheter to slip easily into the more anterior renal pelvis. Ultrasound is thus helpful in identifying the posterior calices, which on fluoroscopy may only be filled with non opacified urine. The ultrasound may be used to give a skin marker and an idea of depth and angle for the puncture before cleaning the skin or it may be used with a sterile sleeve to direct the needle puncture in real-time. A fine needle may be inserted first to inject contrast and opacify the collecting system and then, under fluoroscopic control, a sheathed needle may be inserted into a selected calyx. If obstruction is not severe, intravenous contrast will opacify the system and a single puncture rather than a double puncture technique may be employed. A large hydronephrosis may be rapidly drained by a single puncture, using a needle fitted with a catheter sheath [1]. These are large and rather traumatic and most radiologists prefer to use the Seldinger technique, a small 18-gauge sheathed needle being used followed by the introduction of a 0.35-inch guidewire through the sheath. An 8-Ch teflon facial dilator can then be inserted, allowing a soft 7-Ch pigtail nephrostomy catheter to be introduced over the guidewire. Care should be taken not to inject contrast into a system which is already under pressure and possibly infected as this may cause intravasation and septicaemia. Always exchange the trapped urine for contrast. It may even be wise to delay any contrast study for a day or so to allow an infection to settle. A later nephrostogram can then outline the site and cause of obstruction.

## Percutaneous Nephrolithotomy

The first percutaneous nephrolithotomies (PCNL) were performed by radiologists, using biplane fluoroscopy and basket catheters [2]. In Germany, urologists used tracks already formed by emergency needle nephrostomies to remove obstructing calculi from the pelviureteric junction (PUJ) using cystoscopes [3]. A one-stage PCNL was developed to remove any calculus from a kidney whether or not there was obstruction [4].

A one-stage PCNL should be performed in the X-ray department, ideally using a ceiling-mounted C arm image intensifier. However, it can be carried out on a conventional overcouch or, preferably, undercouch screening table, taking care that the irrigant fluids used during the endoscopic procedures are carefully kept away from the electrical supply. Alternatively, a mobile C arm image intensifier can be used in the operating theatre.

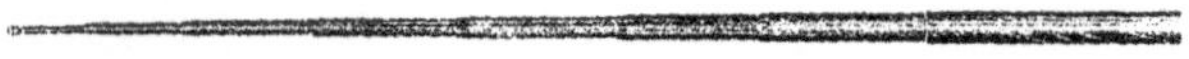

**Fig. 1.** Metallic aerial dilators over long central control rod

Under general anaesthesia, a retrograde catheter is passed up the ureter to the kidney so that dilute contrast and a small amount of methylene blue can be injected to distend the collecting system. The patient is placed in the prone position on the X-ray table and the kidney is punctured as for a needle nephrostomy. A posterior lower pole calix is usually selected as this gives the best access to the pelvicaliceal system. Contrast injected via the ureteric catheter can be use to distend the system just before the puncture and the blue dye aspirated from the needle helps to confirm the correst position immediately so that a guidewire can be inserted. Track dilatation may be performed using telescopic metallic dilators, balloon catheters or Teflon dilators. Metallic aerial dilators have the advantage that they are reusable and thus inexpensive (Fig. 1). They neatly tamponade the track during dilatation, thus minimising bleeding into the collecting system. Care needs to be taken, however, not to advance them too fast, thus damaging the kidney. Serial Teflon dilatation is easy to perform but results in bleeding as the dilators are exchanged. Balloon catheters are attractive to the radiologist as they can tamponade the track prior to the insertion of an operating channel, but they are relatively expensive.

At the end of track dilatation an Amplatz sheath is introduced to act as the endoscopic channel. Through this sheath nephroscopes can be passed into the pelvis and calculi can be removed with grasping forceps. Larger calculi require disintegration with electrohydraulic probes or ultrasound drilling rods [5].

Multiple or complicated branched calculi can be removed as well, either using several tracks or a "Y" track. Two stones in adjacent calices which cannot both be reached from the initial track may require a "Y" puncture, withdrawing from the first calix after removing that stone and puncturing the second calix still using the initial percutaneous track. At open operation multiple radial nephrotomies may be performed for multiple caliceal calculi. In the same way, several percutaneous tracks can be formed to remove multiple stones percu-

taneously. However, the complication rate, though low, does increase with the more complex calculi [6] and extracorporeal shockwave lithotripsy (ESWL) should be used for multiple small stones.

## PCNL or ESWL?

Large staghorn calculi are best treated by a debulking PCNL to remove the central mass of the stone and any caliceal fragments that are easily accessible. A ureteric stent is then inserted via the nephrostomy track and the remaining calculi are treated by ESWL [7]. Clearly, for ESWL to work there must be a freely draining kidney. Patients with narrow-necked calices containing calculi or with a tight PUJ (as in horseshoe kidneys) are best treated by PCNL. Occasionally, hard cystine stones fail to fragment with ESWL and require PCNL. In some cases the waiting list for ESWL or the lack of easy access to a lithotriptor still requires the practice of PCNL. If a patient has severe symptoms, the longer waiting list for treatment by ESWL may be an indication to treat the patient by PCNL and, in view of the shortage of lithotriptors in the UK, PCNL is a very practical alternative.

## Ureteric Stones

Stones in the ureter can be most challenging to the urologist and interventional radiologist. ESWL to stones within the ureter is possible but not as easy or effective as renal pelvic stone ESWL. In practice, stones in the proximal third of the ureter have a trial of lithotripsy. If this fails they may be flushed back into the kidney using a retrograde ureteric catheter. They may then be treated by PCNL under the same anaesthesia [8] or a ureteric stent may be inserted to trap the stone in the renal pelvis for subsequent ESWL. Occasionally, stones in the mid- and distal third of the ureter may be flushed back if they have just dropped down from the kidney. However, if there is any surrounding oedema, it is rarely effective. Most of the stones in the lower ureter are treated by ureteroscopy.

## Percutaneous Pyelolysis

Patients with a PUJ obstruction can have an endoscopic treatment of the obstruction without an open operation. The method developed by Wickham and Kellett [9] is an adaptation of the open operation Davis's intubated pyelotomy.

### Method

Access is gained percutaneously in the same way as for a PCNL. A guidewire is passed into the renal pelvis via the ureteric catheter and brought out to the skin through the percutaneous endoscopic track. This wire safeguards the PUJ and stabilises it throughout the treatment. Using a urethrotome, or purpose-built endoscope with a mounted cutting blade, the PUJ is cut open on the renal side (posterior lateral aspect) of the pelvis, thus being clear of the medial renal artery. Care is required, however, as accessory lower polar vessels may hook under the PUJ. If present, these can be seen with careful endoscopy. The resection is a full-thickness cut through to the retroperitoneal fat and extended 3 cm down the ureter. A tapered catheter is then introduced over the guidewire under fluoroscopic control so that the lysed junction is supported by a 16-Ch catheter - the pelvic portion of the catheter having side holes to drain the kidney and the distal tapered portion of the catheter being positioned halfway down the ureter. This stent is then left in situ with internal or external drainage for 4-6 weeks to allow the PUJ to heal and surrounding fibrosis to form, thus holding the PUJ open. Initial results show a 64%-72% success rate [10, 11] but the technique is still evolving and in view of the minimal invasiveness of the procedure, it is sure to have a role in the management of PUJ obstruction.

An invagination method has been developed from workers in Lyon. A balloon catheter is passed up the ureter over a guidewire and sited just beneath the PUJ. After gaining percutaneous access, this balloon is inflated so that it sits firmly in the proximal ureter. By fixing the distal end of the wire to the catheter with forceps, traction applied to the proximal guidewire (out through the nephrostomy tract) will invaginate the PUJ, producing a much simpler target for the endoscopist to cut the junction [12].

Balloon dilation by the radiologist has been used with extremely floppy and mobile PUJ but the results of irregularly splitting open the junction are probably not as good as pyelolysis.

## Percutaneous Resection of Transitional Cell Tumours

Tumours of the urothelial lining to the pelvicaliceal system can be resected through a percutaneous track. However, the danger of seeding these tumours into the track and spillage of tumour cells into the blood stream means that only low-grade well-differentiated tumours may be treated this way.

The radiologist performs the percutaneous track, carefully selecting a calix which will lead easily to the tumour. It is vital to perform the puncture and dilatation with the least trauma to avoid vascular damage and minimalise any chance of tumour dissemination. The tumour is removed with a resectoscope via an Amplatz sheath and a nephrostomy is inserted at the end to allow the track to heal. An iridium wire can then be intro-

duced to sterilise the track [13]; 3 days later the nephrostomy is removed.

The role of conservative treatment of transitional cell tumours of the upper urinary tract is still under debate [14]. In a review of 28 cases of percutaneous resection [15] the early results were encouraging and low-grade, low-stage tumours should be managed as they would in the bladder. No surgeon would perform a cystectomy for a well-differentiated, noninvasive transitional cell tumour, and the kidney should not be removed for a similar lesion.

## Ureteric Stenting

Ureteric stents may be inserted under local anaesthesia using a percutaneous approach. If a needle nephrostomy is being performed because of obstruction, this is the route of choice if the obstruction can be passed with a guidewire. If the patient is due to have cystoscopy anyway, for example for haematuria, then the retrograde route is the preferred method of choice using the same general anaesthesia.

For antegrade stenting, a puncture through a posterior middle calix [16] facilitates the passage of the stent. The usual approach for a needle nephrostomy is via a lower calix but this may result in a tight angle back through the PUJ to the ureter. Whilst this can be easily negotiated with a cobra catheter and a straight guidewire, insertion of a stent may be difficult. Tortuous bends in the ureter may require patience to negotiate. Usually the combination of a cobra catheter with a straight wire or floppy Bentson or Terumo wire can allow the bends to be passed. By a caterpillar approach, advancing first the guidewire and then the catheter, the ureter is descended and the ureteric orifice is finally crossed.

The cobra catheter may need to be exchanged for a straight, tapered Teflon catheter such as a 7-Ch Van Andel angioplasty catheter and the bend at PUJ may be straightened using a stiff Amplatz wire. Finally, the ureteric stent is pushed down the ureter with careful positioning so that the distal end is through the ureteric orifice, but not irritating the trigone, and the proximal end is coiled in the renal pelvis. The length of stent required can be judged by measuring the length of a catheter required to pass over the guidewire into the bladder. In practice it is rare for anything longer than 22 cm to be required (Fig. 2).

When a needle nephrostomy is being performed for a small steinstrasse obstructing the ureter, it may be possible once the kidney is decompressed to manipulate a guidewire past the stones into the bladder. A 7-Ch Teflon dilator (Van Andel) can then be passed down the ureter over the guide wire and finally a single J stent from the skin to the bladder with side holes from the renal pelvis down to the bladder can be inserted. This al-

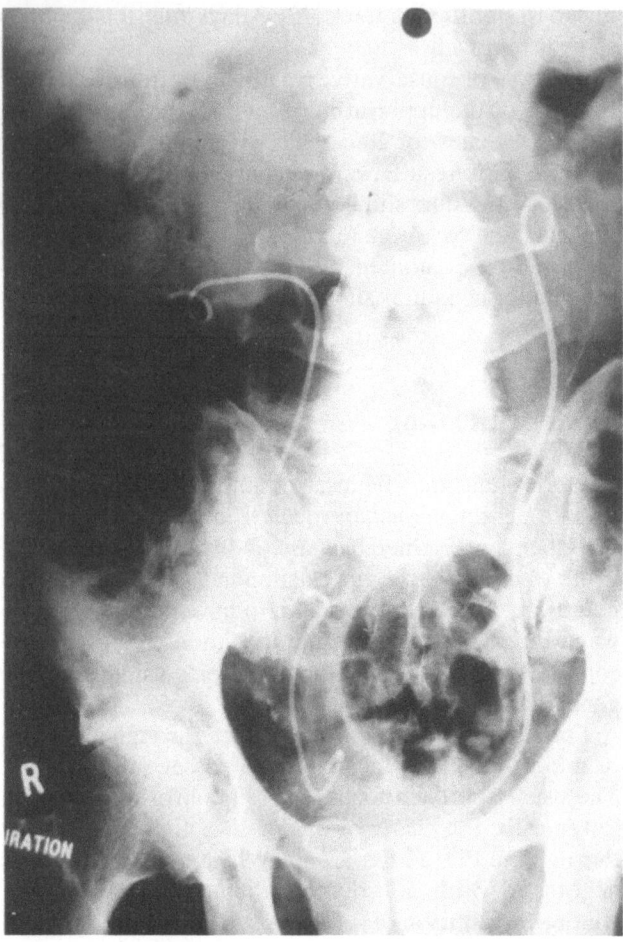

**Fig. 2.** Retroperitoneal fibrosis with aortic aneurysm. Both antegrade stents are too long: *left*, irritating bladder base; *right*, proximal 1 cm still in renal parenchyma

lows the kidney to drain and at the same time causes ureteric dilatation which facilitates the passage of the stone fragments. The advantage of a single J stent is that it can be easily removed through the skin. If it is envisaged that the stent will be left in for any length of time, a JJ ureteric stent can be inserted, which later requires cystoscopic removal by the urologist. To facilitate the insertion of a ureteric stent a stiff wire such as an Amplatz wire allows the pressure of the pushing catheter to be transferred to the ureter.

## Dilatation of Ureteric Strictures

### Benign Strictures

An acute stricture following ureteric trauma may be successfully dilated via a percutaneous track. The results with dilating chronic strictures of more than 3 months' standing are not good but it may be worth attempting before reverting to open surgery.

Once the stricture is reached via a needle nephrostomy, dilute contrast should be injected to outline the extent and shape of the stricture. Most can be passed using a tapered Teflon Van Andel catheter and straight guidewire. Occasionally, tortuous strictures require angled cobra catheters with straight or floppy Bentson wires. Great care is required to avoid perforating the ureter. Hydrostatic dilatation may be of initial help using very dilute contrast. A slippery Terumo wire may also be useful. Once the stricture is passed with a guidewire it can be simply dilated with graduated Van Andel catheters or with balloon catheters. All strictures, once dilated, require stenting for several weeks to allow the urothelium to repair. Restricturing may occur if a stent is not left or if there is a vascular compromise to the ureter as in a transplanted ureteric anastomotic stricture. Results are better with strictures in the proximal rather than the distal ureter and, as already mentioned, the results are far better with early strictures than in chronic strictures. Large stents (> 8 Ch) are more traumatic to the ureter when removed than are small stents but as with pyelolysis, restricturing may occur if the ureter is not adequately stented. One alternative is to insert two parallel ureteric stents over two guidewires after dilatation of the ureteric stricture. This allows good dilatation and excellent drainage around the two stents.

### Malignant Obstruction

Malignant strictures may be dilated and palliative ureteric stents inserted in just the same way as with benign strictures. However, as with the insertion of a needle nephrostomy in a patient with a malignant obstruction, clinical acumen is required to ensure that it is in the patient's best interest to have the obstruction and renal failure relieved.

## Conclusion

The role of the radiologist and that of the urologist are changing rapidly. Interventional radiological techniques using percutaneous tracks to manipulate guidewires and catheters through the urinary tract are presently under external X-ray and ultrasound guidance, but real-time intraluminal ultrasound may lead us closer to the actual target of interest and, together with external ultrasound, may significantly replace X-ray imaging.

Urological endoscopy has led to the development of smaller, more versatile endoscopes which can carry energy through smaller and smaller channels. The two disciplines of interventional radiology and endourology will almost certainly overlap, if not join, as "minimally invasive therapy". At the same time extracorporeal treatments are developing so that not only shock waves can be focused to disintegrate renal calculi but also ultrasound can be used to pinpoint and to treat lesions such as liver metastases from outside the body.

Such focused ultrasound will soon be more than experimental and developing technology will lead to a huge expansion in the field of minimally invasive therapy.

# References

1. Rezneck RH, Tainer LB (1980) Percutaneous nephrostomy. Radiol Clin North Am 22 (2): 393-406
2. Fernstrom I, Johansson B (1976) Percutaneous pyelolithotomy: a new extraction technique. Scand J Urol Nephrol 10: 257-259
3. Alken P, Hutschneiter G, Gunter R (9982) Percutaneous kidney stone removal. Eur Urol 8: 304-311
4. Wickham JEA, Miller RA, Kellett MJ, Payne SR (1984) Percutaneous nephrolithotomy - one stage or two? Br J Urol 56: 582-585
5. Marberger M, Jeyasekharan D (1990) Percutaneous nephrolithotripsy with ultrasound. In: Wickham JEA, Buck AC (eds) Renal tract stone. Livingstone Churchill, Edinburgh, pp 535-545
6. Jones DJ, Russell GL, Kellett MJ, Wickham JEA (1990) The changing practice of percutaneous stone surgery. Review of 1000 cases 1981 -1988. Br J Urol 66: 1-5
7. Eisenberger F, Fuchs G, Muller K, Butt P, Rassweiler J (1985) Extracorporeal shockwave lithotripsy (ESWL) and endourology: an ideal combination for the treatment of kidney stones. World J Urol 3: 41-47
8. Kellett MJ, Wickham JEA, Payne (1985) Combined retrograde and antegrade manipulation for percutaneous nephrolithotomy of ureteric calculi. A push-pull technique. Urology 25: 391-392
9. Wickham JEA, Kellett MJ (1983) Percutaneous pyelolysis. Eur Urol 9: 122-124
10. Ramsay JWA, Miller RA, Kellett MJ, Blackford HM, Wickham JEA, Whitfield HM (1984) Percutaneous pyelolysis: indications, complications and results. Br J Urol 56: 586-588
11. Winkle DC, Joyce AD, Kellett MJ, Wickham JEA (1990) Percutaneous pyelolysis a review. Br J Urol (submitted)
12. Gelet A, Martin X, Dessouki T (1991) Ureteropelvic invagination: reliable technique of endopyelotomy. J Endourology 5: 223-224
13. Woodhouse CRJ, Kellett MJ, Bloom HJG (1986) Percutaneous renal surgery and local radiotherapy in the management of renal pelvic transitional cell carcinoma. Br J Urol 58: 245-249
14. Nurse ED, Woodhouse CRJ, Kellett MJ, Dearniey DP (1989) Percutaneous removal of upper tract tumours. World J Urol 7: 131-134
15. Patel A, Soonawalla P, Shepherd S, Dearniey D, Ketlett M, Woodhouse C (1994) Long term outcome after percutaneous treatment of TCC of the renal pelvis. 12th World Congress of Endourology and SWL (abstr)
16. Baumer MP, Pollack HM (1984) Dilatation of ureteral stenoses: technique and experience in 44 patients. Am J Radiol 143: 789-793

# Management Issues in Radiology

H.M. Saxton

Ash House, Houghton Road, Stockbridge, Hampshire SO20 6LE, UK

## Introduction

The word 'management' has entered the vocabulary of doctors in the UK and other countries with increasing frequency in the past 15 years. To some it causes anxiety, even hostility. Others are quite comfortable with management concepts. So, what is management and why do radiologists need to understand it?

In the UK the imaging department in an average hospital serving a community of, say, 300000 people has an annual budget equivalent to US $ 3-5m, of which 65%-70% is spent on staff salaries. Its capital equipment will have a value of at least $ 5m. This is a considerable resource of people, space and equipment and in many situations the sums involved are much higher still. It hardly needs to be emphasised that in all health care systems such resources should be used as efficiently and effectively as possible. In this context 'efficiently' means that everything is done economically and to the highest standard; 'effectively' means that the right things are done. So the well-managed department will be giving a high-quality service in both clinical and operational terms, and it will be doing so with the least expenditure of resources. Such standards are not achieved by accident and that is why good management is needed.

Radiologists will have little difficulty with the idea of *clinical efficiency*; it is what they have been trained to provide. They try to offer the range of studies needed by clinicians and their patients, to minimise staff and patient irradiation, and to reduce unnecessary investigations. They strive for the production of high-quality images and for accurate reports. Finally, they aim to perform diagnostic and interventional procedures with minimal complications.

Where many radiologists are less successful and what they are in less interested is in ensuring *operational efficiency*. Yet the hallmark of a good radiologist-manager (RM) is an equal interest in and concern for this aspect of their work. He or she will know, for example, that the best performed scan is of much less value to patient and clinician if not performed promptly, or if there are delays in the report being issued or if the films and report cannot be traced. Operational efficiency has therefore to do with such matters as the optimal utilisation of space and equipment; an optimal staffing structure and the economical use of staff; the speedy and efficient handling of films and reports; keeping patient waiting times to a minimum; careful costing of the work of the department; and the production of accurate data on work load. A concern for these matters will help to ensure first class service and also that the department stays within its budget.

At the interface between these two types of efficiency is the question of what each radiologist does. Some are ready to contribute long hours undertaking angiograms or computed tomographic (CT) scans but may be unwilling to give a share of their time to routine plain film reporting. As plain film work constitutes commonly over 80% of an imaging department's caseload, it is essential that this part of a department's work is properly covered and not left to the most junior staff. The hospital community usually looks for a sensible balance between these components of an imaging department's work.

## What Management Involves

In this brief outline I have tried to make the case for taking the management of an imaging department seriously and not assuming that it will just happen. So what is management and what does it involve? A simple definition is 'making things happen through other people'. The first part implies that something should happen as the result of management. This may be something new but can mean equally that the agreed processes of a department happen regularly and reliably because of good decisions in the past. However, to understand the management process properly, let us consider what is needed before a decision can be made about a possible change in some part of a department's working. The procedure, formally or implicitly, will include the following elements:
- Getting information about the issue(s) under discussion

- Agreeing on the department's approach to it after looking at the options
- Planning, forecasting and setting targets
- Organising, coordinating, defining roles and responsibilities
- Motivating all staff and monitoring progress

## 'Through Other People'

The need to work through others is what causes the greatest difficulty for some doctors. The manager's skill at its best should ensure that all his/her colleagues are fully involved and concerned, each ready to suggest or accept changes which will improve the way the service is run and each feeling a valued member of the team. A department which is not a team will seldom function as well as one which has a good team spirit. For this the requirements are:
- An effective leader who selects good team members
- Members who work hard and are ready to make sacrifices for the group
- A shared vision of how the department should be - its philosophy
- Complementary skills and mutual respect
- Agreement on specific aims, i.e. practical targets

It will be obvious that such a situation takes time to achieve and that it requires a patient and determined leader, one who keeps in touch with all who work in the department - what Tom Peters has called 'management by walking about' [1]. This can, for example, make it clear that problems with the portering service are impairing the effective working of the department. Relatively few doctors have the qualities or are interested in such matters and many find it difficult to create the time needed. However, those who do not feel able to take on such tasks should always be ready to support those who do because the greatest problems for the medical manager come from the medical staff. This was well expressed by Professor Warren Bennis [2] when he said that 'leading doctors is a bit like herding cats'. In this context it is of interest to consider the managerial qualities which are desirable:
- The ability to plan and set goals
- Leadership and an ability to motivate
- Care over details
- Breadth of vision coupled with sensitivity
- A capacity to handle numbers, numeracy
- Persistence, determination, and toughness
_ Imagination, flexibility and open-mindedness
- Skill in communication

No one person can have all these qualities. This reinforces the argument for working as a team, for Belbin [3] has stressed that a well-structured team can provide the right mix of abilities to give success in management. So the doctor selecting an assistant should look for qualities which complement his or her own.

## Management Style

This brings us to the point that there are two main management styles, the authoritative and the collaborative. The authoritative style is attractive to some temperaments because it requires little discussion; the manager, who sees himself as the 'boss' will expect his decisions to be accepted. Such a style is increasingly regarded as old-fashioned and unsatisfactory in management circles It may have short-term advantages but it does not produce a cohesive, enthusiastic team and, in the long run, that is what counts. The collaborative approach, by contrast, promotes the initiative and enthusiasm of the team by involving them, giving responsibility where appropriate and encouraging them to contribute as fully as possible. Such a contrast in style has been seen, in the past at least, between the better US departments and some in Europe, with European professors keeping absolute control and American chairmen delegating to and encouraging their staff, taking pride in their achievements.

## Managerial Assistance

It would not be possible for a radiologist to manage a department effectively and give a proper measure of time to radiology without some support: this means a 'business manager' who can act for the RM, seeing that the decisions made are put into effect, interacting with other hospital departments, supervising the work of the clerical and secretarial staff, making sure that the departmental computer is working effectively and so on. Such individuals may have a background in radiography or in general management; their background is less important than their capabilities and their ability to work with the radiologist in charge. As noted, the RM should look for qualities which complement his/her own abilities, rather than looking for someone of similar characteristics.

## The Radiological Manager and the Hospital Management

So far, the functions of an RM have been discussed mainly in terms of the running of the imaging department. It is obvious, however, that the department has to be represented to the hospital as a whole and to its management. This will sometimes mean that members of the department have to be defended from clinicians who are attacking them. It will also mean that the RM has to work with the managers of the hospital, trying to influence their decisions in ways favourable to the department and trying also to secure more resources for it. At times it will also mean that unpleasant decisions taken by the hospital management board must be explained to the department and the consequences implemented.

It is at such times of difficulty that the capabilities of a manager are most strongly tested: the support of the team is then of greatest value.

## Committee Meetings

One of the features of the manager's life which is most disliked by doctors is the frequency of committees. Meetings are, unfortunately, necessary at times but it is true that hospital managers do not realise how much they can disrupt the work of doctors. The more important functions of a committee are:
– Discussing and deciding routine matters
– 'Brainstorming' a particular issue
– Disseminating information
– Getting people involved, giving a 'feel good' effect

Information which does not need to be discussed can be covered by a 'For Information' agenda item or a newsletter. Single issue committees should be called 'task forces' and given a fixed term.

Whenever possible, a committee should be presented with fully worked out issues, with clear options from which to choose. This will help to focus discussion on the most relevant matters. If hospital managers set up too many committees it may be worth asking that the cost of the meeting should be calculated, i.e. the hourly pay of each person involved multiplied by the time spent in committee. This will remind everyone of the need to make meetings really productive.

## Conclusions

There is no doubt that radiologists will experience increasing pressure to contribute to the management of their departments and to the running of their hospitals. These duties should be taken seriously but should not imply an excessive time commitment if they are well organised, if colleagues support them and if effective managerial assistance is provided. Most of us can recognise a clinically effective imaging department without difficulty. The corresponding signs of a well-managed department may be less apparent, though the way patients and visitors are greeted and the appearance of the waiting areas offer clues. In more conventional managerial terms, the signs are:
– Everyone knows to whom he or she is responsible or accountable
– Each person knows their part in the running of the department
– All who are interested are fully aware of what is happening
– Each departmental group, e.g. radiographic technicians, has its own subcommittee with a representative on the main departmental committee
– There is a strategic plan for the next 5 years

To achieve all this will take time and the RM may have, in the words of John Gabbay [4] to provide leadership by 'inspiring', politicking, plotting, cajoling, fighting, bargaining, compromising and persevering'. For those with the right temperament the rewards will be the satisfaction of a department in which it is a pleasure to work and which serves its patients skilfully and well.

## References

1. Peters T (1989) Thriving on chaos. Pan, London, pp 423-432
2. Bennis W (1992) Quoted in Smith, R Leadership and doctors BMJ 305: 137-138
3. Belbin M (1981) Management teams: why some succeed and some fail. Heinemann, Oxford
4. Gabbay J (1988) Opinion: inspiring, politicking, plotting, cojoling BMJ 297: 992

## Further Reading

Burrows M, Dyson R, Jackson P, Saxton H (1994) Management for hospital doctors. Butterworth - Heinemann, Oxford